MRI in Practice

Fourth Edition

Catherine Westbrook

MSc, FHEA, PgC(HE), DCRR, CTC
Senior Lecturer
Anglia Ruskin University
Cambridge
UK

Carolyn Kaut Roth

RT (R) (MR) (CT) (M) (CV), FSMRT
CEO, Imaging Education Associates
Pennsylvania
USA

John Talbot

MSc, FHEA, PgC(HE), DCRR
Senior Lecturer
Anglia Ruskin University
Cambridge
UK

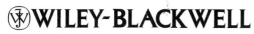

WILEY-BLACKWELL

A John Wiley & Sons, Ltd., Publication

This edition first published 2011
© 1993, 1998 by Blackwell Science
© 2005, 2011 by Blackwell Publishing Ltd

Blackwell Publishing was acquired by John Wiley & Sons in February 2007. Blackwell's publishing program has been merged with Wiley's global Scientific, Technical and Medical business to form Wiley-Blackwell.

Registered office: John Wiley & Sons, Ltd, The Atrium, Southern Gate, Chichester, West Sussex, PO19 8SQ, UK

Editorial offices: 9600 Garsington Road, Oxford, OX4 2DQ, UK
The Atrium, Southern Gate, Chichester, West Sussex, PO19 8SQ, UK
350 Main Street, Malden, MA 02148-5020, USA

For details of our global editorial offices, for customer services and for information about how to apply for permission to reuse the copyright material in this book please see our website at www.wiley.com/wiley-blackwell.

First published 1993
Second edition 1998
Third edition 2005
Fourth edition 2011

Library of Congress Cataloging-in-Publication Data

Westbrook, Catherine.
    MRI in practice / Catherine Westbrook, Carolyn Kaut Roth and John Talbot. – 4th ed.
        p. cm.
    Includes bibliographical references and index.
    ISBN 978-1-4443-3743-3 (pbk. : alk. paper)   1. Magnetic resonance imaging.   I. Roth, Carolyn Kaut.   II. Talbot, John, MSc.   III. Title.
    RC78.7.N83W48 2011
    616.07'548–dc22

                                                                                            2010052328

A catalogue record for this book is available from the British Library.

Set in 10/12 pt Calibri by Toppan Best-set Premedia Limited, Hong Kong

2   2012

Contents

**See the supporting companion website for this book:
www.wiley.com/go/mriinpractice**

CHECK OUT THE
MRI IN
PRACTICE
FOURTH EDITION
Companion Website

Foreword

Cathy Westbrook, John Talbot and Candi Kaut Roth have been teaching magnetic resonance imaging physics for more than twenty years. Two of them have lectured for the SMRT (Society of MR Technologists) and two of them give their own MRI Technologist Course all over the world. They are well known in the MRI community as uber-techs. Thus, at first glance *MRI in Practice* might be seen as a watered down physics book for MRI technologists. However this initial perception could not be further from the truth. This is the fourth edition of an excellent textbook on MR physics which will be useful not only to MRI technologists but also to radiology residents and attendings who want to get seriously involved with MRI. This book provides an excellent framework for MRI for graduate students as well as nonradiologist attendings who want to get involved with MRI research.

The beauty of this book is that it starts simple for the beginning MRI technologist but goes into more than enough detail to satisfy senior technologists and radiologists specializing in MRI and teaching radiology residents. For example, the ranges of TRs and TEs for a T1- or T2-weighted sequence are given for the beginning technologist who just wants a cookbook. But the discussion rapidly evolves into pulse sequence diagrams for gradient echo, conventional spin echo, and fast/turbo spin echo. The discussion of fast spin echo leads naturally into an excellent discussion of K space which avoids its sometimes-threatening Fourier transform origins and uses an analogy of a chest of drawers. This discussion of K space is necessary to understand parallel imaging, 'half Nex' imaging (partial Fourier in phase), 'fractional echo' (partial Fourier in frequency), and echo planar imaging and its applications, perfusion, diffusion, and diffusion tensor imaging. It is necessary to understand motion artefact suppression techniques like PROPELLER and BLADE which cover K space radially rather than in the usual Cartesian/rectilinear fashion.

Another example is their discussion of receiver bandwidth, a primary determinant of signal-to-noise. For the beginner, they give typical numerical values. But then they go on from there to discuss the Nyquist theorem and Nyquist frequency as well as the effect of bandwidth on chemical shift artefact, field of view, and echo sampling time.

The book is beautifully illustrated and features weblinks to animated sequences which further help explain the intricacies of MRI. Even though I have been teaching and writing about MRI physics for over three decades I found numerous examples where the authors' explanations were better than what I have been using – and which I now intend to adopt! In summary, this is an excellent, easy-to-understand book on MRI physics which will benefit almost anyone who reads it. I heartily recommend *MRI in Practice*!

William G. Bradley, Jr, MD, PhD, FACR
Professor and Chair
Department of Radiology
University of California, San Diego

Preface to the Fourth Edition

MRI in Practice has become one of the bestselling books in its genre. First published in 1993, it was pioneering in that it was written by radiographers rather than physicists or radiologists and it attempted to provide a basic understanding of magnetic resonance imaging (MRI) physics to the clinical masses. These MRI practitioners are not always interested in complex mathematics but just want to know how it essentially 'all works' and how to manipulate parameters to acquire the best images. When *MRI in Practice* was first published, it is fair to say that it attracted some criticism, mainly for being too simplistic. However, it quickly became a bestseller and I received many messages from grateful readers who found the book a life saver. Some commented that after reading *MRI in Practice*, subjects that had eluded them for years were suddenly understandable as though a 'light had been switched on in their head'.

Over the years, *MRI in Practice* has grown from strength to strength. Despite other books coming onto the market, its readership has increased. It has been translated into several languages and is used by tens of thousands of readers from all over the world. The accompanying *MRI in Practice* course is now 18 years old. John Talbot and I teach the course and it is based on the book. We deliver this course about 20 times a year, in 14 countries, and have met thousands of MRI practitioners, many of whom have joined our *MRI in Practice* community.

The last edition of *MRI in Practice* saw the book emerge in glorious technicolor and this edition goes one step further. In response to feedback from the readers, Chapters 3 and 5 have been given a gentle rewrite to more clearly explain topics such as sampling, data acquisition and the latest sequences. Some of the diagrams have been overhauled and the glossary has been updated. However, the main change in this edition is the online element of the book. This provides some 3D animations from the *MRI in Practice* course with accompanying explanatory text that really make the book come alive. The online element also contains many questions and answers so that readers can test what they have learned. The online presence of the book is something I hope to develop further in the future, so that MRI practitioners can use *MRI in Practice* 'on the go'.

I hope that the many fans of *MRI in Practice* around the world continue to enjoy and learn from it. A big thank you to all of you for your continued support and loyalty.

Catherine Westbrook

Useful websites

www.mrieducation.com (for details about *MRI in Practice*, the course)
Check out the *MRI in Practice* iphone app in the iTunes store

Acknowledgments

Many thanks to John Talbot for his excellent diagrams and animations for the online element of this edition.

A big thank you to my family, Toni, Adam, Ben and Maddie, and my mum and sister in the USA for their continued love and support.

CW

1

Basic principles

Introduction

The basic principles of magnetic resonance imaging (MRI) form the foundation for further understanding of this complex subject. It is important that these ideas are fully grasped before moving on to areas that are more complicated. There are essentially two ways of explaining the fundamentals of MRI: classically and via quantum physics. Any discussion requires both, so we have attempted to integrate the two versions. Within this chapter, the properties of atoms and their interactions with magnetic fields, excitation and relaxation are discussed.

Atomic structure

All things are made of **atoms**, including the human body. Atoms are very small. Half a million lined up together are narrower than a human hair. Atoms are organized in **molecules**, which are two or more atoms arranged together. The most abundant atom in the body is **hydrogen**. This is most commonly found in molecules of water (where two hydrogen atoms are arranged with one oxygen

MRI in Practice, Fourth Edition. Catherine Westbrook, Carolyn Kaut Roth, John Talbot.
© 2011 Blackwell Publishing Ltd. Published 2011 by Blackwell Publishing Ltd.

atom, H_2O) and fat (where hydrogen atoms are arranged with carbon and oxygen atoms; the number of each depends on the type of fat).

The atom consists of a central nucleus and orbiting **electrons** (Figure 1.1). The nucleus is very small, one millionth of a billionth of the total volume of an atom, but it contains all the atom's mass. This mass comes mainly from particles called **nucleons**, which are subdivided into **protons** and **neutrons**. Atoms are characterized in two ways. The **atomic number** is the sum of the protons in the nucleus. This number gives an atom its chemical identity. The **mass number** is the sum of the protons and neutrons in the nucleus. The number of neutrons and protons in a nucleus are usually balanced so that the mass number is an even number. In some atoms, however, there are slightly more or fewer neutrons than protons. Atoms of elements with the same number of protons but a different number of neutrons are called **isotopes**. Nuclei with an odd mass number (a different number of protons to neutrons) are important in MRI (*see* later).

Electrons are particles that spin around the nucleus. Traditionally this is thought of as being analogous to planets orbiting around the sun. In reality, electrons exist around the nucleus in a cloud; the outermost dimension of the cloud is the edge of the atom. The position of an electron in the cloud is not predictable as it depends on the energy of an individual electron at any moment in time (physicists call this Heisenberg's Uncertainty Principle). The number of electrons, however, is usually the same as the number of protons in the nucleus.

Protons have a positive electrical charge, neutrons have no net charge and electrons are negatively charged. So atoms are electrically stable if the number of negatively charged electrons equals the number of positively charged protons. This balance is sometimes altered by applying external energy to knock out electrons from the atom. This causes a deficit in the number of electrons compared with protons and causes electrical instability. Atoms in which this has occurred are called **ions**.

Motion in the atom

Three types of motion are present within the atom (Figure 1.1). These are:

- electrons spinning on their own axis
- electrons orbiting the nucleus
- the nucleus itself spinning about its own axis.

The principles of MRI rely on the spinning motion of specific nuclei present in biological tissues. This spin derives from the individual spins of protons and neutrons within the nucleus. Pairs of subatomic particles automatically spin in opposite directions but at the same rate as their partners. In nuclei that have an even mass number, i.e. the number of protons equals the number of neutrons, half spin in one direction and half in the other. The nucleus itself has no net spin. However, in nuclei with odd mass numbers, i.e. where the number of neutrons is slightly more or less than the number of protons, spin directions are not equal and opposite, so the nucleus itself has a net spin or **angular momentum**. These are known as **MR active nuclei.**

MR active nuclei

MR active nuclei are characterized by their tendency to align their axis of rotation to an applied magnetic field. This occurs because they have angular momentum or spin and, as they contain

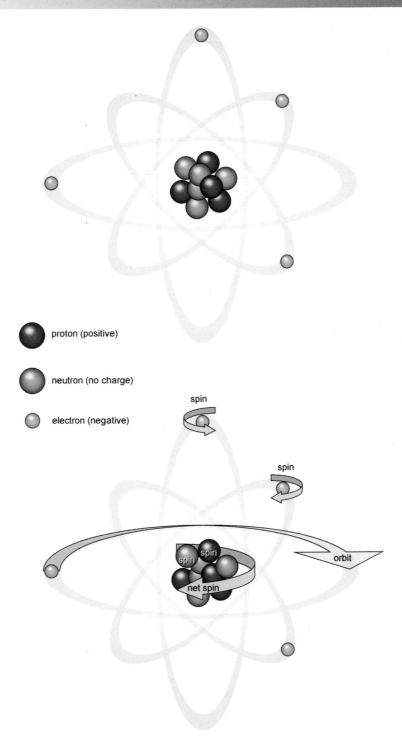

Figure 1.1 The atom.

positively charged protons, they possess electrical charge. The law of electromagnetic induction (set out by Michael Faraday in 1833) refers to three individual forces – motion, magnetism and charge – and states that if two of these are present, then the third is automatically induced. MR active nuclei that have a net charge and are spinning (motion), automatically acquire a **magnetic moment** and can align with an external magnetic field.

Important examples of MR active nuclei, together with their mass numbers are listed below:

hydrogen	1
carbon	13
nitrogen	15
oxygen	17
fluorine	19
sodium	23
phosphorus	31

Although neutrons have no net charge, their subatomic particles are not evenly arranged over the surface of the neutron and this imbalance enables the nucleus in which the neutron is situated to be MR active as long as the mass number is odd. Alignment is measured as the total sum of the nuclear magnetic moments and is expressed as a vector quantity. The strength of the total magnetic moment is specific to every nucleus and determines the sensitivity to magnetic resonance.

The hydrogen nucleus

The isotope of the hydrogen nucleus called **protium** is the MR active nucleus used in clinical MRI. This contains a single proton (atomic and mass number 1). It is used because hydrogen is very abundant in the human body, and because its solitary proton gives it a relatively large magnetic moment. Both of these characteristics enable utilization of the maximum amount of available magnetization in the body. From now on in this book when the terms spin, nucleus or hydrogen nucleus are used we are referring to this particular isotope of hydrogen.

The hydrogen nucleus as a magnet

The laws of electromagnetism state that a magnetic field is created when a charged particle moves. The hydrogen nucleus contains one positively charged proton that spins, i.e. it moves. Therefore the hydrogen nucleus has a magnetic field induced around it and acts as a small magnet. The magnet of each hydrogen nucleus has a north and a south pole of equal strength. The north/south axis of each nucleus is represented by a magnetic moment and is used in the classical theory of the principles of MRI. The magnetic moment of each nucleus has vector properties, i.e. it has size and direction and is denoted by an arrow. The direction of the vector designates the direction of the magnetic moment, and the length of the vector designates the size of the magnetic moment as in Figure 1.2.

Alignment

In the absence of an applied magnetic field, the magnetic moments of the hydrogen nuclei are randomly orientated. However, when placed in a strong static external magnetic field (shown as

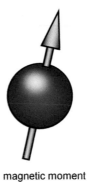

magnetic moment

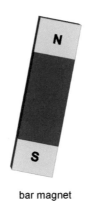

bar magnet

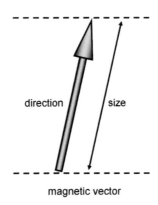

magnetic vector

Figure 1.2 The magnetic moment of the hydrogen nucleus.

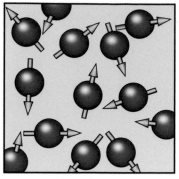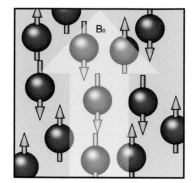

random alignment
no external field

alignment
external magnetic field

Figure 1.3   Alignment – classical theory.

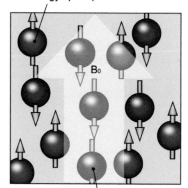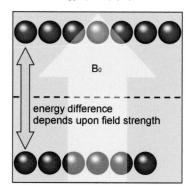

low energy spin-up nucleus

low energy spin-up population

high energy spin-down nucleus

high energy spin-down population

Figure 1.4   Alignment – quantum theory.

a white arrow on Figure 1.3 and termed B_0), the magnetic moments of the hydrogen nuclei align with this magnetic field. Some of the hydrogen nuclei align parallel with the magnetic field (in the same direction), while a smaller number of the nuclei align anti-parallel to the magnetic field (in the opposite direction) as in Figure 1.3.

Quantum theory (first discovered by Max Planck in 1900) describes the properties of electro-magnetic radiation in terms of discrete quantities of energy called quanta. Applying quantum theory to MRI, hydrogen nuclei possess energy in two discrete quantities or populations termed low and high (Figure 1.4). Low-energy nuclei align their magnetic moments parallel to the external field (shown as a white arrow on Figure 1.4) and are termed **spin-up** nuclei (shown in blue in Figure 1.4). High-energy nuclei align their magnetic moments in the anti-parallel direction and are termed **spin-down** nuclei (shown in red in Figure 1.4).

Learning point: magnetic moments

It is the magnetic moments of the hydrogen nuclei that align with B_o not the hydrogen nuclei themselves. In addition they are only capable of aligning in one of two directions; parallel or anti-parallel to B_o. This is because they represent the only two possible energy states of hydrogen. The hydrogen nucleus itself does not change direction but merely spins on its axis.

The factors affecting which hydrogen nuclei align parallel and which align anti-parallel are determined by the strength of the external magnetic field and the thermal energy level of the nuclei. Low thermal energy nuclei do not possess enough energy to oppose the magnetic field in the anti-parallel direction. High thermal energy nuclei, however, do possess enough energy to oppose this field, and as the strength of the magnetic field increases, fewer nuclei have enough energy to do so. The thermal energy of a nucleus is mainly determined by the temperature of the patient. In clinical applications this cannot be significantly altered and is not important. This is called **thermal equilibrium**. Under these circumstances it is the strength of the external field that determines the relative quantities of spin-up to spin-down nuclei.

In thermal equilibrium there are always fewer high-energy nuclei than low-energy nuclei, therefore the magnetic moments of the nuclei aligned parallel to the magnetic field cancel out the smaller number of magnetic moments aligned anti-parallel. As there is a larger number aligned parallel, there is always a small excess in this direction that produces a net magnetic moment (Figure 1.5). Other MR active nuclei also align with the magnetic field and produce their own small net magnetic moments.

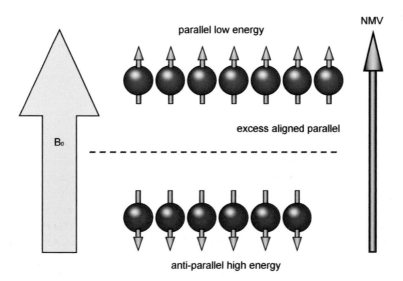

Figure 1.5   The net magnetization vector.

These magnetic moments are not used in clinical MRI because they do not exist in enough abundance in the body to be imaged adequately, as their net magnetic moments are very small. The net magnetic moment of hydrogen, however, produces a significant magnetic vector that is used in clinical MRI. This is called the **net magnetization vector** (**NMV**) and reflects the relative balance between spin-up and spin-down nuclei.

Learning point: NMV vs field strength

When a patient is placed in the bore of the magnet, the magnetic moments of hydrogen nuclei within the patient align parallel and anti-parallel to B_0. A small excess line up parallel to B_0 and constitute the NMV of the patient (Figure 1.5). The energy difference between the two populations increases as B_0 increases. At high field strengths fewer nuclei have enough energy to join the high-energy population and align their magnetic moments in opposition to the stronger B_0 field. This means that the magnitude of the NMV is larger at high field strengths than low field strengths, resulting in improved signal. This is discussed further in Chapter 4.

Summary

- The net magnetic moment of the patient is called the net magnetization vector (NMV)
- The static external magnetic field is called B_0
- The interaction of the NMV with B_0 is the basis of MRI
- The unit of B_0 is Tesla or gauss. 1 Tesla (T) is the equivalent of 10 000 gauss (G)

Precession

Each hydrogen nucleus is spinning on its axis as in Figure 1.6. The influence of B_0 produces an additional spin or wobble of the magnetic moments of hydrogen around B_0. This secondary spin is called **precession** and causes the magnetic moments to follow a circular path around B_0. This path is called the **precessional path** and the speed at which they wobble around B_0 is called the **precessional frequency**. The unit of precessional frequency is megahertz (MHz) where 1 Hz is one cycle or rotation per second and 1 MHz is one million cycles or rotations per second.

Combining Figure 1.6 with what we now know about quantum physics, it is possible to appreciate that there are two populations of hydrogen nuclei: some high-energy, spin-down nuclei and a greater number of low-energy, spin-up hydrogen nuclei. The magnetic moments of all these nuclei precess around B_0 on a circular precessional path (Figure 1.7).

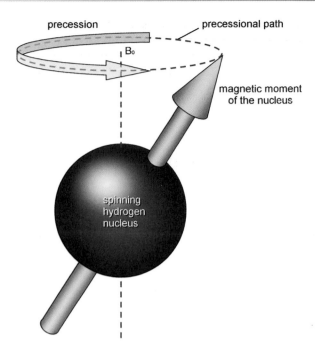

Figure 1.6   Precession.

The Larmor equation

The value of the precessional frequency is governed by the Larmor equation. The Larmor equation states that:

$$\omega_0 = B_0 \times \lambda$$

where:

ω_0 is the precessional frequency
B_0 is the magnetic field strength of the magnet
λ is the gyromagnetic ratio.

The gyromagnetic ratio expresses the relationship between the angular momentum and the magnetic moment of each MR active nucleus. It is constant and is expressed as the precessional frequency of a specific MR active nucleus at 1 T. The unit of the gyromagnetic ratio is therefore MHz/T.
 The gyromagnetic ratio of hydrogen is 42.57 MHz/T. Other MR active nuclei have different gyromagnetic ratios, so have different precessional frequencies at the same field strength. In addition, hydrogen has a different precessional frequency at different field strengths. For example:

- at 1.5 T the precessional frequency of hydrogen is 63.86 MHz (42.57 MHz × 1.5 T)
- at 1.0 T the precessional frequency of hydrogen is 42.57 MHz (42.57 MHz × 1.0 T)
- at 0.5 T the precessional frequency of hydrogen is 21.28 MHz (42.57 MHz × 0.5 T).

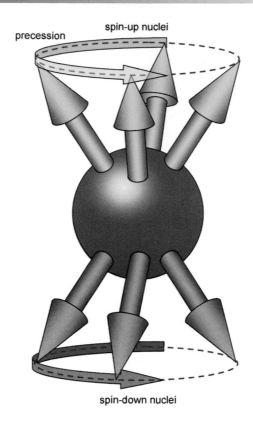

Figure 1.7 Precession of the spin-up and spin-down populations.

The precessional frequency is often called the **Larmor frequency**, because it is determined by the Larmor equation.

Learning point: the Larmor equation

The Larmor equation tells us two important facts:

1. All MR active nuclei have their own gyromagnetic constant so that when they are exposed to the same field strength, they precess at different frequencies, i.e. hydrogen precesses at a different frequency to either fluorine or carbon, which are also MR active nuclei. This allows us to specifically image hydrogen and ignore the other MR active nuclei in the body. The way in which this is done is discussed later.
2. As the gyromagnetic ratio is a constant of proportionality, B_o is proportional to the Larmor frequency. Therefore if B_o increases, the Larmor frequency increases and vice versa.

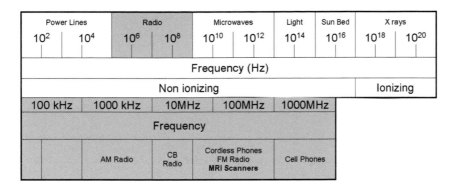

Figure 1.8   The electromagnetic spectrum.

Resonance

Resonance is a phenomenon that occurs when an object is exposed to an oscillating perturbation that has a frequency close to its own natural frequency of oscillation. When a nucleus is exposed to an external perturbation that has an oscillation similar to its own natural frequency, the nucleus gains energy from the external force. The nucleus gains energy and resonates if the energy is delivered at exactly the same precessional frequency. If energy is delivered at a different frequency to that of the Larmor frequency of the nucleus, resonance does not occur.

Energy at the precessional frequency of hydrogen at all field strengths in clinical MRI corresponds to the **radio frequency (RF)** band of the electromagnetic spectrum (Figure 1.8). For resonance of hydrogen to occur, an **RF pulse** of energy at exactly the Larmor frequency of hydrogen must be applied. Other MR active nuclei that have aligned with B_0 do not resonate, because their precessional frequencies are different to that of hydrogen. This is because their gyromagnetic ratios are different to that of hydrogen.

The application of an RF pulse that causes resonance to occur is termed **excitation**. This absorption of energy causes an increase in the number of spin-down hydrogen nuclei populations as some of the spin-up (shown in blue in Figure 1.9) nuclei gain energy via resonance and become high-energy nuclei (shown in red in Figure 1.9). The energy difference between the two populations corresponds to the energy required to produce resonance via excitation. As the field strength increases, the energy difference between the two populations also increases so that more energy (higher frequencies) are required to produce resonance.

The results of resonance

One of the results of resonance is that the NMV moves out of alignment away from B_0. This occurs because some of the low-energy nuclei are given enough energy via resonance to join the high-energy population. As the NMV reflects the balance between the low and high-energy populations, resonance causes the NMV to no longer lie parallel to B_0 but at an angle to it. The angle to which the NMV moves out of alignment is called the **flip angle** (Figure 1.10). The magnitude of the flip angle depends on the amplitude and duration of the RF pulse. Usually the flip angle is

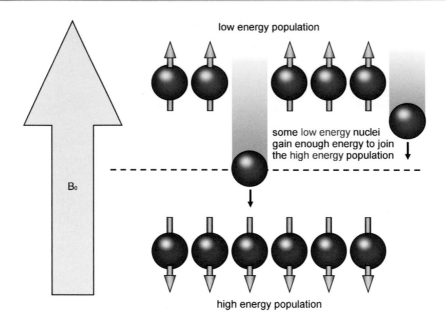

Figure 1.9 Energy transfer during excitation.

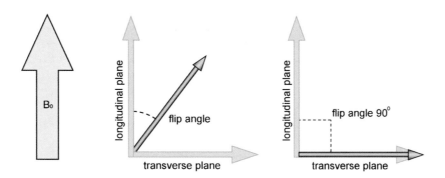

Figure 1.10 The flip angle.

90°, i.e. the NMV is given enough energy by the RF pulse to move through 90° relative to B_0. However, as the NMV is a vector, even if flip angles other than 90° are used, there is always a component of magnetization in a plane perpendicular to B_0.

- B_0 is now termed the **longitudinal plane**.
- The plane at 90° to B_0 is termed the **transverse plane**.

With a flip angle of 90° the nuclei are given sufficient energy so that the longitudinal NMV is completely transferred into a transverse NMV. This transverse NMV rotates in the transverse plane at the Larmor frequency. When flip angles less than 90° are used, only a portion of the NMV is

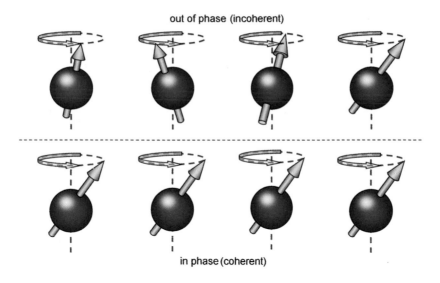

out of phase (incoherent)

in phase (coherent)

Figure 1.11   In phase (coherent) and out of phase (incoherent).

transferred to the transverse plane. This represents a smaller number of low-energy spins becoming high-energy spins as a result of excitation. If flip angles greater than 90° are used, this represents a larger number of high-energy spins to low-energy spins. The NMV merely reflects the balance between the spin-up to spin-down populations.

The other result of resonance is that the magnetic moments of hydrogen nuclei move into phase with each other. **Phase** is the position of each magnetic moment on the precessional path around B_0. Magnetic moments that are **in phase** (or **coherent**) are in the same place on the precessional path around B_0 at any given time. Magnetic moments that are **out of phase** (or **incoherent**) are not in the same place on the precessional path. When resonance occurs, all the magnetic moments move to the same position on the precessional path and are then in phase (Figure 1.11).

Learning point: the watch analogy

The terms frequency and phase are used many times in this book and it is important to understand the difference between them and how they relate to each other. The easiest analogy is the hour hand on an analogue watch. **Frequency** is the time it takes the hour hand to make one revolution of the watch face, i.e. 12 hours. The unit of frequency is hertz (Hz), where 1 Hz is one cycle or rotation per second. Using the watch analogy, the frequency of the hour hand is $1/43200\,s = 0.0000231\,Hz$ as it moves around the watch face once every 12 hours. The **phase** of the hour hand, measured in degrees or radians, is the time on the watch, e.g. 1 o'clock, 2 o'clock, which corresponds to its position around the watch face when you look to see what time it is (Figure 1.12).

The phase of the hour hand depends on its frequency. If the frequency is correct then the hour hand always tells the correct time. If the watch goes fast or slow, i.e. the frequency either increases or decreases, then the watch tells an incorrect time. There are 360 degrees in a circle, so 360 possible phase positions. However, there are an infinite number of frequencies.

Imagine a room full of people with watches that tell perfect time who are asked to synchronize their watches at 12 noon. One hour later, all their watches will say 1 o'clock because they have kept perfect time. They are in phase or coherent because they all tell the same time and their hour hands are all at the same place on the watch face at the same time. However, if after synchronization the watches on the left-hand side of the room go fast for one hour and the watches on the right-hand side of the room go slow for one hour, then at 1 o'clock they will be telling different times. The watches on the left-hand side of the room will be telling a time greater than 1 o'clock, e.g. 1.15 pm, and those on the right-hand side of the room will be telling a time less than 1 o'clock, e.g. 12.45 pm. Therefore the watches are out of phase or incoherent because they tell different times and their hours hands are not at the same place on the watch face at the same time. How much they are out of phase depends on their relative frequencies between 12 noon and 1 o'clock.

If the difference in frequencies is large then the difference in phase is greater than if the frequency difference is small. Phase and frequency are therefore connected. In this context the frequency of the hour hand is related to its change of phase over time. In other contexts used later in this book, frequency is a change of phase over distance. We refer to the watch analogy many times in this book. Look out for the watch symbol in the margin.

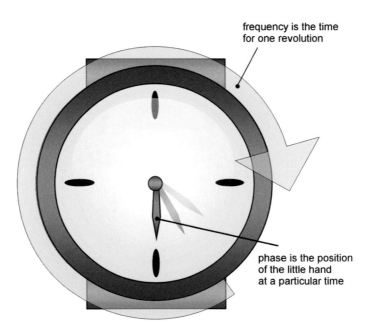

frequency is the time
for one revolution

phase is the position
of the little hand
at a particular time

Figure 1.12   Phase and frequency.

Summary

- For resonance of hydrogen to occur, RF at exactly the Larmor frequency of hydrogen must be applied
- The result of resonance is magnetization in the transverse plane that is in phase or coherent
- This in phase or coherent transverse magnetization precesses at the Larmor frequency

The MR signal

As a result of resonance, in phase or coherent magnetization precesses at the Larmor frequency in the transverse plane. Faraday's law of electromagnetic induction states that if a receiver coil or any conductive loop is placed in the area of a moving magnetic field, i.e. the magnetization precessing in the transverse plane, a voltage is induced in this receiver coil. The **MR signal** is produced when coherent (in phase) magnetization cuts across the coil. Therefore the coherent moving transverse magnetization produces magnetic field fluctuations inside the coil that induce an electrical voltage in the coil. This voltage constitutes the MR signal. The frequency of the signal is the same as the Larmor frequency – the magnitude of the signal depends on the amount of magnetization present in the transverse plane (Figure 1.13).

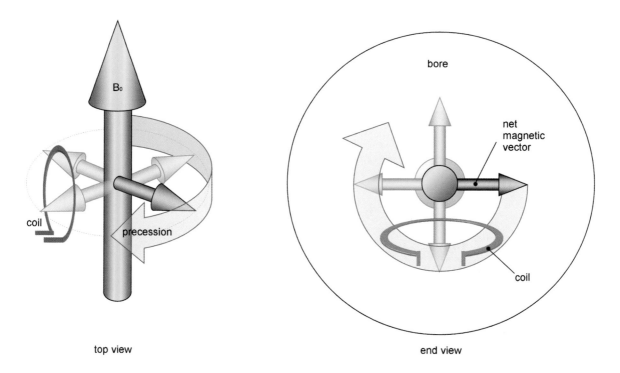

Figure 1.13 Generation of the signal.

Refer to animations 1.1 and 1.2 on the supporting companion website for this book: www.wiley.com/go/mriinpractice

The free induction decay signal (FID)

When the RF pulse is switched off, the NMV is again influenced by B_0 and it tries to realign with it. To do so, the hydrogen nuclei must lose the energy given to them by the RF pulse. The process by which hydrogen loses this energy is called **relaxation.** As relaxation occurs, the NMV returns to realign with B_0 because some of the high-energy nuclei return to the low-energy population and align their magnetic moments in the spin-up direction.

- The amount of magnetization in the longitudinal plane gradually increases – this is called **recovery**.
- At the same time, but independently, the amount of magnetization in the transverse plane gradually decreases – this is called **decay.**

As the magnitude of transverse magnetization decreases, so does the magnitude of the voltage induced in the receiver coil. The induction of reduced signal is called the free induction decay (FID) signal.

Relaxation

During relaxation hydrogen nuclei give up absorbed RF energy and the NMV returns to B_0. At the same time, but independently, the magnetic moments of hydrogen lose coherency due to dephasing. Relaxation results in recovery of magnetization in the longitudinal plane and decay of magnetization in the transverse plane.

- The recovery of longitudinal magnetization is caused by a process termed **T1 recovery**.
- The decay of transverse magnetization is caused by a process termed **T2 decay**.

T1 recovery

T1 recovery is caused by the nuclei giving up their energy to the surrounding environment or lattice, and it is termed **spin lattice relaxation**. Energy released to the surrounding lattice causes the magnetic moments of nuclei to recover their longitudinal magnetization (magnetization in the longitudinal plane). The rate of recovery is an exponential process, with a recovery time constant called the **T1 relaxation time**. This is the time it takes 63% of the longitudinal magnetization to recover in the tissue (Figure 1.14).

T2 decay

T2 decay is caused by the magnetic fields of neighbouring nuclei interacting with each other. It is termed **spin-spin relaxation** and results in decay or loss of coherent transverse magnetization (magnetization in the transverse plane). The rate of decay is also an exponential process, so that the **T2 relaxation time** of a tissue is its time constant of decay. It is the time it takes 63% of the transverse magnetization to be lost (37% remains) (Figure 1.15).

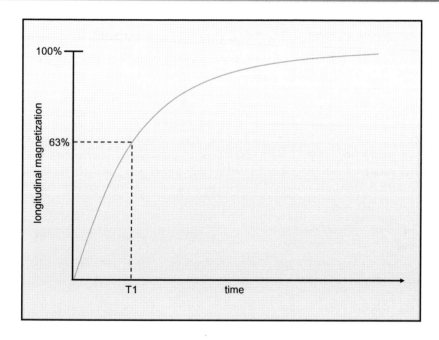

Figure 1.14   The T1 recovery curve.

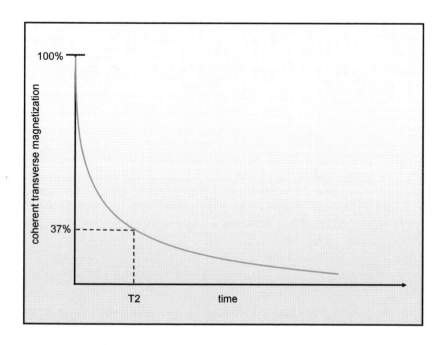

Figure 1.15   The T2 decay curve.

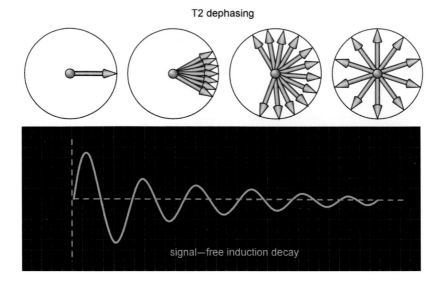

Figure 1.16 Dephasing and free induction decay (FID).

Summary

- T1 relaxation results in the recovery of longitudinal magnetization due to energy dissipation to the surrounding lattice
- T2 relaxation results in the loss of coherent transverse magnetization due to interactions between the magnetic fields of adjacent nuclei
- A signal or voltage is only induced in the receiver coil if there is coherent magnetization in the transverse plane, that is, in phase (Figure 1.16)

Learning point: vectors

The NMV is a vector quantity. It is created by two components at 90° to each other. These two components are magnetization in the longitudinal plane and magnetization in the transverse plane (Figure 1.17). Before resonance, there is full longitudinal magnetization parallel to B_o. After the application of the RF pulse and assuming a flip angle of 90°, the NMV is flipped fully into the transverse plane. There is now full transverse magnetization and zero longitudinal magnetization.

Once the RF pulse is removed, the NMV recovers. As this occurs, the longitudinal component of magnetization grows again, while the transverse component decreases (shown later in Figure 2.1). As the received signal amplitude is related to the magnitude of the coherent transverse component, the signal in the coil decays as relaxation takes place.

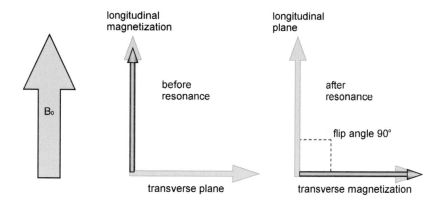

Figure 1.17   Longitudinal and transverse magnetization.

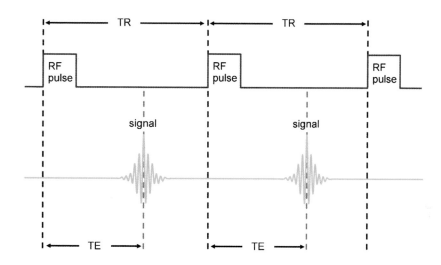

Figure 1.18   A basic pulse sequence.

The magnitude and timing of the RF pulses form part of **pulse sequences**, which are the basis of contrast generation in MRI.

Pulse timing parameters

A very simplified pulse sequence is a combination of RF pulses, signals and intervening periods of recovery (Figure 1.18). It is important to note that a pulse sequence as shown diagrammatically in Figure 1.18 merely shows in simple terms the separate timing parameters used in more complicated sequences, i.e. TR and TE.

A pulse sequence consists of several time periods: the main ones are outlined below.

- The **repetition time (TR)** is the time from the application of one RF pulse to the application of the next RF pulse for each slice and is measured in milliseconds (ms). The TR determines the amount of longitudinal relaxation that is allowed to occur between the end of one RF pulse and the application of the next. TR thus determines the amount of T1 relaxation that has occurred when the signal is read.
- The **echo time (TE)** is the time from the application of the RF pulse to the peak of the signal induced in the coil and is also measured in ms. The TE determines how much decay of transverse magnetization is allowed to occur. TE thus controls the amount of T2 relaxation that has occurred when the signal is read.

The basic principles of signal creation have now been described.

For questions and answers on this topic please visit the supporting companion website for this book: www.wiley.com/go/ mriinpractice

The application of RF pulses at certain repetition times and the receiving of signals at predefined echo times produce contrast in MRI images. This concept is discussed fully in the next chapter.

2

Image weighting and contrast

Introduction

All clinical diagnostic images must demonstrate contrast between normal anatomical features and between anatomy and any pathology. If there is no contrast difference, it is impossible to detect abnormalities within the body. One of the main advantages of MRI compared with other imaging modalities is the excellent soft tissue discrimination of the images. The contrast characteristics of each image depend on many variables, and it is important that the mechanisms that affect image contrast in MRI are understood.

Image contrast

The factors that affect image contrast in diagnostic imaging are usually divided into two categories.

- **Intrinsic contrast parameters** are those that cannot be changed because they are inherent to the body's tissues.
- **Extrinsic contrast parameters** are those that can be changed.

MRI in Practice, Fourth Edition. Catherine Westbrook, Carolyn Kaut Roth, John Talbot.
© 2011 Blackwell Publishing Ltd. Published 2011 by Blackwell Publishing Ltd.

For example, in X-ray imaging, intrinsic contrast parameters include the density of structures the X-ray beam passes through and is attenuated by, while extrinsic contrast parameters include the exposure factors set by the X-ray technician. Both of these determine X-ray image contrast. In MRI there are several parameters in each group.

Intrinsic contrast parameters are:

- T1 recovery time
- T2 decay time
- proton density
- flow
- apparent diffusion coefficient (ADC).

All these are inherent to the body's tissues and cannot be changed. T1 recovery time, T2 decay time and proton density are discussed in this chapter. Flow and ADC are discussed in Chapters 6 and 12.

Extrinsic contrast parameters are:

- TR
- TE
- flip angle
- TI
- turbo factor/echo train length
- b value.

These are all selected at the operator console. The parameters selected depend on the pulse sequence used. TR and TE were discussed in Chapter 1. The others are described in Chapters 5 and 12.

Contrast mechanisms

An MR image has contrast if there are areas of high signal (white on the image) and areas of low signal (dark on the image). Some areas have an intermediate signal (shades of gray in between white and black). The NMV can be separated into the individual vectors of the tissues present in the patient, such as fat, cerebrospinal fluid (CSF) and muscle.

A tissue has a high signal if it has a large transverse component of coherent magnetization at time TE. If there is a large component of coherent transverse magnetization the amplitude of the signal received by the coil is large, resulting in a bright area on the image. A tissue returns a low signal if it has a small transverse component of coherent magnetization at time TE. If there is a small component of transverse coherent magnetization, the amplitude of the signal received by the coil is small, resulting in a dark area on the image.

Images obtain contrast mainly through the mechanisms of T1 recovery, T2 decay and proton or spin density. T1 recovery and T2 decay were discussed in Chapter 1. The **proton density** of a tissue is the number of mobile hydrogen protons per unit volume of that tissue. The higher the proton density of a tissue, the more signal available from that tissue. T1 and T2 relaxation depend on three factors:

- *The inherent energy of the tissue.* If the inherent energy is low, then the molecular lattice is more able to absorb energy from hydrogen nuclei. Tissues with a low inherent energy are like sponges that can easily absorb energy from hydrogen nuclei during relaxation. The reverse is true in tissues with a high inherent energy that cannot easily absorb energy from hydrogen nuclei. These tissues are like kitchen paper, which is less able to absorb energy during relaxation. This is especially important in T1 relaxation processes, which rely on energy exchange between the hydrogen nuclei and the molecular lattice (spin lattice).

- *How closely packed the molecules are.* In tissues where molecules are closely spaced, there is more efficient interaction between the magnetic fields of neighboring hydrogen nuclei. The reverse is true when molecules are spaced apart. This is especially important in T2 decay processes, which rely on the efficiency of interactions between the magnetic fields of neighbouring hydrogen nuclei (spin-spin).
- *How well the molecular tumbling rate matches the Larmor frequency of hydrogen.* If there is a good match between the two, energy exchange between hydrogen nuclei and the molecular lattice is efficient. (This is similar to resonance, where energy exchange occurs most efficiently when energy is applied at the same frequency as the Larmor frequency of hydrogen.) When there is a bad match, energy exchange is not as efficient.

Relaxation in different tissues

As discussed in Chapter 1, T1 relaxation and T2 decay are exponential processes with time constants T1 and T2, which represent the time it takes for 63% of the total magnetization to be regained in the longitudinal plane via spin lattice energy transfer (T1), or lost in the transverse plane via spin–spin interactions (T2). This section relates the exponential curves to relaxation processes within tissues.

Generally, the two extremes of contrast in MRI are fat and water (Figure 2.1). In this book fat vectors are drawn in yellow and water vectors in blue.

Fat and water

Fat molecules contain atoms of hydrogen arranged with carbon and oxygen. They consist of large molecules called lipids that are closely packed together and whose molecular tumbling rate is relatively slow. Water molecules contain two hydrogen atoms arranged with one oxygen atom (H_2O). Its molecules are spaced apart and their molecular tumbling rate is relatively fast. The oxygen in water tends to steal the electrons away from around the hydrogen nucleus. This renders it more available to the effects of the main magnetic field.

In fat, the carbon does not take the electrons from around the hydrogen nucleus. They remain in an electron cloud, protecting the nucleus from the effects of the main field. The Larmor frequency of hydrogen in water is higher than that of hydrogen in fat. Hydrogen in fat recovers more rapidly along the longitudinal axis than water and loses transverse magnetization faster than in water. Subsequently, fat and water appear differently in MR images.

T1 recovery in fat

T1 recovery occurs due to nuclei giving up their energy to the surrounding environment. Fat has a low inherent energy and can easily absorb energy into its lattice from hydrogen nuclei. The slow

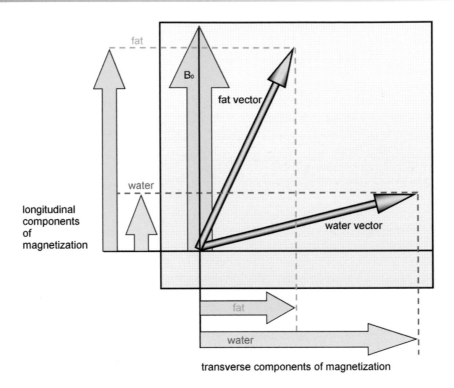

longitudinal
components
of
magnetization

transverse components of magnetization

Figure 2.1   The magnitude of transverse magnetization vs amplitude of signal.

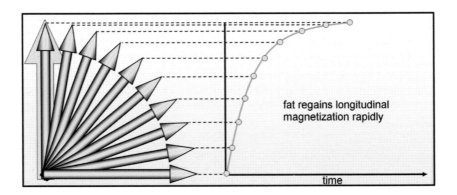

fat regains longitudinal
magnetization rapidly

time

Figure 2.2   T1 recovery in fat.

molecular tumbling in fat allows the recovery process to be relatively rapid, because the molecular tumbling rate matches the Larmor frequency and allows efficient energy exchange from hydrogen nuclei to the surrounding molecular lattice. This means that the magnetic moments of fat nuclei are able to relax and regain their longitudinal magnetization quickly. The NMV of fat realigns rapidly with B_0 so the T1 time of fat is short (Figure 2.2).

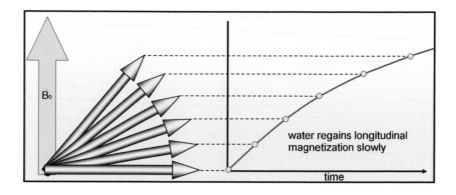

Figure 2.3   T1 recovery in water.

T1 recovery in water

T1 recovery occurs due to nuclei giving up the energy acquired from the RF excitation pulse to the surrounding lattice. Water has a high inherent energy and cannot easily absorb energy into its lattice from hydrogen nuclei. In water, molecular mobility is high, resulting in less efficient T1 recovery because the molecular tumbling rate does not match the Larmor frequency and does not allow efficient energy exchange from hydrogen nuclei to the surrounding molecular lattice. The magnetic moments of water take longer to relax and regain their longitudinal magnetization. The NMV of water takes longer to realign with B_0 and so the T1 time of water is long (Figure 2.3).

T2 decay in fat

T2 decay occurs as a result of the magnetic fields of the nuclei interacting with each other. This process is efficient in hydrogen in fat as the molecules are packed closely together and therefore spin–spin interactions are more likely to occur. As a result spins dephase quickly and the loss of transverse magnetization is rapid. The T2 time of fat is therefore short (Figure 2.4).

T2 decay in water

T2 decay in water is less efficient than in fat, as the molecules are spaced apart and spin–spin interactions are less likely to occur. As a result, spins dephase slowly and the loss of transverse magnetization is gradual. The T2 time of water is therefore long (Figure 2.5).

T1 contrast

As the T1 time of fat is shorter than that of water, the fat vector realigns with B_0 faster than the water vector. The longitudinal component of magnetization of fat is therefore larger than that of water. After a certain TR that is shorter than the total relaxation times of the tissues, the next RF excitation pulse is applied. The RF excitation pulse flips the longitudinal components of magnetization of both fat and water into the transverse plane (assuming a 90° pulse is applied)

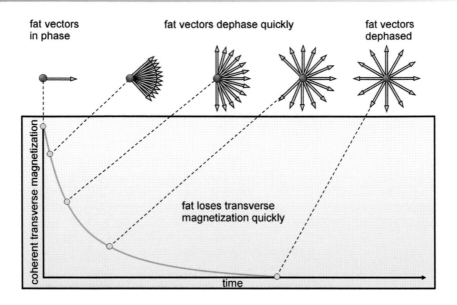

Figure 2.4   T2 decay in fat.

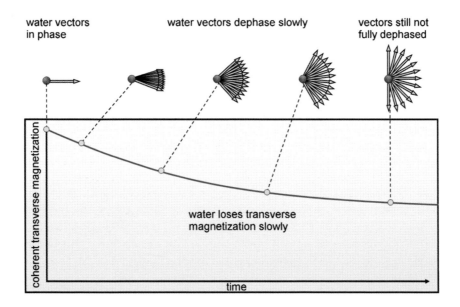

Figure 2.5   T2 decay in water.

as in Figure 2.6. As there is more longitudinal magnetization in fat before the RF pulse, there is more transverse magnetization in fat after the RF pulse. Fat therefore has a high signal and appears bright on a T1 contrast image. As there is less longitudinal magnetization in water before the RF pulse, there is less transverse magnetization in water after the RF pulse. Water therefore has a low signal and appears dark on a T1 contrast image. Such images are called **T1 weighted images** (*see* Figures 2.23 and 2.26).

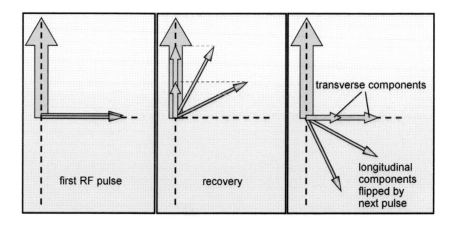

Figure 2.6   T1 contrast generation.

T2 contrast

The T2 time of fat is shorter than that of water, so the transverse component of magnetization of fat decays faster. The magnitude of transverse magnetization in water is large. Water has a high signal and appears bright on a T2 contrast image. However, the magnitude of transverse magnetization in fat is small. Fat therefore has a low signal and appears dark on a T2 contrast image (Figure 2.7). Such images are called **T2 weighted images** (*see* Figure 2.25).

Proton density contrast

Proton density contrast refers to differences in signal intensity between tissues that are a consequence of their relative number of mobile hydrogen protons per unit volume. To produce contrast due to the differences in the proton densities between the tissues, the transverse component of magnetization must reflect these differences. Tissues with a high proton density (e.g. brain tissue) have a large transverse component of magnetization (and therefore a high signal) and are bright on a proton density contrast image. Tissues with a low proton density (e.g. cortical bone) have a small transverse component of magnetization (and therefore a low signal) and are dark on a proton density contrast image (*see* Figure 2.24). Proton density contrast is always present and depends on the patient and the area being examined. It is the basic MRI contrast and is called **proton density weighting.**

Summary

- Fat has a short T1 and T2 time
- Water has a long T1 and T2 time
- To produce high signal, there must be a large component of coherent magnetization in the transverse plane to induce a large signal in the coil
- To produce a low signal, there must be a small component of coherent magnetization in the transverse plane to induce a small signal in the coil

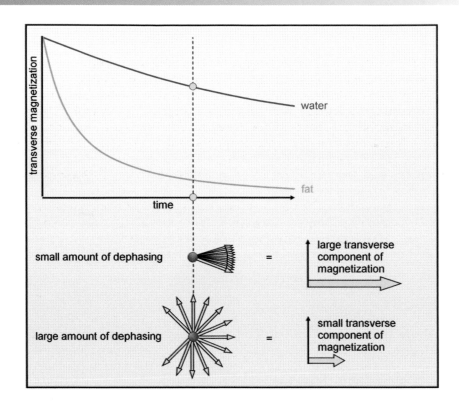

Figure 2.7 T2 contrast generation.

Table 2.1 T1 and T2 relaxation times of brain tissue at 1T.

Tissue	T1 time (ms)	T2 time (ms)
Water	2500	2500
Fat	200	100
Cerebrospinal fluid	2000	300
White matter	500	100

- T1 weighted images are characterized by bright fat and dark water
- T2 weighted images are characterized by bright water and dark fat
- Proton density weighted images are characterized by areas with high proton density (bright) and areas with low proton density (dark)
- The T1 and T2 relaxation times of a tissue, although inherent to that tissue, are dependent on the field strength of the magnet. As field strength increases, tissues take longer to relax. Table 2.1 shows the T1 and T2 relaxation times of brain tissue at 1T

Weighting

All the intrinsic contrast parameters listed at the beginning of this chapter simultaneously affect image contrast and would therefore produce images of mixed contrast. This means that when reading an image it would be very difficult to determine the relative contribution of each param-eter to the contrast observed. This makes image interpretation very challenging. So we need to *weight* image contrast towards one of the parameters and away from the others. This is done by using our understanding of how extrinsic contrast parameters control the relative contribution of each intrinsic contrast parameter. Flow and ADC are discussed in later chapters and are controlled in a specialized way. The other types of weighting mechanisms (T1, T2 and proton density) are discussed here.

To demonstrate either T1, proton density or T2 contrast, specific values of TR and TE are selected for a given pulse sequence. The selection of appropriate TR and TE weights an image so that one contrast mechanism *predominates* over the other two.

T1 weighting

A T1 weighted image is one where the contrast depends predominantly on the differences in the T1 times between fat and water (and all the tissues with intermediate signal). Because the TR controls how far each vector recovers before the slice is excited by the next RF pulse, to achieve T1 weighting the TR must be short enough so that neither fat nor water has sufficient time to fully return to B_0. If the TR is too long, both fat and water return to B_0 and recover their longitu-dinal magnetization fully. When this occurs, T1 relaxation is complete in both tissues and the differences in their T1 times are not demonstrated (Figure 2.8).

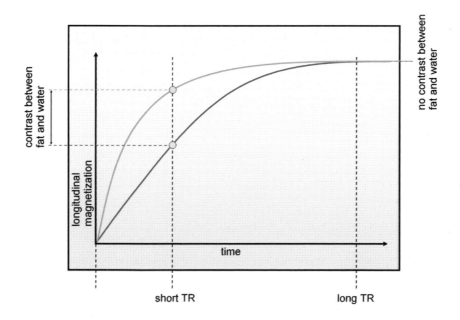

Figure 2.8   The T1 differences between fat and water.

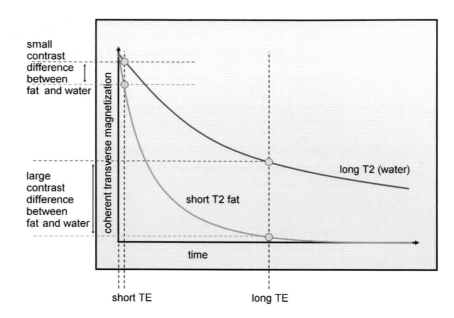

Figure 2.9 The T2 differences between fat and water.

- *TR* controls the amount of *T1 weighting.*
- For *T1* weighting the *TR* must be *short.*

Refer to animation 2.1 on the supporting companion website for this book: www.wiley.com/go/mriinpractice

T2 weighting

A T2 weighted image is one where the contrast predominantly depends on the differences in the T2 times between fat and water (and all the tissues with intermediate signal). The TE controls the amount of T2 decay that is allowed to occur before the signal is received. To achieve T2 weighting, the TE must be long enough to give both fat and water time to decay. If the TE is too short, neither fat nor water has had time to decay, and therefore the differences in their T2 times are not demonstrated (Figure 2.9).

- *TE* controls the amount of *T2 weighting.*
- For *T2* weighting the *TE* must be *long.*

Proton density weighting

A proton density image is one where the difference in the numbers of mobile hydrogen protons per unit volume in the patient is the main determining factor in forming image contrast. Proton density weighting is always present to some extent. To achieve proton density weighting, the effects of T1 and T2 contrast must be diminished so that proton density weighting can dominate. A long TR allows both fat and water to fully recover their longitudinal magnetization and so diminishes T1 weighting. A short TE does not give fat or water time to decay and so diminishes T2 weighting.

In any image, the contrast due to the inherent proton density together with T1 and T2 mechanisms occur simultaneously and contribute to image contrast. To weight an image so that one process is dominant, the other processes must be diminished.

Learning point: the heat analogy

The mechanisms of weighting are well described using an analogy of a gas oven that has two knobs labeled TR and TE. The TR knob controls the amount of T1 contrast; the TE knob controls the amount of T2 contrast. The TR knob turns the heat up or down on T1 contrast. The TE knob turns the heat up or down on T2 contrast.

Turning the *TR knob down*, turns the *heat up on T1 contrast*, i.e. T1 contrast is increased. Turning the *TE knob up*, turns the *heat up on T2 contrast*, i.e. T2 contrast is increased. To weight an image in a particular direction we need to turn the heat up on one intrinsic contrast parameter and the heat down on the others.

For example, for *T1 weighting* turn the heat up on T1 and the heat down on T2 so the image is weighted towards T1 contrast and away from T2 contrast (proton density depends on the relative number of protons and cannot be changed for a given area).

- To turn the heat up on T1 contrast the TR is short (TR knob down).
- To turn the heat down on T2 the TE is short (TE knob down) (Figure 2.10).

For *T2 weighting* turn the heat up on T2 and the heat down on T1. In this way the image is weighted towards T2 contrast and away from T1 contrast (proton density depends on the relative number of protons and cannot be changed for a given area).

- To turn the heat up on T2 contrast the TE is long (TE knob up).
- To turn the heat down on T1 contrast the TR is long (TR knob up) (Figure 2.11).

For *PD weighting* turn the heat down on T1 and the heat down on T2. In this way proton density contrast predominates.

- To turn the heat down on T1 contrast the TR is long (TR knob up).
- To turn the heat down on T2 the TE is short (TE knob down) (Figure 2.12).

The heat analogy is used elsewhere in this book. Look out for the heat symbol in the margin.

T2* decay

When the RF excitation pulse is removed, the relaxation and decay processes occur immediately. T2* decay is the decay of the FID following the RF excitation pulse. This decay is faster than T2 decay since it is a combination of two effects:

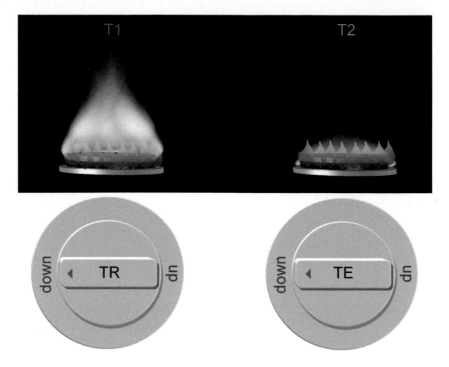

Figure 2.10   T1 weighting and the heat analogy.

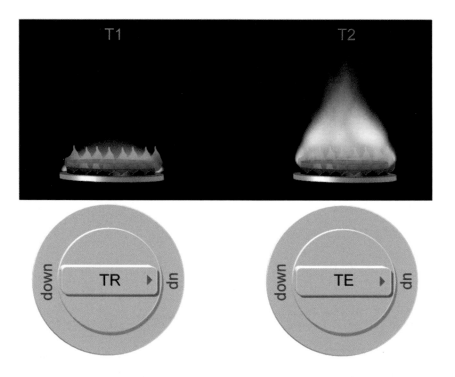

Figure 2.11   T2 weighting and the heat analogy.

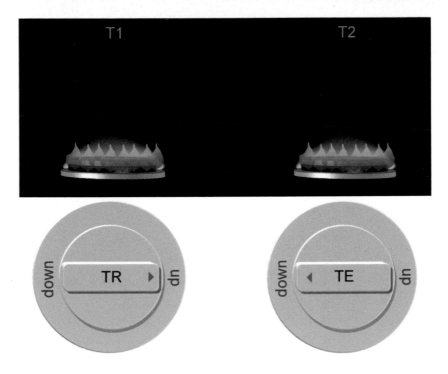

Figure 2.12   Proton density weighting and the heat analogy.

Learning point: saturation

Whenever the NMV is pushed beyond 90° it is said to be **partially saturated**. When the NMV is pushed to a full 180° it is said to be **fully saturated**. If partial saturation of the fat and water vectors occurs, T1 weighting results. If, however, saturation of the fat and water vectors does not occur, proton density weighting results. To understand this, the processes of T1 recovery should be reviewed.

Look at Figure 2.13. Before the application of the first RF pulse, the fat and water vectors are aligned with B_0. When the first 90° RF pulse is applied, the fat and water vectors are flipped into the transverse plane. The RF pulse is then removed, and the vectors begin to relax and return to B_0. Fat has a shorter T1 than water and so returns to B_0 faster than water. If the TR is shorter than the T1 of the tissues, the next (and all succeeding) RF pulses flip the vectors beyond 90° and into partial saturation because their recovery was incomplete. The fat and water vectors are saturated to different degrees because they were at different points of recovery before the 90° flip. The transverse component of magnetization for each vector is therefore different.

The transverse component of fat is greater than that of water because its longitudinal component recovers to a greater degree before the next RF pulse is applied, and so more longitudinal magnetization is available to be flipped into the transverse plane. The fat vector therefore generates a higher signal than water – fat is bright and water is dark. A T1 weighted image results.

Now look at Figure 2.14. If the TR is longer than the T1 times of the tissues, both fat and water fully recover before the next (and all succeeding) RF pulses are applied. Both vectors are flipped directly into the transverse plane and are not saturated. The magnitude of the transverse component of magnetization for fat and water depends only on their individual proton densities, rather than the rate of recovery of their longitudinal components. Tissues with a high proton density are bright, while tissues with a low proton density are dark. A proton density weighted image results. Clearly the flip angle (how far the RF excitation pulse moves the vectors via resonance) has a significant impact on saturation effects. This is discussed in more detail later.

- T2 decay itself
- dephasing due to magnetic field **inhomogeneities**.

Inhomogeneities are areas within the magnetic field that do not exactly match the external magnetic field strength. Some areas have a magnetic field strength slightly less than the main magnetic field (shown in blue in Figure 2.15), while other areas have a magnetic field strength slightly more than the main magnetic field (shown in red in Figure 2.15).

As the Larmor equation states, the Larmor frequency of a nucleus is proportional to the magnetic field strength it experiences. If a nucleus lies in an area of inhomogeneity with higher field strength, the precessional frequency of the nucleus increases, i.e. it speeds up. However, if a nucleus lies in an area of inhomogeneity with lower field strength, the precessional frequency of the nucleus decreases, i.e. it slows down. This is shown in Figure 2.15. This relative acceleration and deceleration as a result of magnetic field inhomogeneities and differences in the precessional frequency in certain tissues, causes immediate dephasing of the spins and produces a FID as shown in Figure 2.15. This dephasing is predominantly responsible for T2* decay. The rate of dephasing due to inhomogeneities is an exponential process.

Learning point: inhomogeneities

Do you remember the watch analogy in Chapter 1? The change of phase of magnetic moments due to inhomogeneities in the field is exactly the same as several watches telling different times because the frequencies of their hour hands are different.

Introduction to pulse sequences

Dephasing caused by inhomogeneities produces a rapid loss of coherent transverse magnetization and therefore signal, so that it reaches zero before most tissues have had time to attain their T1 or T2 relaxation times. To measure relaxation times and produce an image with good contrast we need to regenerate the signal. There are two ways of doing this – by using an additional 180° RF

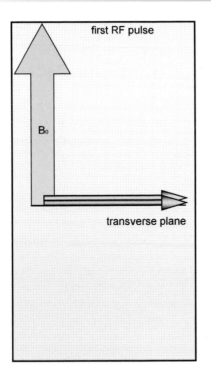

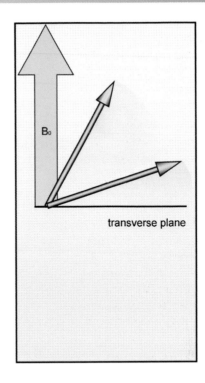

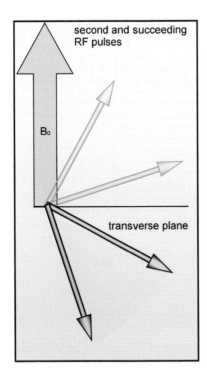

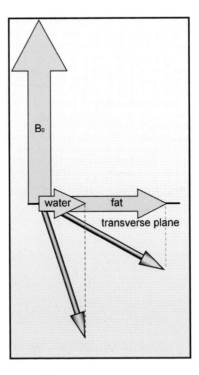

Figure 2.13   Saturation with a short TR.

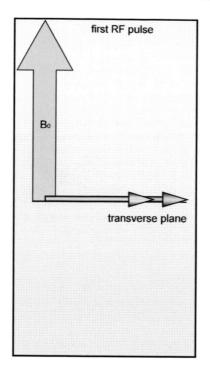

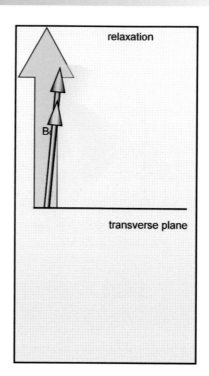

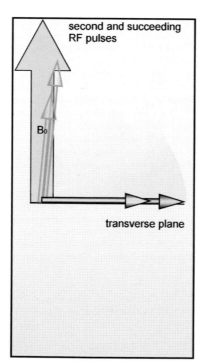

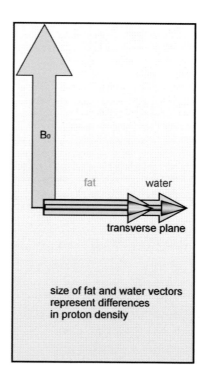

Figure 2.14   No saturation with a long TR.

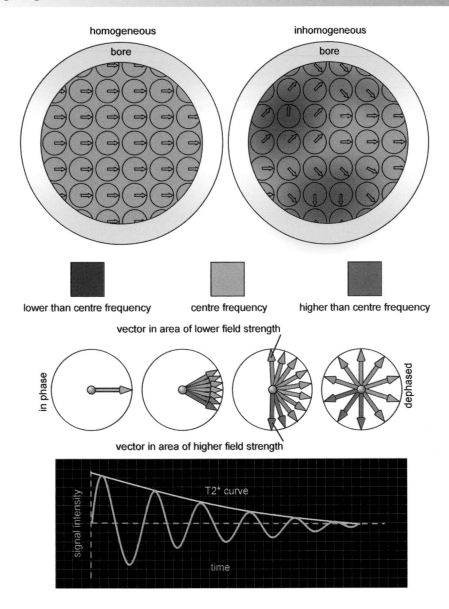

Figure 2.15   T2* decay and field inhomogeneities.

pulse or by using gradients. Sequences that use a 180° pulse to regenerate signal are called **spin echo pulse sequences**; those that use a gradient are called **gradient echo pulse sequences**. These are now discussed in more detail.

The spin echo pulse sequence

The **spin echo pulse sequence** commonly uses a 90° excitation pulse to flip the NMV into the transverse plane. The NMV precesses in the transverse plane inducing a voltage in the receiver

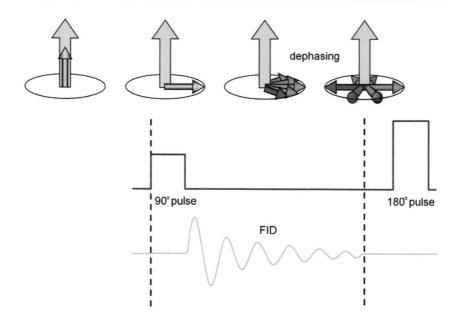

Figure 2.16   T2* dephasing.

coil. The precessional paths of the magnetic moments of the nuclei are translated into the transverse plane. When the 90° RF pulse is removed, a free induction decay signal (FID) is produced. T2* dephasing occurs almost immediately, and the signal decays. A 180° RF pulse is then used to compensate for this dephasing (Figure 2.16).

Refer to animation 2.2 on the supporting companion website for this book: www.wiley.com/go/mriinpractice

The 180° RF pulse is an RF pulse that has sufficient energy to move the NMV through 180°. The T2* dephasing causes the magnetic moments to dephase or 'fan out' in the transverse plane. The magnetic moments are now out of phase with each other, i.e. they are at different positions on the precessional path at any given time. The magnetic moments that slow down form the trailing edge of the fan (shown in blue in Figure 2.17). The magnetic moments that speed up form the leading edge of the fan (shown in red in Figure 2.17). The 180° RF pulse flips these individual magnetic moments through 180° (a bit like flipping a pancake). They are still in the transverse plane, but now the magnetic moments that formed the trailing edge before the 180° pulse form the leading edge. Conversely, the magnetic moments that formed the leading edge before the 180° pulse now form the trailing edge (as shown in the bottom half of Figure 2.17). The red spin that formed the leading edge before the 180° pulse now forms the trailing edge. The blue spin that formed the trailing edge before the 180° pulse now forms the leading edge.

The direction of precession remains the same, and so the trailing edge begins to catch up with the leading edge. At a specific time later, the two edges are superimposed. The magnetic moments

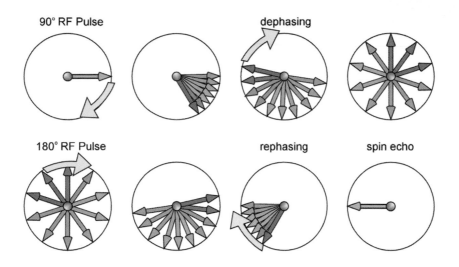

Figure 2.17   180° rephasing.

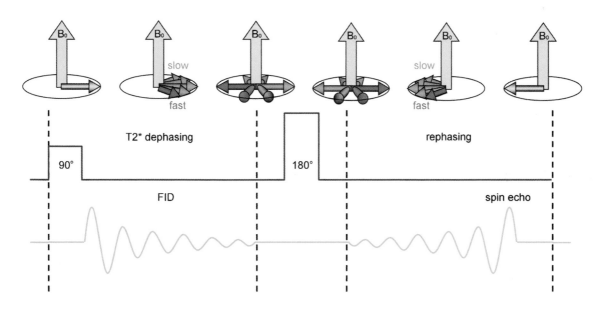

Figure 2.18   A basic rephasing sequence.

are now momentarily in phase because they are momentarily at the same place on the precessional path. At this instant, there is transverse magnetization in phase, and so a maximum signal
is induced in the coil. This signal is called a **spin echo**. The spin echo now contains T1 and T2
information as T2* dephasing has been reduced and more time has been allowed for tissues to
reach their T1 and T2 relaxation times (Figure 2.18).

Learning point: the Larmor Grand Prix

An easy way to understand 180° rephasing is to imagine three cars on a circular racetrack. The cars relate to three magnetic moments and the circular racetrack to the precessional path of the magnetic moments. The cars have varying speeds; one is a racing car, one a family saloon and one a tractor (see Figure 2.19).

At the sound of the start gun the cars set off around the track. Very shortly, the racing car pulls ahead of the family car, which in turn sprints ahead of the tractor. They are now out of phase with each other, as they are in a different place on the track to each other at a given time. The longer the race is allowed to run, the more dephasing between the vehicles occurs.

The starting gun is fired again. The starting gun now refers to the 180° RF pulse. On hearing the gun, the cars turn around through 180° and head back towards the start line again. The racing car is now at the back, because it traveled furthest at the beginning of the race. The tractor is at the front because it traveled slower at the beginning of the race. The family saloon is somewhere in between. Assuming the cars travel back to the start line at exactly the same speed as they traveled out at the beginning of the race, the racing car and family saloon catch up with the tractor, and are at exactly the same place at the same time when they get back to the start line. So they are back in phase, and if they were magnetic moments they would generate a spin echo at this point. The time taken for the cars to complete the whole race (from the starting line to the point where they turn around and back to the starting line again) corresponds to the TE.

Timing parameters in spin echo

TR is the time between each 90° excitation pulse for each slice. TE is the time between the 90° excitation pulse and the peak of the spin echo (Figure 2.20). The time taken to rephase after the application of the 180° RF pulse equals the time to dephase when the 90° RF pulse was withdrawn. This time is called the **TAU** time. The TE is therefore twice the TAU. Look at Figure 2.20 and note the symmetry of the spin echo. As spins gradually come into phase, the signal gradually builds, reaching a peak at the TE when all the spins are in phase. However, the fast spins soon overtake the slow ones and dephasing occurs again. This results in a gradual loss of signal, which mirrors the gradual growth before the peak of the echo. This accounts for its symmetry.

In most spin echo pulse sequences, more than one 180° RF pulse can be applied after the 90° excitation pulse. Each 180° pulse generates a separate spin echo that can be received by the coil and used to create an image. Although any number of echoes can be created, spin echo sequences are typically used generating either one or two echoes.

Spin echo using one echo

This pulse sequence can be used to produce T1 weighted images if a short TR and TE are used (Figure 2.21). One 180° RF pulse is applied after the 90° excitation pulse. The single 180° RF

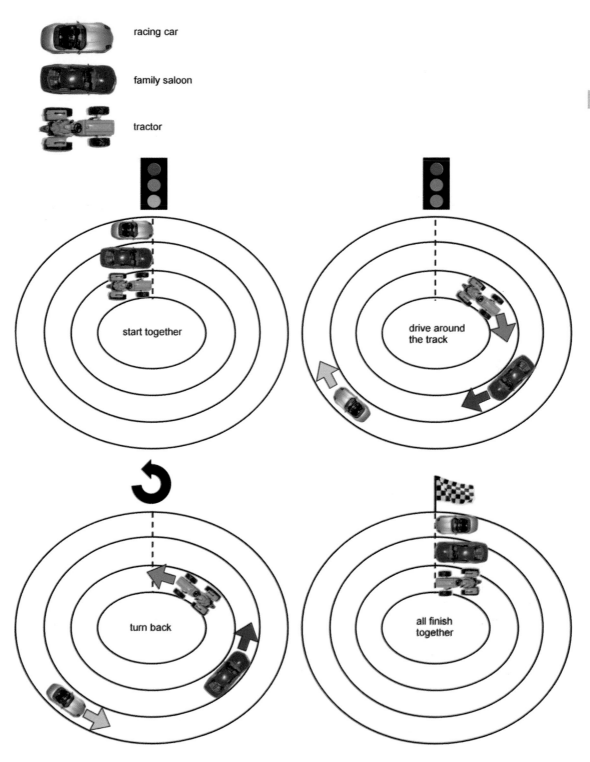

racing car

family saloon

tractor

start together

drive around
the track

turn back

all finish
together

Figure 2.19   The Larmor Grand Prix.

Refer to animation 2.3 on the supporting companion website for this book: www.wiley.com/go/mriinpractice

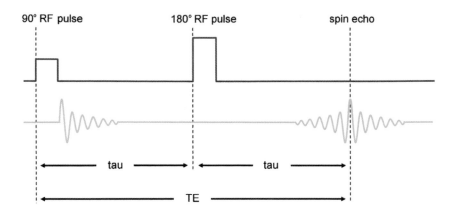

Figure 2.20   TAU.

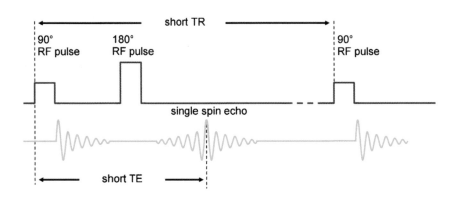

Figure 2.21   Spin echo with one echo.

pulse generates a single spin echo. The timing parameters used are selected to produce a T1 weighted image. A short TE ensures that the 180° RF pulse and subsequent echo occur early, so that only a little T2 decay has occurred. The differences in the T2 times of the tissues do not dominate the echo and its contrast. A short TR ensures that the fat and water vectors have not fully recovered, and so the differences in their T1 times dominate the echo and its contrast (Figure 2.23).

Spin echo using two echoes

This can be used to produce both a proton density and a T2 weighted image in the TR time (Figure 2.22). The first spin echo is generated early by selecting a short TE. Only a little T2 decay has occurred and so T2 differences between the tissues are minimized in this echo. The

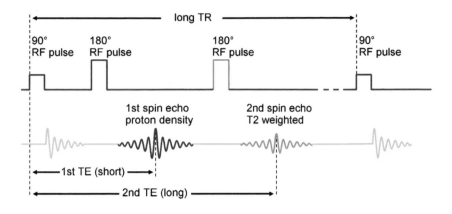

Figure 2.22   Spin echo with two echoes.

second spin echo is generated much later by selecting a long TE. A significant amount of T2 decay has now occurred, and so the differences in the T2 times of the tissues are maximized in this echo. The TR selected is long, so that T1 differences between the tissues are minimized. The first spin echo therefore has a short TE and a long TR and is proton density weighted. The second spin echo has a long TE and a long TR and is T2 weighted. Figure 2.23 shows a T1 weighted image; Figure 2.24 shows a proton density weighted image; and Figure 2.25 shows a T2 weighted image.

Summary

- Spin echo pulse sequences produce either T1, T2 or proton density weighting
- TR controls the T1 weighting (see the heat analogy)
- Short TR maximizes T1 weighting
- Long TR maximizes proton density weighting
- TE controls the T2 weighting
- Short TE minimizes T2 weighting
- Long TE maximizes T2 weighting

Typical values of TR and TE

Long TR   2000 ms
Short TR   300–700 ms
Long TE   60 ms+
Short TE   10–25 ms

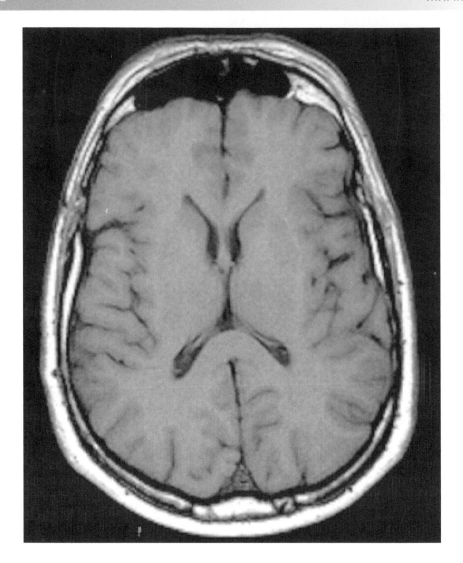

Figure 2.23   Axial T1 weighted spin echo image through the brain.

Learning point:
understanding weighting

Understanding image weighting is a fundamental skill in MRI. One of the basic rules is to look for the water content in the image, and if it has a high signal the image is likely to be T2 weighted and have been acquired with a long TE. If water has a low signal it is likely to be T1 weighted and have been acquired with a short TR, but depending on the area of the body, some proton density images have dark water. Fat is an unreliable marker as it can be bright on many types of weighting depending on the pulse sequence used.

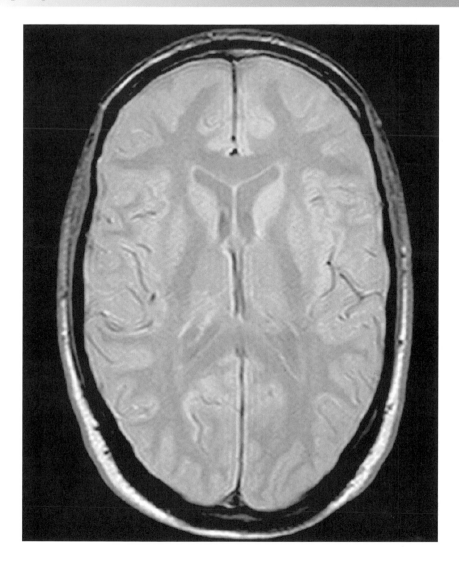

Figure 2.24   Axial PD weighted spin echo image through the brain.

To demonstrate the variables in image contrast, look at Figure 2.26. It was acquired using a standard spin echo sequence and is a T1 weighted image so the contrast is predominantly due to differences in the T1 recovery times of the tissues. It has contrast we would expect from an image acquired with a short TR and TE, e.g. fat in the scalp and bony marrow of the clivus is bright and water in the CSF is dark. However, looking more closely it is clear that not all areas of high signal are fat and not all areas of low signal are water. For example, the area labeled A, which has a high signal, is not fat but slow-flowing blood in the superior sagittal sinus. The area labeled B, which has a low signal, is not water but air in the sphenoid sinus. Although this image is predominantly T1 weighted, there are also flow and proton density affects contributing to image contrast. Now look at Figures 2.24 and 2.25 and see if you can identify areas that demonstrate contrast not typical of the weighting shown.

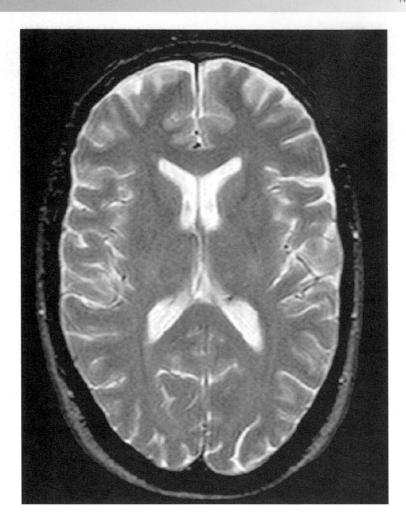

Figure 2.25 Axial T2 weighted spin echo image through the brain.

The gradient echo pulse sequence

A gradient echo pulse sequence uses an RF excitation pulse that is variable, and therefore flips the NMV through any angle (not just 90°). A transverse component of magnetization is created, the magnitude of which is less than in spin echo, where all the longitudinal magnetization is converted to the transverse plane. When a flip angle other than 90° is used, only part of the longitudinal magnetization is converted to transverse magnetization, which precesses in the transverse plane and induces a signal in the receiver coil (Figure 2.27).

After the RF pulse is withdrawn, the FID signal is immediately produced due to inhomogeneities in the magnetic field and T2* dephasing therefore occurs. The magnetic moments within the transverse component of magnetization dephase, and are then rephased by a gradient. A gradient causes a change in the magnetic field strength within the magnet and is discussed in more detail later. The gradient rephases the magnetic moments so that a signal is received by the coil, which contains T1 and T2 information. This signal is called a **gradient echo.**

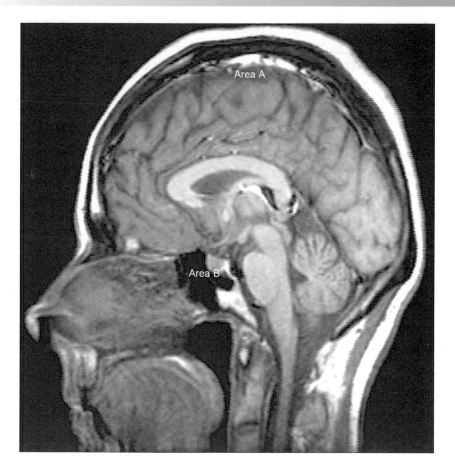

Figure 2.26 Midline sagittal T1 weighted spin echo image through the brain.

Gradients

Gradients perform many tasks, which are explored fully in Chapter 3. **Magnetic field gradients** are generated by coils of wire situated within the bore of the magnet. The law of electromagnetic induction states that when charge moves through a gradient coil, a magnetic field (or gradient field as it is now known) is induced around it. This gradient field interacts with the main static magnetic field, so that the magnetic field strength along the axis of the gradient coil is altered in a linear way. The middle of the axis of the gradients remains at the field strength of the main magnetic field. This is called **magnetic isocentre**.

The magnetic field strength increases relative to isocentre in one direction of the gradient axis because the magnetic field produced by the gradient adds to the main magnetic field (shown in red on Figure 2.28). It decreases relative to isocentre in the other direction of the gradient axis because the magnetic field produced by the gradient subtracts from the main magnetic field (shown in blue in Figure 2.28). Whether a gradient field adds or subtracts from the main magnetic field depends on the direction of current passing through the gradient coils. This is called the **polarity** of the gradient.

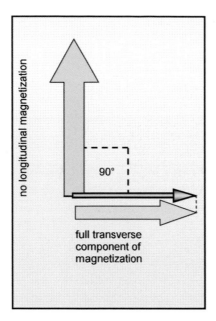 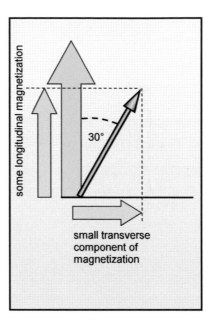

Figure 2.27   How the flip angle controls the amplitude of the signal.

When a gradient is switched on, the magnetic field strength along its axis is sloped or graded. The Larmor equation states that the precessional frequency of the magnetic moments increases or decreases depending on the magnetic field strength they experience at different points along the gradient (Figure 2.28).

The precessional frequency increases when the magnetic field increases and decreases when the magnetic field decreases. Magnetic moments experiencing an increased field strength due to the gradient speed up, i.e. their precessional frequency increases. Magnetic moments experiencing a decreased magnetic field strength slow down, i.e. their precessional frequency decreases. As gradients cause nuclei to speed up or slow down, they can be used to either dephase or rephase their magnetic moments.

How gradients dephase

Look at Figure 2.29. With no gradient applied, all spins precess at the same frequency as they experience the same field strength (in reality they do not because of inhomogeneities in the field, but these changes are relatively small compared with those imposed by a gradient). A gradient is applied to coherent (in phase) magnetization (all the magnetic moments are in the same place at the same time). The gradient alters the magnetic field strength experienced by the coherent magnetization. Depending on their position along the gradient axis some of the magnetic moments speed up and some slow down. Thus the magnetic moments fan out or dephase because their frequencies have been changed by the gradient (*see* the watch analogy in Chapter 1).

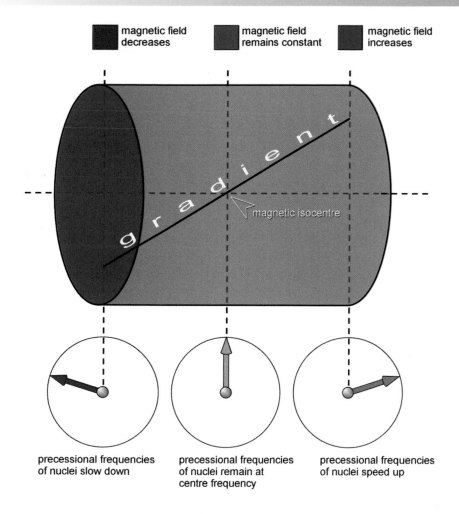

Figure 2.28   The gradients.

The trailing edge of the fan (shown in blue) consists of nuclei that have slowed down, because they are situated on the gradient axis that has a lower magnetic field strength relative to isocentre. The leading edge of the fan (shown in red) consists of nuclei that have sped up because they are situated on the gradient axis that has a higher magnetic field strength relative to isocentre. The magnetic moments of the nuclei are therefore no longer in the same place at the same time and so the magnetization has been dephased by the gradient. Gradients that dephase are called **spoilers**.

How gradients rephase

Look at Figure 2.30. A gradient is applied to incoherent (out of phase) magnetization. The magnetic moments have fanned out due to T2* dephasing and the fan has a trailing edge consisting of slow

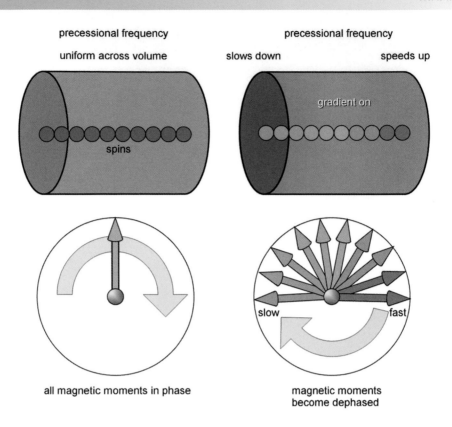

precessional frequency
uniform across volume

precessional frequency
slows down   speeds up

gradient on

spins

all magnetic moments in phase

magnetic moments
become dephased

slow   fast

Figure 2.29   How gradients dephase.

nuclei (shown in blue), and a leading edge consisting of faster nuclei (shown in red). A gradient is then applied, so that the magnetic field strength is altered in a linear fashion along the axis of the gradient. The direction of this altered field strength is such that the slow nuclei in the trailing edge of the fan experience an increased magnetic field strength and speed up.

In Figure 2.30 the blue spins are experiencing the red, 'high end' of the gradient. The faster nuclei in the leading edge of the fan experience a decreased magnetic field strength and slow down. In Figure 2.30 the red spins are experiencing the blue 'low end' of the gradient. After a short period of time, the slow nuclei have sped up sufficiently to meet the faster nuclei that are slowing down. When the two meet, all the magnetic moments are in the same place at the same time and have been rephased by the gradient. A maximum signal is therefore induced in the receiver coil and this signal is called a gradient echo. Gradients that rephase are called **rewinders**.

The advantages of gradient echo pulse sequences

Since gradients rephase faster than 180° RF pulses, the minimum TE is much shorter than in spin echo pulse sequences, and so the TR can also be reduced. The TR can also be decreased because flip angles other than 90° are used. With low flip angles, full recovery of the longitudinal magnetization occurs sooner than with large flip angles. The TR can therefore be shortened without producing saturation. The TR plays an important part in the time of the scan (*see* Chapter 3), so

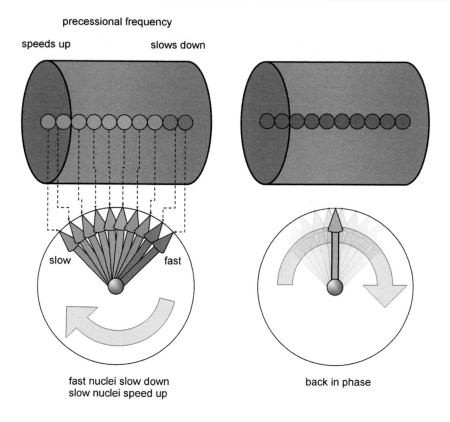

precessional frequency

speeds up   slows down

slow   fast

fast nuclei slow down
slow nuclei speed up

back in phase

Figure 2.30   How gradients rephase.

as the TR is reduced, the scan time is also reduced. Gradient echo pulse sequences are therefore usually associated with much shorter scan times than spin echo pulse sequences.

The disadvantages of gradient echo pulse sequences

The most important disadvantage is that there is no compensation for magnetic field inhomogeneities. Gradient echo pulse sequences are therefore very susceptible to magnetic field inhomogeneities. Gradient echo pulse sequences contain magnetic susceptibility artefact (*see* Chapter 7). As the T2* effects are not eliminated, in gradient echo imaging T2 weighting is termed T2* weighting and T2 decay is termed T2* decay.

Timing parameters in gradient echo

As in spin echo, the TR is the time between each RF excitation pulse, while the TE is the time from the excitation pulse to the peak of gradient echo. Although not a timing parameter, in gradient echo sequences the flip angle is an extrinsic contrast parameter that is changed to affect image contrast. Its value, combined with the TR, determines whether T1 effects are maximized or minimized.

Weighting and contrast in gradient echo

The TR, TE and flip angle affect image weighting and contrast, and the TR (and therefore the scan time) can be much shorter than in spin echo pulse sequences. As the TR controls that amount of T1 recovery that has been allowed to occur before the application of the next RF pulse, a short TR usually produces T1 weighting and never permits a T2 or proton density weighted image to be obtained. To give gradient echo imaging more flexibility, the flip angle is usually reduced to less than 90°. If the flip angle is less than 90°, it does not take the NMV as long to recover full longitudinal magnetization as it does with a larger flip angle, and so the TR can be shortened to reduce the scan time without producing saturation.

In gradient echo pulse sequences, the TR and the flip angle control the amount of T1 relaxation that has occurred before the next RF pulse is applied. The TE controls the amount of T2* decay that has occurred before the gradient echo is received by the coil. Apart from the added variable of the flip angle, the rules of weighting in gradient echo are exactly the same as in spin echo (*see* the heat analogy in Chapter 1).

T1 weighting in gradient echo

To obtain a T1 weighted image, the differences in the T1 times of the tissues are maximized and the differences in the T2 times of the tissues are minimized. To maximize T1 differences, neither the fat nor water vectors must have had time to recover full longitudinal magnetization before the next RF pulse is applied. To avoid full recovery, the flip angle is large and the TR short, so that the fat and water vectors are still in the process of relaxing when the next RF is applied. To minimize T2* differences, the TE is short so that neither fat nor water has had time to decay (Figure 2.31).

T2* weighting in gradient echo

To obtain a T2* weighted image, the differences in the T2* times of the tissues are maximized and the differences in the T1 times are minimized. To maximize T2* decay, the TE is long so that the fat and water vectors have had time to decay sufficiently to show their decay differences. To minimize T1 recovery, the flip angle is small and the TR long enough to permit full recovery of the fat and water vectors. In this way, T1 differences are not demonstrated. In practice, small flip angles produce such little transverse magnetization that the TR can be kept relatively short and full recovery still has time to occur (Figure 2.32).

Proton density weighting in gradient echo

To obtain a proton density weighted image both T1 and T2* processes are minimized so that the differences in proton density of the tissues can be demonstrated. To minimize T2* decay, the TE is short so that neither the fat nor the water vectors have had time to decay. To minimize T1 recovery, the flip angle is small and the TR long enough to permit full recovery of longitudinal magnetization.

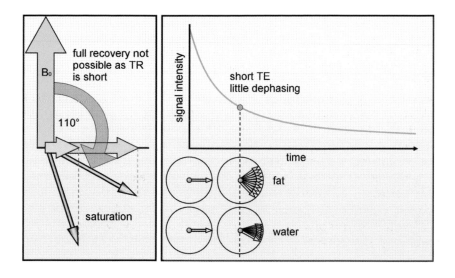

Figure 2.31   T1 weighting in gradient echo.

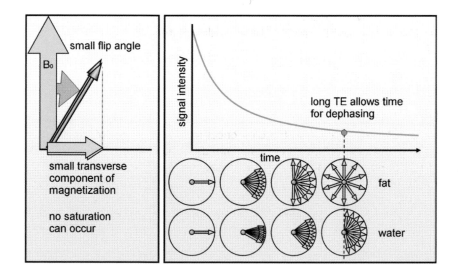

Figure 2.32   T2* weighting in gradient echo.

Learning point: weighting and gradient echo using the heat analogy

For T1 weighting turn the heat up on T1 and the heat down on T2*. Flip angle and TR control T1 contrast, TE controls T2* contrast (proton density depends on the relative number of protons and cannot be changed for a given area).

- To turn the heat up on T1 contrast the TR is short (TR knob down) and the flip angle is high.
- To turn the heat down on T2* the TE is short (TE knob down) (Figure 2.33).

For T2 weighting* turn the heat up on T2* and the heat down on T1. Flip angle and TR control T1 contrast, TE controls T2* contrast (proton density depends on the relative number of protons and cannot be changed for a given area).

- To turn the heat up on T2* contrast the TE is long (TE knob up).
- To turn the heat down on T1 contrast the TR is long (TR knob up) and the flip angle is low (Figure 2.34).

For PD weighting turn the heat down on T1 and the heat down on T2*. In this way proton density contrast predominates.

- To turn the heat down on T1 contrast the TR is long (TR knob up) and the flip angle low.
- To turn the heat down on T2* the TE is short (TE knob down) (Figure 2.35).

Look at Figures 2.36 and 2.37. Both were acquired using a gradient echo sequence and the same TR. To change the weighting, one other parameter has been altered. Is it the flip angle or TE?

To answer this question, first determine their weighting. Figure 2.36 is clearly T2* weighted as CSF has a high signal. Figure 2.37 is more difficult to interpret. Although CSF is darker than on Figure 2.36 and could be thought to be T1 weighted, the hydrated intervertebral discs have a high signal, which we would not expect on a T1 weighted image. Therefore this image is proton density weighted. As neither image is T1 weighted, neither was acquired with a high flip angle. Both have a low flip angle and – as the TR is the same – the parameter that has changed is the TE.

In Figure 2.37, low flip angles have minimized saturation and therefore T1 contrast and a short TE has minimized T2* contrast, resulting in a proton density weighted image. Figure 2.36 has also been acquired with a low flip angle minimizing T1 contrast, but has a long TE maximizing T2* contrast resulting in a T2* weighted image. The parameter that has been changed is therefore the TE.

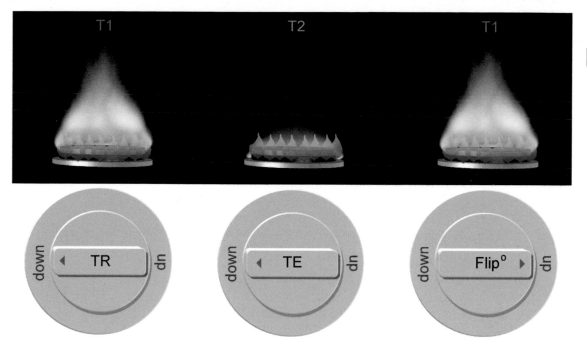

Figure 2.33 T1 contrast in gradient echo and the heat analogy.

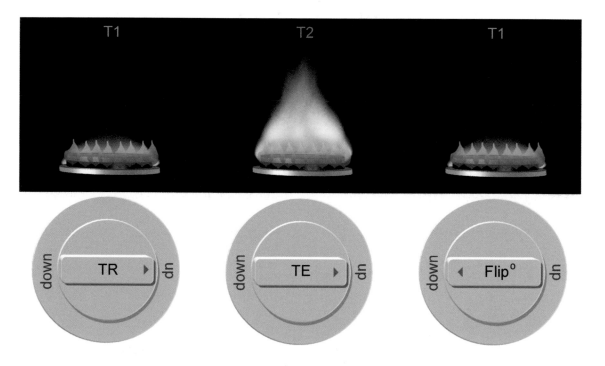

Figure 2.34 T2* contrast in gradient echo and the heat analogy.

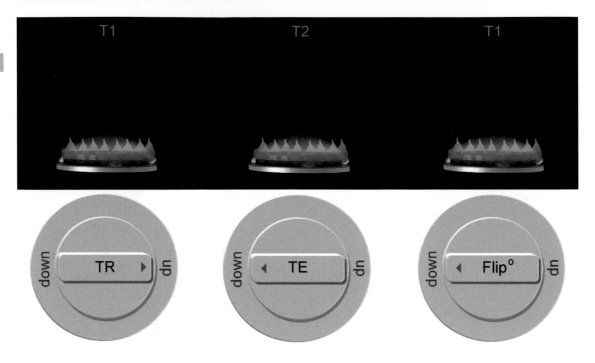

Figure 2.35   PD contrast in gradient echo and the heat analogy.

Summary

- Gradient echo pulse sequences use a gradient to rephase the magnetic moments
- Variable flip angles are used
- The TE can be much shorter than in spin echo imaging
- Gradients do not eliminate effects from magnetic field inhomogeneities

Typical values in gradient echo imaging

Long TR	100 ms+
Short TR	less than 50 ms
Short TE	1–5 ms
Long TE	15–25 ms
Low flip angles	5–20°
Large flip angles	70°+

Table 2.2 summarizes the differences between spin echo and gradient echo. Table 2.3 gives the parameters used in gradient echo. Signal creation and how it can be manipulated to produce image contrast has now been discussed. In the next chapter, the process of image formation is described.

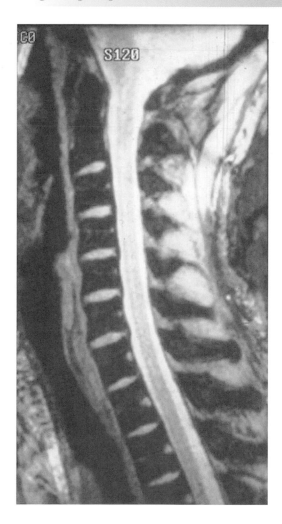

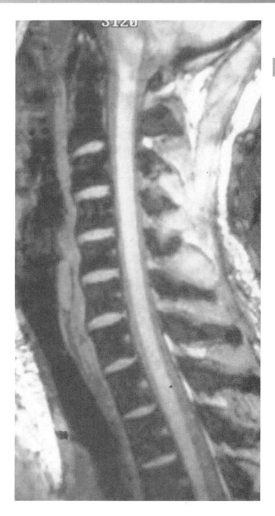

Figure 2.36   Midline sagittal T2 *
weighted gradient echo through the
cervical spine.

Figure 2.37   Midline sagittal PD
weighted gradient echo through the
cervical spine.

Table 2.2   Summary of the differences between parameters used in spin echo and gradient
echo.

Sequence	TR	TE	Flip angle
Spin echo	long 2000 ms+	long 70 ms+	90°
	short 300–700 ms+	short 10–30 ms+	90°
Gradient echo	long 100 ms+	long 15–25 ms	small 5°–20°
	short less than 50 ms	short less than 5 ms	medium 30°–45°
			large 70°+

Table 2.3   Parameters used in gradient echo.

Weighting	TR	TE	Flip angle
T1	short	short	large
T2	long	long	small
Proton density	long	short	small

 For questions and answers on this topic please visit the supporting companion website for this book: www.wiley.com/go/ mriinpractice

3

Encoding and image formation

ENCODING

Introduction

As previously described, for resonance to occur RF must be applied at 90° to B_0 at the precessional frequency of hydrogen. The RF pulse gives hydrogen nuclei energy so that transverse magnetization is created. The RF pulse also puts the individual magnetic moments of hydrogen into phase. The resultant coherent transverse magnetization precesses at the Larmor frequency of hydrogen in the transverse plane. A voltage or signal is therefore induced in the receiver coil that is positioned in the transverse plane. This signal has a frequency equal to the Larmor frequency of hydrogen, regardless of the origin of signal in the patient.

The system must be able to locate signal spatially in three dimensions, so that it can position each signal at the correct point on the image. To do this, it first locates a slice. Once a slice is selected, the signal is located or **encoded** along both axes of the image. These tasks are performed by gradients.

MRI in Practice, Fourth Edition. Catherine Westbrook, Carolyn Kaut Roth, John Talbot.

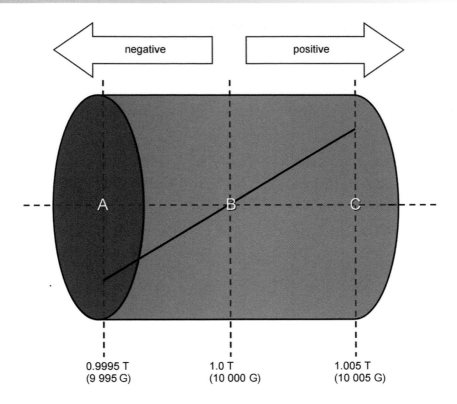

negative   positive

0.9995 T   1.0 T   1.005 T
(9 995 G)   (10 000 G)   (10 005 G)

Figure 3.1   Gradients and changing field strength.

Gradients

The mechanisms of gradients were introduced in Chapter 2 and are further discussed in Chapter 9. To recap, gradients are alterations to the main magnetic field and are generated by coils of wire located within the bore of the magnet through which current is passed. The passage of current through a gradient coil induces a gradient (magnetic) field around it, which either subtracts from, or adds to, the main static magnetic field B_0. The magnitude of B_0 is altered in a linear fashion by the gradient coils, so that the magnetic field strength and therefore the precessional frequency experienced by nuclei situated along the axis of the gradient can be predicted (Figure 3.1). This is called **spatial encoding**.

Look at Figure 3.1. A gradient has been applied that increases the magnetic field strength towards the right-hand side of the magnet (shown in red) and decreases it towards the left-hand side (blue). The change in magnetic field strength is linear, and with this particular amplitude, at point A a nucleus experiences a field of 0.9995 T, a nucleus at point B (isocentre) experiences exactly 1 T, and at point C a nucleus experiences a field of 1.005 T. In all gradient diagrams in this book, magnetic fields higher than isocentre are shown in red and those lower, in blue.

Nuclei that experience an increased magnetic field strength due to the gradient speed up, i.e. their precessional frequency increases, while nuclei that experience a lower magnetic field strength due to the gradient slow down, i.e. their precessional frequency decreases. Therefore the position of a nucleus along a gradient can be identified according to its precessional frequency.

Table 3.1   Frequency changes along a linear gradient.

Position along gradient	Field strength	Larmor frequency
At isocentre	10 000 G	42.5700 MHz
1 cm negative to isocentre	9999 G	42.5657 MHz
2 cm negative to isocentre	9998 G	42.5614 MHz
1 cm positive to isocentre	10 001 G	42.5742 MHz
2 cm positive to isocentre	10 002 G	42.5785 MHz
10 cm negative to isocentre	9990 G	42.5274 MHz

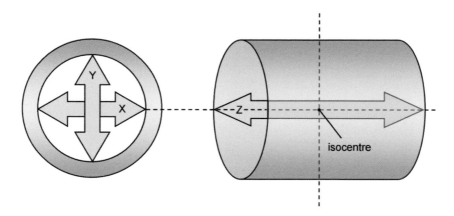

Figure 3.2   Gradient axes in a typical superconducting system.

Table 3.1 gives the frequency changes along a linear gradient that alters the magnetic field strength by 1 G/cm at a main field strength of 1 T.

There are three gradient coils situated within the bore of the magnet, and these are named according to the axis along which they act when they are switched on. Figure 3.2 shows these directions in a typical superconducting magnet. However, some manufacturers may use a different system.

- The *Z gradient* alters the magnetic field strength along the Z- (*long*) axis of the magnet.
- The *Y gradient* alters the magnetic field strength along the Y- (*vertical*) axis of the magnet.
- The *X gradient* alters the magnetic field strength along the X- (*horizontal*) axis of the magnet.

The magnetic isocentre is the center point of the axis of all three gradients, and the bore of the magnet. The magnetic field strength and therefore the precessional frequency remain unaltered here even when the gradients are applied.

Permanent magnets (*see* Chapter 9) have different axes. The Z-axis is vertical, not horizontal, as shown in Figure 3.2. The magnetic field strength at the isocentre is always the same as B_0 (e.g.

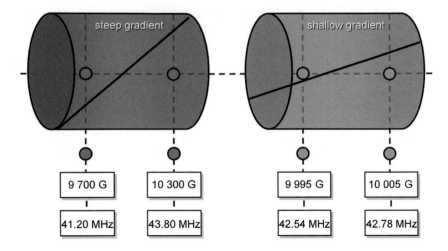

Figure 3.3   Steep and shallow slopes.

1.5 T, 1.0 T, 0.5 T), even when the gradients are switched on. When a gradient coil is switched on, the magnetic field strength is either subtracted from or added to B_0 relative to isocentre. The slope of the resulting magnetic field is the amplitude of the magnetic field gradient and it determines the rate of change of the magnetic field strength along the gradient axis. Steep gradient slopes alter the magnetic field strength between two points more than shallow gradient slopes. Steep gradient slopes therefore alter the precessional frequency of nuclei between two points, more than shallow gradient slopes (Figure 3.3).

It is convenient (for easy mathematics) to now use the unit gauss to describe magnetic field strength rather than tesla where 1.0 T is equal to 10 000 G. Gauss is the unit used to show the relative change in field strength between two points in Figure 3.3.

Gradients perform many important tasks during a pulse sequence as previously described in Chapter 2. Can you remember what these are? Gradients can be used to either dephase or rephase the magnetic moments of nuclei. Gradients also perform the following three main tasks in encoding.

- **Slice selection** – locating a slice within the scan plane selected.
- Spatially locating (encoding) signal along the long axis of the anatomy – this is called **frequency encoding**.
- Spatially locating (encoding) signal along the short axis of the anatomy – this is called **phase encoding**.

Slice selection

When a gradient coil is switched on, the magnetic field strength, and therefore the precessional frequency of nuclei located along its axis, is altered in a linear fashion. Therefore a specific point along the axis of the gradient has a specific precessional frequency (*see* Figure 3.3), and nuclei situated within a slice have a particular precessional frequency. A slice can therefore be selectively excited, by transmitting RF with a band of frequencies coinciding with the Larmor frequencies of spins in a particular slice as defined by the slice select gradient. Resonance of nuclei within the slice occurs because RF appropriate to that position is transmitted. However, nuclei situated in other slices along the gradient do not resonate, because their precessional frequency is different due to the presence of the gradient (Figure 3.4).

Learning point: slice selection and the tuning fork analogy

Look at Figure 3.4 in which tuning forks are used to illustrate how slice selection is performed. In the top diagram a gradient has been applied to change the magnetic field strength from low (blue) to high (red). Imagine we are trying to select slice A. With this particular amplitude of gradient the spins in this slice have a precessional frequency of 41.20 MHz when the gradient is switched on. Spins on either side of this slice have a different frequency because the gradient has changed the field strength across the bore of the magnet. Without the gradient all spins would precess at the same frequency and therefore we would not be able to differentiate them. As the gradient has been applied, however, the precessional frequency of spins has changed across the bore, so that along the Z-axis spins in different slices precess at different frequencies.

This is analogous to having tuning forks tuned to different frequencies located across the Z-axis of the magnet. To produce resonance and excite spins in slice A, an RF excitation pulse that matches the precessional frequency of spins in slice A, i.e. 41.20 MHz, must be applied. Doing so causes resonance just in spins in slice A; spins in other slices do not resonate because they are precessing at different frequencies. To produce the same affect in slice B (bottom diagram) an RF excitation pulse with a frequency of 43.80 MHz must be applied to produce resonance in spins in slice B. In this example, axial slices are being excited (assuming the patient is lying either supine or prone on the scan table) by applying the slice select gradient during the application of the excitation pulse.

The scan plane selected determines which of the three gradients performs slice selection during the excitation pulse (Figure 3.5). Typically they are as follows (although some manufacturers may vary).

- The *Z gradient* alters the field strength and precessional frequency along the Z-axis of the magnet and therefore selects axial slices.
- The *X gradient* alters the field strength and the precessional frequency along the X-axis of the magnet and therefore selects sagittal slices.
- The *Y gradient* alters the field strength and the precessional frequency along the Y-axis of the magnet and therefore selects coronal slices.
- Oblique slices are selected using two gradients in combination.

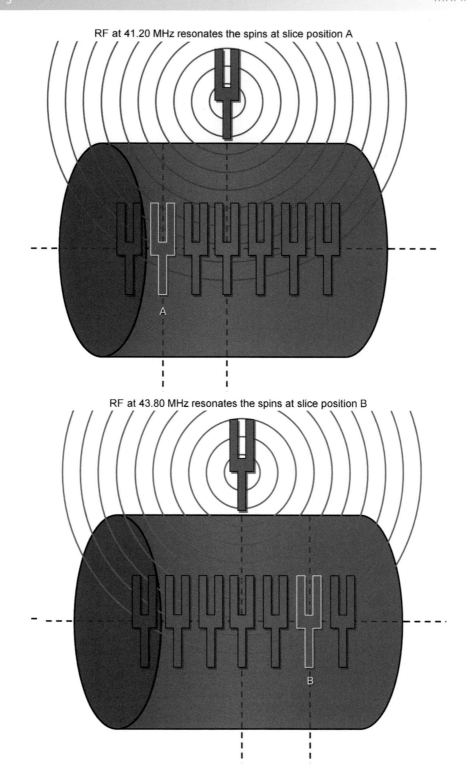

Figure 3.4   Slice selection.

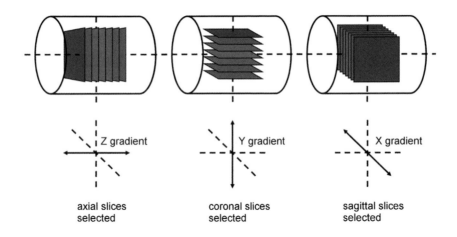

axial slices   coronal slices   sagittal slices
selected   selected   selected

Figure 3.5   X, Y and Z as slice selectors.

Slice thickness

To give each slice a thickness, a 'band' of nuclei must be excited by the excitation pulse. The slope of the slice select gradient determines the difference in precessional frequency between two points on the gradient. Steep gradient slopes result in a large difference in precessional frequency between two points on the gradient, while shallow gradient slopes result in a small difference in precessional frequency between the same two points. Once a certain gradient slope is applied, the RF pulse transmitted to excite the slice must contain a range of frequencies to match the difference in precessional frequency between two points. This frequency range is called the **bandwidth**, and as the RF is being transmitted at this point it is specifically called the **transmit bandwidth** (Figure 3.6).

- To achieve *thin slices*, a steep slice select slope and/or *narrow transmit bandwidth* is applied.
- To achieve *thick slices*, a shallow slice select slope and/or *broad transmit bandwidth* is applied.

In practice, the system automatically applies the appropriate gradient slope and transmit bandwidth according to the thickness of slice required. The slice is excited by transmitting RF at the center frequency corresponding to the precessional frequency of nuclei in the middle of the slice, and the bandwidth and gradient slope determine the range of nuclei that resonate on either side of the center.

The gap between the slices is determined by the gradient slope and by the thickness of the slice. The size of the gap is important in reducing image artefact (*see* Chapter 7). In spin echo pulse sequences, the slice select gradient is switched on during the application of the 90° excitation pulse and during the 180° rephasing pulse, to excite and rephase each slice selectively (Figure 3.7). In gradient echo pulse sequences, the slice select gradient is switched on during the excitation pulse only. The significance of this is explored in Chapter 6.

Frequency encoding

Once a slice has been selected, the signal coming from it must be located along both axes of the image. The signal is usually located along the long axis of the anatomy by a process known as

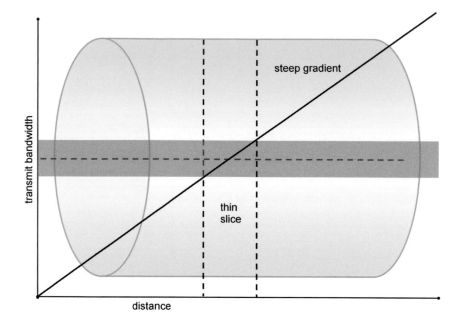

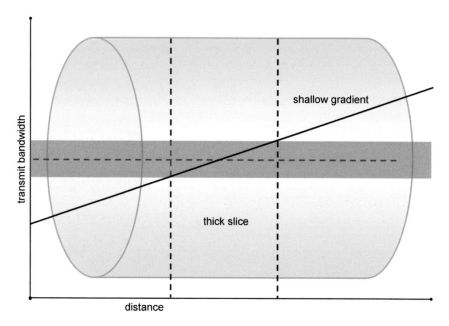

Figure 3.6   Transmit bandwidth, gradient slope and slice thickness.

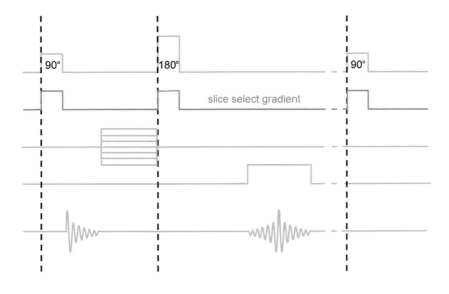

Figure 3.7   Timing of slice selection in a pulse sequence.

frequency encoding. When the frequency encoding gradient is switched on, the magnetic field strength, and therefore the precessional frequency of signal along the axis of the gradient, is altered in a linear fashion. The gradient therefore produces a frequency difference or shift of signal along its axis. The signal can now be located along the axis of the gradient according to its frequency (Figure 3.8).

Learning point:
the keyboard analogy

Within the echo many different frequencies are present. This is because initially spins with a range of frequencies are excited and rephased within each slice. This is what gives a slice its thickness. In addition, the phase encoding gradient produces a change of phase across the slice that remains when the gradient is switched off. Finally, the application of the frequency encoding gradient produces a change of frequency across the remaining axis of the slice. This frequency change depends on the spatial location of frequencies along the frequency encoding gradient.

   In some ways the result is similar to a piano keyboard. Each key is tuned to produce a certain note when pressed. Different notes are characterized by the fact that they resonate a piano wire at different frequencies so that note A, for example, has a different frequency to note B. Each note has a different position or spatial location on the keyboard. Experienced pianists, on hearing a particular note, will know which key has been pressed and where on the keyboard it is located. In other words, they have spatially located that key by its frequency. This is the basis of spatial encoding.

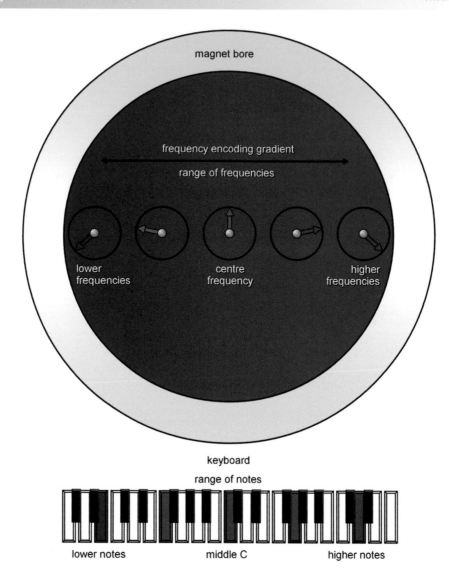

Figure 3.8 Frequency encoding.

The operator can select the direction of frequency encoding so that it encodes the signal along the long axis of the anatomy. It may help to refer to the images in Chapter 2 to work out which gradient was used for each spatial encoding function. Always remember the patient is usually lying supine along the Z-axis while on the table (in a superconducting system). Using this standard, it is easy to work out the long and short axis of anatomy.

- In *coronal* and *sagittal* images, the long axis of the anatomy lies along the Z-axis of the magnet and therefore, the *Z gradient* performs frequency encoding.
- In *axial* images, the long axis of the anatomy usually lies along the horizontal axis of the magnet and therefore, the *X gradient* performs frequency encoding. However, in imaging of

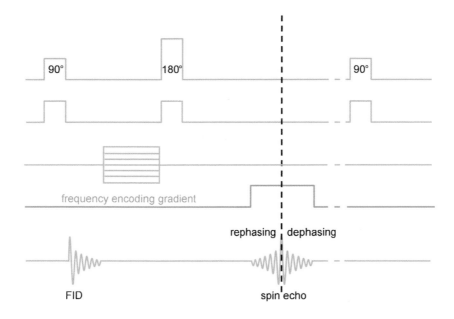

Figure 3.9   Timing of frequency encoding in a pulse sequence.

the head, the long axis of the anatomy usually lies along the anterior posterior axis of the magnet, so in this case the *Y gradient* performs frequency encoding.

The frequency encoding gradient is switched on when the signal is received and is often called the **readout gradient**. The echo is usually centered in the middle of the frequency encoding gradient, so that the gradient is switched on during the rephasing and dephasing part of the echo and the peak (Figure 3.9). Typically, the frequency encoding gradient is switched on for 8 ms, during 4 ms of rephasing and 4 ms of dephasing of the echo. The steepness of the slope of the frequency encoding gradient determines the size of the anatomy covered along the frequency encoding axis during the scan. This is called the frequency **field of view (FOV)**.

Phase encoding

Signal must now be located along the remaining short axis of the image and this localization of signal is called phase encoding. When the phase encoding gradient is switched on, the magnetic field strength and therefore the precessional frequency of nuclei along the axis of the gradient is altered. As the speed of precession of the nuclei changes, so does the accumulated phase of the magnetic moments along their precessional path. Nuclei that have sped up due to the presence of the gradient move further around their precessional path than if the gradients had not been applied. Nuclei that have slowed down due to the presence of the gradient move further back around their precessional path than if the gradient had not been applied.

Learning point: phase encoding and the watch analogy

The watch analogy referred to in Chapter 1 is a very easy way of understanding how phase encoding works. Imagine a watch telling the time of 12 o'clock. The hour and minute hand are both located over the number 12. Assume that the position of the hour hand at this point is equivalent to the phase of a magnetic moment of a nucleus experiencing B_0. When the phase encoding gradient is switched on, the magnetic field strength, precessional frequency and phase of the magnetic moments of nuclei change according to their position along the gradient. Magnetic moments of nuclei experiencing a higher field strength gain phase, i.e. move further around the watch to say 4 o'clock, because they travel faster while the gradient is switched on. Magnetic moments of nuclei experiencing a lower field strength lose phase, i.e. move back around the watch to say 8 o'clock, because they travel slower while the gradient is switched on. Magnetic moments of nuclei at isocentre do not experience a changed field strength and their phase remains unchanged, i.e. 12 o'clock (Figure 3.10).

There is now a phase difference or shift between magnetic moments of nuclei positioned along the axis of the gradient. When the phase encoding gradient is switched off, the magnetic field strength experienced by the nuclei returns to the main field strength B_0 and therefore the precessional frequency of all the nuclei returns to the Larmor frequency. However, the phase difference between the nuclei remains. The nuclei travel at the same speed (frequency) around their precessional paths, but their phases or positions on the watch are different because a gradient was previously switched on. This difference in phase between the nuclei is used to determine their position along the phase encoding gradient.

The phase encoding gradient is usually switched after the application of the excitation pulse (Figure 3.11). The steepness of the slope of the phase encoding gradient determines the degree of phase shift between two points along the gradient (Figure 3.12).

A steep phase encoding gradient causes a large phase shift between two points along the gradient, for example 8 o'clock and 4 o'clock, while a shallow phase encoding gradient causes a smaller phase shift between the same two points along the gradient, for example 10 o'clock and 2 o'clock, as shown in Figure 3.12.

Figure 3.13, Table 3.2 and the following list summarize the essential concepts of spatial encoding.

- The phase encoding gradient alters the phase along the remaining axis of the image, which is usually the short axis of the anatomy.
- In coronal images the short axis of the anatomy usually lies along the horizontal axis of the magnet, therefore the X gradient performs phase encoding.

71

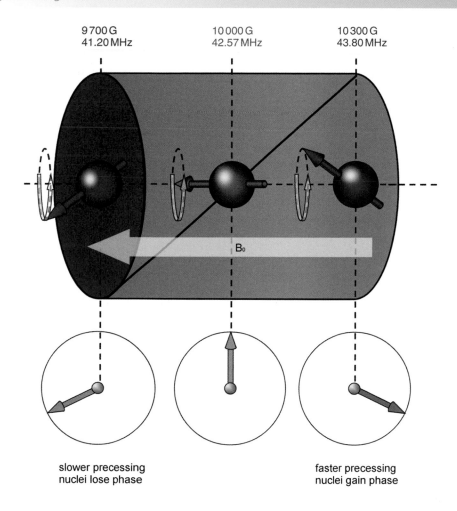

Figure 3.10   Phase encoding.

- In sagittal images the short axis of the anatomy usually lies along the vertical axis of the magnet, therefore the Y gradient performs phase encoding.
- In axial images the short axis of the anatomy usually lies along the vertical axis of the magnet, therefore the Y gradient performs phase encoding. However, when imaging the head, the short axis of the anatomy lies along the horizontal axis of the magnet and therefore the X gradient performs phase encoding.

Summary

- The slice select gradient is switched on during the 90° and 180° pulses in spin echo pulse sequences, and during the excitation pulse only in gradient echo pulse sequences
- The slope of the slice select gradient determines the slice thickness and slice gap (along with the transmit bandwidth)

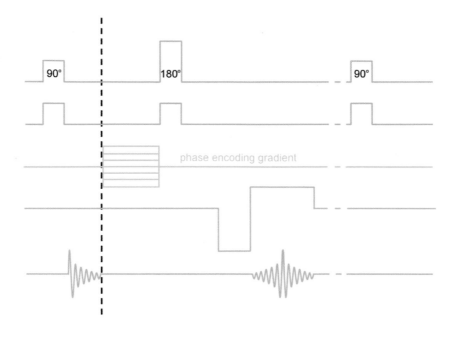

Figure 3.11   Timing of phase encoding in a pulse sequence.

- The phase encoding gradient is switched on after the excitation pulse
- The slope of the phase encoding gradient determines the degree of phase shift along the phase encoding axis. This determines the phase matrix (*see* later)
- The frequency encoding gradient is switched on during the collection of the signal (the echo)
- The amplitude of the frequency encoding gradient determines the frequency FOV dimension
- The timing of all these gradient functions during a pulse sequence is shown in Figure 3.14

Learning point: using the watch analogy to understand spatial encoding

The watch analogy is a good way of remembering how all gradients encode. Imagine two people wearing watches that are synchronized and tell perfect time. They walk into the MRI scan room for 15 minutes. The magnetic field of the scanner affects the timekeeping of the watches because it magnetizes the hands of the watches. The person standing nearest to the magnet is affected the most because the magnetic field here is strongest. The person standing furthest away is affected to a lesser degree because the magnetic field here is less strong.

   If they then walk out of the room so they are no longer affected by the magnetic field, a stranger will be able to tell which person was standing nearer to the magnet and which was standing further away simply by looking at their watches. This is because the hands of the watch of the person standing closer to the magnet will be more out of phase from the synchronized time than the watch of the person standing further away. In other words, the stranger has used the frequency and phase shift of the hands of the watch, produced as a result of applying a magnetic field to the watches, to spatially encode the relative positions of each person while they were in the room.

Sampling

This is a difficult subject and one you may need some time to learn. However, it is important to grasp this concept as it affects several parameters selected at the console.

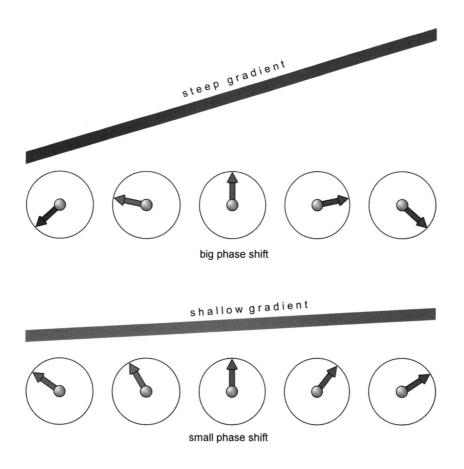

Figure 3.12   Steep and shallow phase gradients.

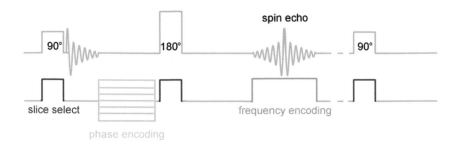

Figure 3.13 Gradient timing in a spin echo pulse sequence.

Table 3.2 Gradient axes in orthogonal imaging (some manufacturers vary).

Plane	Slice selection	Phase encoding	Frequency encoding
Sagittal	X	Y	Z
Axial (body)	Z	Y	X
Axial (head)	Z	X	Y
Coronal	Y	X	Z

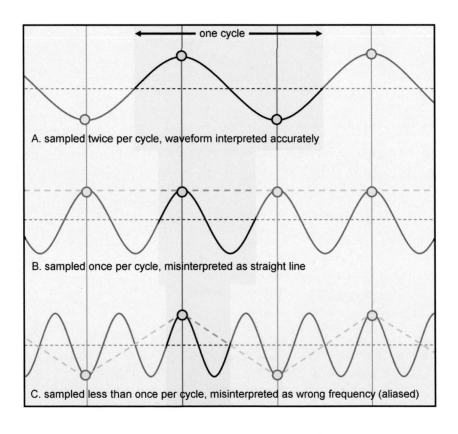

Figure 3.14 The Nyquist theorem.

Refer to animation 3.1 on the supporting companion website for this book: www.wiley.com/go/mriinpractice

The frequency encoding gradient is switched on while the system reads frequencies present in the signal and samples or digitizes them. It is therefore sometimes called the readout gradient. The duration of the readout gradient is called the **sampling time** or **acquisition window** (referred to as *acquisition window* from now on). Every time a sample is taken, this is stored as a **data point**. During the acquisition window, the system samples or digitizes frequencies up to 2048 different times (using current technology) and therefore acquires up to 2048 data points. The **sampling rate** or **sampling frequency** (referred to as the *sampling frequency* from now on) is the rate at which frequencies are sampled or digitized during the acquisition window *per second*, i.e. the number of samples or data points that are acquired per second. This parameter therefore has the unit Hz, i.e. if one data point is acquired per second, the sampling frequency is 1 Hz. The number of data points collected during the acquisition window is determined by the frequency matrix, so if the frequency matrix is 256, then 256 data points must be acquired during the acquisition window. Therefore the sampling frequency, the frequency matrix and the duration of the acquisition window are related to each other.

Learning point: sampling using the sprinter analogy

This difficult concept is perhaps better understood by using the following analogy. Imagine you have been asked to take a certain number of photographs of a sprinter during a race. You would have to find out the following before you could start:

- how many photographs you must take in total
- how many photographs *per second* your camera can take
- how long the race is.

Each photograph is equivalent to a data point as it is effectively a sample or measurement showing the position of the runner's arms and legs at particular points in the race.

- The number of photographs you end up with at the end of the race is equivalent to the *frequency matrix* (*see* later).
- The time you have available to take the photographs is the length of the race. This is equivalent to the *acquisition window*.
- How many photographs per second you take is equivalent to the *sampling frequency*.

For example, if the sampling frequency is one photograph/s and the race is 10 s long, 10 photographs can be taken, so using this example a frequency matrix of 10 would be achieved thus:

- the sampling frequency is 1/s (1 Hz)
- the number of samples taken is 10
- the acquisition window is 10 s.

The sampling frequency thus determines how many data points can be acquired during the acquisition window and therefore the frequency matrix that can be achieved. It is important therefore that all three parameters (sampling frequency, frequency matrix and acquisition window) are selected appropriately by the operator. The frequency matrix is an obvious user-selectable parameter but what about the sampling frequency and acquisition window? How do we select these parameters and what should these values be?

Sampling frequency

First let us explore the sampling frequency more closely. We have learned that this determines the number of samples taken or data points acquired per second. It therefore also determines the time interval between each sample. This is called the **sampling interval** and is calculated thus:

$$\text{sampling interval} = 1/\text{sampling frequency}.$$

Using the sprinter analogy above:

$$\text{sampling interval} = 1/1 \text{ photographs per s} = 1\,\text{s},$$

i.e. the time interval between each photograph being taken is 1 s.

If the sampling frequency increases, then from the equation above it is easy to see that the sampling interval decreases, i.e. the time interval between each photograph gets shorter so we would able to take 10 photographs in a much shorter period of time. For example, if we used a camera that could take two photographs per second then the sampling interval would be 0.5 s and we could acquire 10 photographs in 5 s instead of 10 s.

In MRI the sampling frequency is determined by the **Nyquist theorem**. This tells us how fast to sample a frequency or frequencies in order to digitize accurately. An echo contains many different frequencies, some of which represent signal frequencies and some that represent noise (*see* Chapter 4). The Nyquist theorem states that when digitizing a signal with a range of analogue frequencies (frequencies represented as a waveform), the highest frequency must be sampled at least twice as fast to accurately digitize or represent it. In other words, the sampling frequency must be at least twice the highest frequency in the signal.

Look at Figure 3.14. Sampling once per cycle or at the same frequency as the frequency we are trying to digitize results in a representation of a straight line or an absent frequency in the data (middle diagram). Sampling at less than once per cycle represents a completely incorrect frequency that leads to an artefact called **aliasing** (bottom diagram) (*see* Chapter 7). Sampling twice per cycle or at twice the frequency we are trying to digitize results in correct representation of that frequency in the data (top diagram). As long as the highest frequency present is sampled twice it will be represented correctly in the data. Lower frequencies are sampled more often at the same sampling frequency and are also represented accurately in the data.

It would seem therefore that the higher the sampling frequency the better, as this would mean a more accurate representation of the original analogue frequencies. However, due to time constraints, the sampling frequency must be limited. Therefore the sampling frequency is ideally kept at just twice the highest frequency in the echo. In this way aliasing is avoided while sampling in the most time efficient manner. The sampling frequency therefore determines the maximum frequency that can be sampled. This maximum frequency is called the **Nyquist frequency**. Therefore if the Nyquist theorem is obeyed exactly:

sampling frequency $= 2 \times$ Nyquist frequency.

The sampling frequency is not, however, a parameter we directly select at the MR console, but we do select another parameter that, when the Nyquist theorem is obeyed exactly, has the same *numerical value* as the sampling frequency. This is called the **receive bandwidth**. The receive bandwidth is the range of frequencies we wish to sample or digitize during readout. The bandwidth is determined by applying a filter on the frequency encoding gradient. This is achieved by selecting the center frequency and defining the upper and lower limits of frequencies to be digitized on either side of the center frequency of the echo. Therefore a receive bandwidth of 32 KHz represents 16 KHz above the center frequency to 16 KHz below the center frequency. Therefore if the Nyquist theorem is obeyed exactly:

receive bandwidth $= 2 \times$ the highest frequency (Nyquist frequency).

Hence when sampling at exactly twice per cycle (i.e. obeying Nyquist exactly), the receive bandwidth and the sampling frequency are both equal to $2 \times$ Nyquist frequency. Therefore although the receive bandwidth and the sampling frequency are different entities, they are given the same numerical value and, as the receive bandwidth is a user-selectable parameter, it can be used to determine the sampling frequency.

For example, if the receive bandwidth is 32 KHz, the Nyquist frequency is 16 KHz. If the Nyquist theorem is obeyed exactly, the sampling frequency must be 32 KHz (16 KHz $\times$ 2). A sampling frequency of 32 KHz means that 32 000 samples or data points are acquired per second. This means that a data point is acquired every 0.00003125 s (the sampling interval).

When the receive bandwidth is increased, the highest frequency in the echo also increases. To sample this higher frequency accurately, the sampling frequency must also increase (if this does not occur, aliasing results). So if the receive bandwidth is increased to 64 KHz, this means that the Nyquist frequency is 32 KHz and the sampling frequency must be twice this, i.e. 64 KHz which is identical to the receive bandwidth. Using a sampling frequency of 64 KHz means that 64 000 data points are acquired per second so that the sampling interval becomes much shorter (half as short as 0.00003125 s). Hence we would be able to acquire the data points needed in half the normal time, i.e. the duration of the acquisition window would halve. The opposite would be true if the receive bandwidth is decreased.

Acquisition window

The acquisition window is not directly selected at the MR console. However, as the echo is usually centered in the middle of this window (i.e. the peak of the echo corresponds to the middle of the application of the frequency encoding gradient) the duration of the acquisition window indirectly affects the TE (which of course is selectable at the console). For example, if the frequency encoding gradient is switched on for 8 ms (i.e. the acquisition window is 8 ms) then the peak of the echo occurs after 4 ms. If the acquisition window is increased, the frequency encoding gradient is switched on for longer. Hence the peak of the echo occurs later, increasing the time from the peak of the echo to the RF excitation pulse that created it (i.e. TE increased). The opposite is true if the acquisition window is decreased.

Learning point: the relationship between TE, receive bandwidth and frequency matrix

The receive bandwidth, frequency matrix and minimum TE we are permitted to select in a protocol are related to one another and have a significant impact on data acquisition. To understand this more clearly let us recap.

- The receive bandwidth determines the range or frequencies we wish to digitize during the acquisition window and has the same numerical value as the sampling frequency when Nyquist principles are applied.
- The sampling frequency determines the number of data points acquired per second.
- The frequency matrix determines the number of data points we must collect during the acquisition window.
- The minimum TE is affected by the duration of the acquisition window because the echo is usually centered in the middle of this window.

Suppose we wish to take 10 photographs of our sprinter but with a camera that only takes a photograph every 2 s instead of every 1 s. We still require 10 photographs of the sprinter to work out exactly how he was running during the race. One of the ways to achieve this is to make the race twice as long, i.e. the race takes 20 s instead of 10 s. The same would be true if we needed 20 photographs instead of 10 – assuming we are taking one photograph per second, to achieve this we would have to double the length of the race.

Now let us use some actual MR parameters. For example, if a frequency matrix of 256 is required, 256 data points must be collected and stored during the acquisition window. If a receive bandwidth of 32 KHz is selected, the sampling frequency is also 32 KHz. This means that 32 000 data points are collected per second. As the sampling interval is 1/sampling frequency, a data point is acquired every 0.00003125 s. Therefore to acquire 256 data points the acquisition window must be 256×0.00003125 s or 8 ms. Hence the frequency encoding gradient must be switched on for 8 ms to allow enough time for 256 data points to be acquired when sampling once every 0.00003125 s or at a sampling frequency of 32 KHz.

If the receive bandwidth is halved to 16 KHz, the sampling frequency also halves to 16 KHz and so 16 000 data points are acquired per second. If the acquisition window is still 8 ms, only 128 data points can be collected instead of the required 256. To collect the necessary data points at that bandwidth, the acquisition window must be doubled to 16 ms and results in a 4 ms increase in the minimum permissible TE, i.e. the peak of the echo moves to occur in the middle of the longer acquisition window.

For example, if the minimum TE was 10 ms using a bandwidth of 32 KHz and a frequency matrix of 256, by halving the receive bandwidth to 16 KHz the minimum TE increases to 14 ms (Figure 3.15). There are occasions when changing the receive bandwidth is desirable and when the resultant change in TE becomes significant. These considerations are discussed later.

In addition, increasing the frequency matrix has the same effect. Using the example above, if the frequency matrix is increased to 512, then 512 data points are required and frequencies must be sampled 512 times during the acquisition window. If the receive bandwidth is maintained at 32 KHz then the acquisition window and therefore the minimum TE must be increased to attain the required number of data points. Table 3.3 outlines this more clearly. The default is shown in the top line where an acquisition window of 8 ms is used with a 32 KHz bandwidth when acquiring a frequency matrix of 256. If the bandwidth is halved, not enough data points are acquired (128 instead of the required 256). To solve this, the acquisition window is doubled to 16 ms, which increases the TE by 4 ms (as the peak of the echo is situated in the middle of the acquisition window as shown in Figure 3.15). The same occurs if a frequency matrix of 512 is required. The acquisition window must be doubled at acquire 512 data points. This also increases the TE by 4 ms.

DATA COLLECTION AND IMAGE FORMATION

Introduction

The application of all the gradients selects an individual slice and produces a frequency shift along one axis of the slice, and a phase shift along the other. The system can now locate an individual

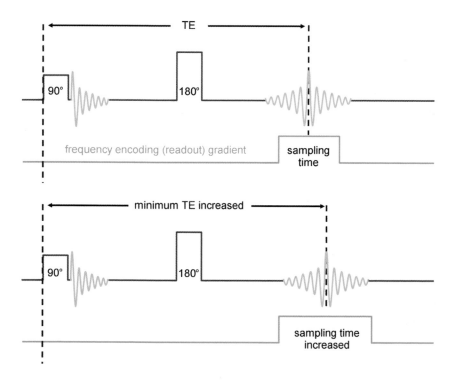

Figure 3.15   Sampling time (acquisition window) and the TE.

Table 3.3   Receive bandwidth, acquisition window and frequency matrix.

Frequency matrix	Receive bandwidth	Acquisition window
256	32 KHz	8 ms
128	16 KHz	8 ms
256	16 KHz	16 ms
512	32 KHz	16 ms

signal within the image by measuring the number of times the magnetic moments cross the receiver coil (frequency) and their position around their precessional path (phase). This information now has to be translated on to the image. When data of each signal position are collected, the information is stored as data points in the array processor of the system computer. The data points are stored in **K space**.

K space description

Figure 3.16 illustrates K space for *one slice*. K space is rectangular in shape and has two axes perpendicular to each other. The frequency axis of K space is horizontal and is centered in the middle of several horizontal lines. The phase axis of K space is vertical and is centered in

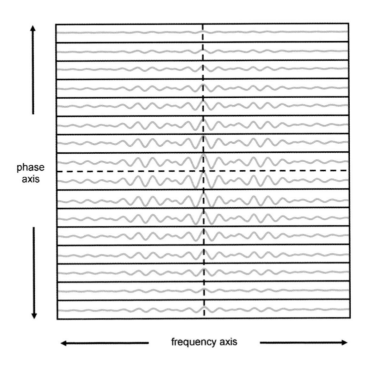

Figure 3.16   K space – axes.

the middle of K space perpendicular to the frequency axis. K space is a spatial frequency domain, i.e. where information about the frequency of a signal and where it comes from in the patient is stored. In other words, it is where information of frequencies in space or distance is stored. In this context frequency is defined as phase change over distance (in other contexts it is the change of phase over time, *see* the watch analogy in Chapter 1) and the unit of phase is radians (a unit of degrees in a circle). The unit of K space is therefore radians per cm.

Learning point: the chest of drawers

K space is analogous to a chest of drawers. Look at Figure 3.17, in which K space with its lines parallel to the phase axis are illustrated. These lines look like drawers in a chest of drawers, which, like K space, is a storage device. The number of drawers corresponds to the number of lines of K space that must be filled with data points to complete the scan. The number of lines or drawers to be filled equals the phase matrix selected, i.e. if a phase matrix of 256 is selected then 256 lines or drawers must be filled with data points to complete the scan. As we will see shortly, the number of data points in each line or drawer corresponds to the frequency matrix selected. The chest of drawers analogy is referred to many times in this book. Look out for the chest of drawers symbol in the margin.

K space filling

Lines of K space are usually numbered with the lowest number near to the central axis (e.g. lines +/− 1,2,3) and the highest numbers towards the outer edges (e.g. +/−128,127,126) (Figure 3.18). The lines in the top half of K space are called positive lines, those in the bottom half are called negative lines. This is because the line to be filled with data in a given TR is determined by the polarity and slope of the phase gradient. Positive polarity phase encoding slopes are associated

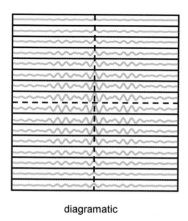

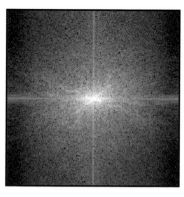

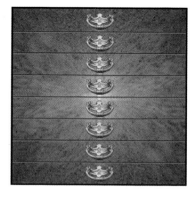

diagramatic   data   the chest of drawers

Figure 3.17   K space – the chest of drawers.

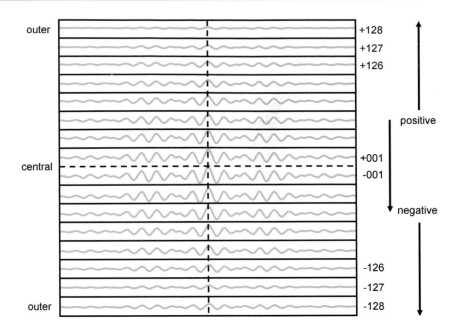

Figure 3.18   K space characteristics.

with lines in the top half of K space, whereas negative polarity phase encoding slopes are associated with lines in the bottom half of K space.

As previously discussed, the phase gradient is usually altered every TR. This is necessary to fill different lines of K space with data. If the phase encoding gradient is not changed, then the same line is filled every TR. As the number of lines filled determines the phase matrix, not changing the phase encoding gradient results in an image with only one pixel in the phase direction of the image. Therefore we need to alter both the polarity and the slope of the phase gradient every TR to give the image resolution in the phase direction.

The phase gradient therefore picks which line of K space or which drawer is filled with data in a particular TR period. Positive polarity phase gradients pick lines in the top half of K space; negative polarity gradients pick lines in the bottom half. In addition, the slope of the phase gradient determines which line is selected. Steep gradients, both positive and negative, select the most **outer lines**, while shallow gradients select the **central lines**. As the slope of the phase gradient decreases from its steepest amplitude, so the lines through K space are stepped down from the most outer lines to the more central lines (Figure 3.19). Usually K space is filled in a linear fashion from top to bottom or bottom to top, although as we will see later, there are many different permutations. Using the linear filling model and the chest of drawers analogy, let us look more closely at exactly what happens during a pulse sequence.

Look at Figure 3.20, showing a typical spin echo sequence. The top half of the diagram shows when gradients are applied to each slice during the pulse sequence. The bottom half shows the equivalent areas of K space, drawn as a chest of drawers.

The slice select gradient is applied during the excitation and rephasing pulses to selectively excite and rephase a slice. The slope of the slice select gradient determines which slice is excited or which chest of drawers is to be selected. Each slice has its own area of K space, or chest of drawers.

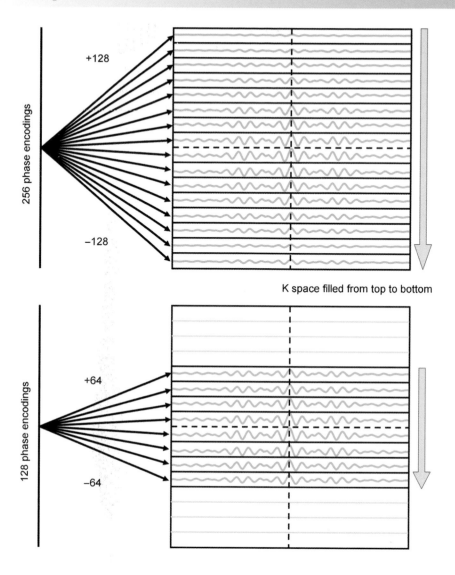

Figure 3.19   K space – phase matrix and the number of drawers.

N.B. Although three chests of drawers are shown in Figure 3.20, they do not represent K space for three separate slices in this diagram. In Figure 3.20, each chest of drawers represents the same slice at three different times in the sequence when each of the three gradients are switched on.

The phase encoding gradient is then applied. This determines which line or drawer to fill with data. Normally K space is filled linearly with line +128 filled first (assuming a 256 matrix has been selected), followed by line +127, and so on. In Figure 3.20, lines +128 and +127 have already been filled, so the next line to fill is line +126. To open this drawer, the phase encoding gradient must be applied positively and steeply corresponding to line +126. Application of this gradient selects line +126 in K space.

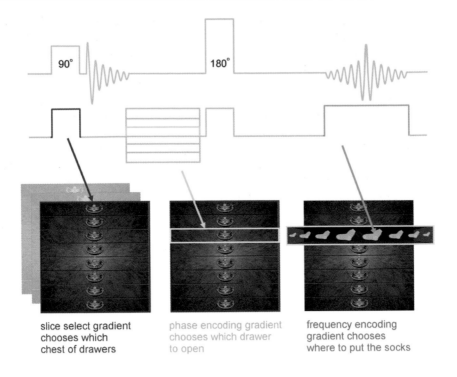

slice select gradient
chooses which
chest of drawers

phase encoding gradient
chooses which drawer
to open

frequency encoding
gradient chooses
where to put the socks

Figure 3.20   K space filling in a spin echo sequence.

Refer to animation 3.2 on the supporting companion website for this book: www.wiley.com/go/mriinpractice

The frequency encoding gradient is now switched on. The amplitude of this determines the FOV in the frequency direction of the image. During application of the frequency encoding gradient, frequencies in the echo are digitized to acquire data points which fill the line of K space selected by the phase encoding gradient. These data points are laid out in a line of K space (or in a drawer in the chest of drawers) during the sampling time or acquisition window, usually from left to right. The number of data points collected determines the frequency matrix of the image, e.g. 256. When sampling is completed, the frequency encoding gradient switches off and the slice select is applied again, to a different amplitude than before, to excite and rephase slice 2. This is equivalent to walking up to chest of drawers 2 (not shown in Figure 3.20).

The phase encoding gradient is applied again to the same polarity and amplitude as for slice 1, filling line +126 for chest of drawers or slice 2. The process is repeated for slice 3 with line +126 being filled for each area of K space or each chest of drawers. All this happens within the TR period. This is why the TR determines how many slices are permitted. Longer TRs result in more time to individually excite, rephase, phase and frequency encode slices. If the TR is short there is less time to do this, so fewer slices are possible.

Once line +126 has been filled for all three slices, the TR is repeated. The slice gradient again selects chest of drawers 1, but this time a different line of K space is filled or different drawer is filled from that filled in the previous TR period. If the linear K space filling model is used, line +125 is filled (or the next drawer down from line +126). To do this the phase encoding gradient must be switched on positively but less steeply than in previous TR period. This opens drawer +125 and when readout occurs, data points are laid out in that drawer during application of the frequency encoding gradient. When this has been completed, the slice select gradient is applied again to select slice 2. The same amplitude and polarity of phase gradient is applied to open drawer +125 for slice or chest of drawers 2. This process is repeated for all the slices.

As the pulse sequence continues, every TR the phase encoding amplitude is gradually decreased to step down through the lines of K space. To fill the bottom lines the phase gradient is switched negatively and gradually increased every TR to progressively fill the outer lines. If a 256 phase matrix has been selected then once 256 lines have been filled the scan is over. In linear K space filling, this means that either the system starts at line +128 and works its way down through 256 lines of K space or it starts at line −128 and works its way up. The central frequency axis corresponds to line 0 (and to fill this line the phase encoding gradient is not switched on at all). Therefore if a 256 phase matrix is selected the system fills 128 lines in the top half of K space, line 0 and 127 lines in the bottom half of K space (+128 to −127). The reverse is true if it starts at −128.

This is the most common type of K space filling method, although there are many others. These are discussed later. The process of data acquisition results in a grid of data points. The number of data points horizontally in each line equals the frequency matrix, e.g. 512, 256, 1024, etc. ; the number of data points vertically corresponds to the phase matrix selected, e.g. 128, 256, 384, 512, etc. (Figure 3.21).

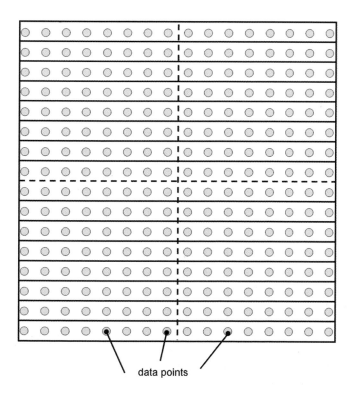

data points

Figure 3.21   Data points.

Learning point: an important fact about K space

It is very important to understand that *K space is not the image*. That is to say, data stored in the top line do not end up being the top of the image. Each data point contains information for the *whole slice*, as the frequencies that represent it come from the whole echo and the echo comes from the whole slice. Later we will look at some examples to prove this point.

To produce an image from the acquired data points we need to complete a mathematical process called **Fast Fourier transform** or FFT.

Fast Fourier transform (FFT)

The mathematics of FFT are well beyond the scope of this book but are described in its basic context here. An MR image consists of a matrix of pixels, the number of which is determined by the number of lines filled in K space (phase matrix) and the number of data points in each line (frequency matrix). As a result of FFT, each pixel is allocated a color on a grayscale corresponding to the amplitude of specific frequencies coming from the same spatial location as represented by that pixel. Each data point contains phase and frequency information from the whole slice at a particular time during readout. In other words, frequency amplitudes are represented in the time domain. The FFT process mathematically converts this to frequency amplitudes in the frequency domain. This is necessary because gradients spatially locate signal according to their frequency, not their time.

Learning point: FFT and the keyboard analogy

Look at Figure 3.22. In the top diagram there is one frequency represented decaying over time. The FFT process converts this single frequency to show its *amplitude*. In the bottom diagram two frequencies are represented and FFT converts them into their separate amplitudes. The MR signal contains many different frequencies. In addition to this, each frequency has a different amplitude depending on whether the tissue it comes from is returning high or low signal intensity. Using the keyboard analogy previously described, an MR signal is a chord where several frequencies or notes are played at once. In addition, each key is pressed to a different degree – some are pressed softly, others are pressed hard. The soft keys are analogous to frequencies in tissues returning a low signal, the hard keys to frequencies returning a high signal. By sampling the frequencies in the MR signal and performing FFT, the MR system can tell exactly which keys have been pressed and how hard they have been pressed. In other words, it has converted frequencies in the echo decaying over time into different frequencies and their relative amplitudes.

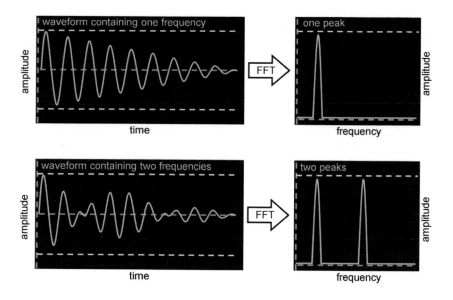

Figure 3.22   Fast Fourier transform.

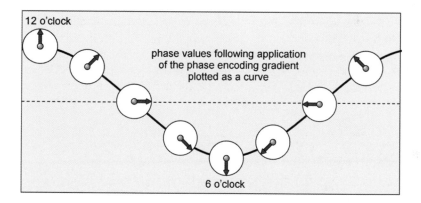

Figure 3.23   The phase curve.

As the FFT process deals in frequencies the system must be able to convert the phase shift information produced as a result of applying the phase encoding gradient into a frequency. This is not as difficult as it sounds. The watch analogy explains how frequency is a change of phase over *time*. However by applying the phase encoding gradient over a distance across the bore of the magnet, a change of phase over *distance* is produced. This is extrapolated as a frequency by creating a sine wave formed from connecting all the phase values associated with a certain phase shift (Figure 3.23). This sine wave has a frequency or **pseudo-frequency** (as it has been indirectly obtained) that depends on the degree of phase shift produced by the gradient. Steep phase encoding gradients produce large phase shifts across a given distance in the patient and result in high pseudo-frequencies, while low amplitude phase gradients produce small phase shifts across the same distance and result in low pseudo-frequencies (Figure 3.24). There are some significant implications from this in optimizing image quality. These are discussed later.

steep phase encoding gradient, pseudo-frequency 1

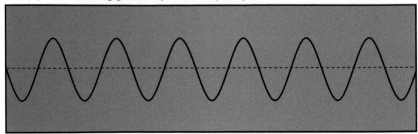

shallow phase encoding gradient, pseudo-frequency 2

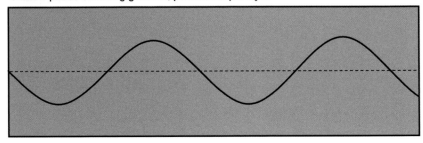

Figure 3.24   Pseudo-frequencies.

Learning point: why does the phase gradient have to change?

You will remember that we need to change the amplitude of the phase encoding gradient to fill different lines of K space and therefore give phase resolution to our image. Another way of looking at this is that by changing the phase gradient and therefore the pseudo-frequency, the data 'look different' than in the previous TR period. This is how the system knows to place these data points in a new line of K space. If the data looked the same every TR, then the system would place the data in the same line every TR and the resultant image would have a resolution of only 1 pixel in the phase direction. The frequency data cannot be changed from one TR to the next because, in order to do this, we would have to alter the slope of the frequency encoding gradient every TR. This is turn would change the size of the frequency FOV every TR, which is obviously not acceptable. The slice encoding data also cannot be changed every TR because this would mean altering the slope of the slice select gradient applied to a particular slice every TR. This in turn would change the slice thickness of a particular slice every TR, which again is not acceptable. The only gradient slope we can change is the phase encoding gradient and by doing so we alter the phase information in a line of data points. This is what the system needs to place this 'different' data in a different line of K space and thus provide phase resolution.

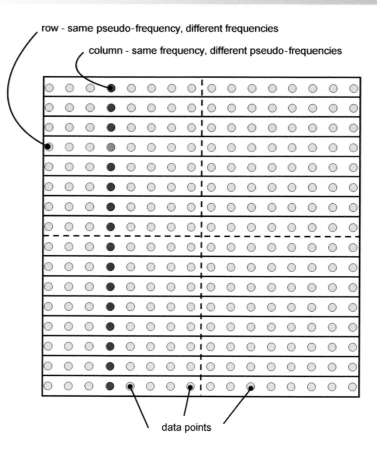

Figure 3.25   Columns and rows in K space.

Therefore before FFT each data point contains frequency information from frequency encoding and pseudo-frequency information from phase encoding.

- *In each line* of K space the pseudo-frequency data in each data point are unchanged because they result from a particular slope of phase encoding gradient. The frequency data, however, are different in each data point as each data point was acquired at a different time during readout when the frequency encoding gradient was on.
- *In each column* of K space the frequency data are unchanged because each data point in the column was acquired at the same time during readout. The pseudo-frequency data, however, are different because each data point was acquired with a different slope of phase encoding gradient (Figure 3.25). This means that in every voxel, spins are phase shifted to a different extent every TR. This phase shift is mapped along the vertical phase axis of K space and is used to spatial encode signal into every voxel along the phase axis of the image.

The FFT process differentiates these different types of data in two dimensions (i.e. horizontally across each line and vertically down each column). It then converts the data into signal amplitude vs its frequency and is therefore able to calculate the grayscale associated with every pixel in the

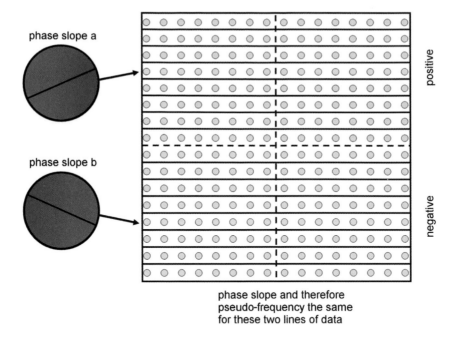

phase slope and therefore
pseudo-frequency the same
for these two lines of data

Figure 3.26   K space symmetry – phase.

two-dimensional matrix of the image, i.e. if signal with a discrete value of frequency and pseudo-frequency at a certain spatial location has high amplitude it is allocated a bright pixel. If signal with a discrete value of frequency and pseudo-frequency at a certain spatial location has low amplitude it is allocated a dark pixel. This process is completed for every area of K space, chest of drawers or slice, and displays the image on the operator's monitor (Figure 3.25).

Important facts about K space

(1) *K space is not the image.* In other words, data points in the top line of K space do not result in the top of the image. In fact, every data point contains information from the whole slice.

(2) *Data are symmetrical in K space.* This means that data in the top half of K space are identical to those in the bottom half. This is because the slope of phase gradient required to select a particular line in one half of K space is identical to that required to select the same line in the opposite side of K space. Although the polarity of gradient is different, because the slope is the same, the pseudo-frequency in each line is also the same (Figure 3.26). In addition, data on the left side of K space are identical to data on the right. That is because as data points are laid out in a line during readout they are placed sequentially from left to right as the echo is rephasing, reaching its peak and dephasing, with the peak of the echo corresponding to the central vertical axis of K space. As echoes are symmetrical features, frequency data digitized from the echo are the same on one side as they are on the other (Figure 3.27). The resultant symmetry is called **conjugate symmetry** and is used to reduce scan times in many imaging options (*see* later).

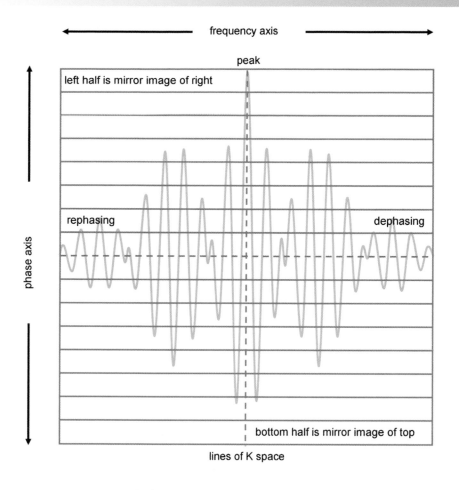

Figure 3.27   K space symmetry – frequency.

(3) *Data acquired in the central lines contribute signal and contrast, while data acquired in the outer lines contribute resolution.* As previously described, the central lines of K space are filled using shallow phase encoding slopes and the outer lines are filled using steep phase encoding slopes. Shallow slopes result in low pseudo-frequencies because of small phase shifts. To produce signal the magnetic moments of nuclei must be coherent or in phase. By minimizing phase shifts, the resultant signal has a high signal amplitude and contributes largely to signal and contrast in the image. Steep slopes result in high pseudo-frequencies because of large phase shifts. The resultant signal therefore has relatively low signal amplitude and does not contribute signal and contrast in the image (Figure 3.28). However, large phase shifts mean that two points close together in the patient are likely to have a phase difference and will thus be differentiated from each other. Therefore outer lines of K space, while not contributing signal, provide resolution. Conversely, central lines, which are filled as a result of small phase shifts, do not provide resolution as two points close together in the patient are unlikely to have different phase values and therefore cannot be differentiated from each other.

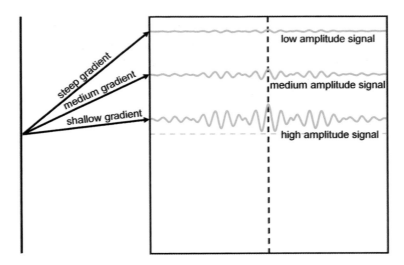

low amplitude signal

medium amplitude signal

high amplitude signal

steep gradient

medium gradient

shallow gradient

Figure 3.28   Phase gradient amplitude vs signal amplitude.

To summarize:

- The *central* portion of K space contains data that have *high signal* amplitude and low resolution.
- The *outer* portion of K space contains data that have *low signal* amplitude and high resolution.

Signal and resolution are important image quality factors and are discussed in Chapter 4. If all K space is filled during an acquisition then both signal and resolution are obtained and displayed in the image. However, as we will see later, there are many different permutations of K space filling whereby the relative proportion of central to outer lines filled is altered. Under these circumstances image quality can be significantly affected. It is also worth noting that when the phase matrix is reduced the outer lines are dropped and the central lines of K space are still filled with data. For example, if the phase matrix is reduced to 128 then lines +64 to −63 (including line 0) are filled, which are the signal producing lines of K space, rather than fill lines +128 to zero (Figure 3.29). This is because as a general rule signal is more important than resolution in the image. When resolution is also required, this is achieved by increasing the proportion of outer lines that contain resolution data.

Learning point: K space, resolution and signal

Figure 3.30 shows an image acquired using all K space. Both resolution and signal are seen on the image. Figure 3.31 illustrates what happens if an image is created out of data from the outer edges of K space. This image has good resolution in that the detail of the hair and eyes are well shown but there is very little signal. Figure 3.32 shows what happens if an image is created from data in the center of K space only. The resultant image has excellent signal but poor resolution. This example also demonstrates that K space is not the image. If it were, the image in Figure 3.31 would lose its nose and Figure 3.32 would show only the nose. Both images, however, show all the image, even though only a small percentage of the total number of data points in K space was used in their creation.

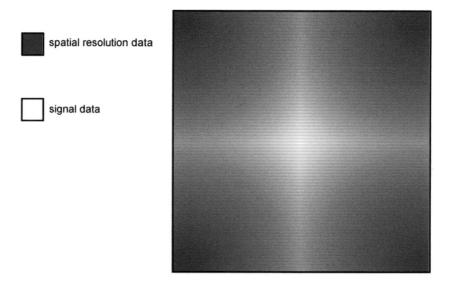

spatial resolution data

signal data

Figure 3.29   K space – signal and resolution.

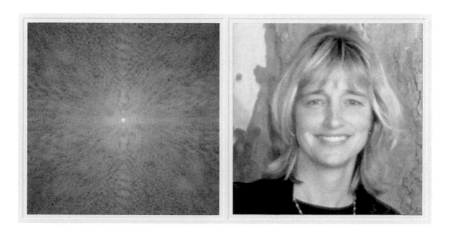

Figure 3.30   K space using all data.

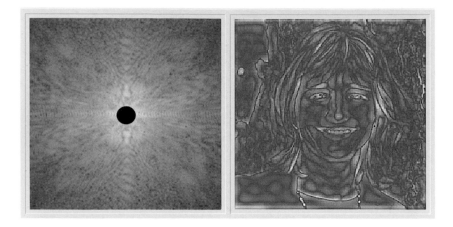

Figure 3.31   K space using resolution data only.

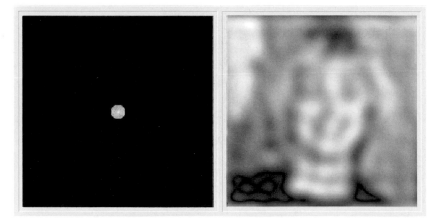

Figure 3.32   K space using signal data only.

(4) *The scan time is the time to fill K space.* The parameters that affect scan time in a typical acquisition are:

- repetition time (TR)
- phase matrix
- number of excitations (NEX).

Repetition time. Every TR each slice is selected, phase encoded and frequency encoded. Slices are not selected together but sequentially, i.e. slice 1 is selected and encoded and frequencies from its echo digitized. Then the next slice is selected, encoded and digitized, and so on. This is why the maximum number of slices available depends on the TR. Longer TRs allow more slices to be selected, encoded and digitized than short TRs. A TR of, say, 500 ms may allow for 15 slices, while a TR of 2000 ms may allow for 40 slices.

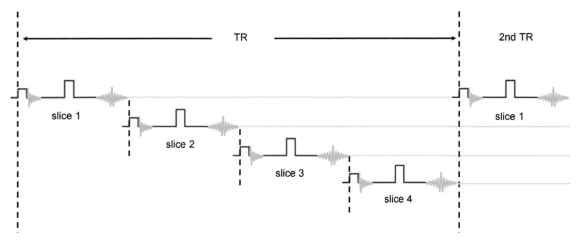

95

Figure 3.33   TR vs number of slices.

Learning point: what is the TR?

It is important to understand that although the TR is defined as the time between excitation pulses, it is *not* the time between each excitation pulse, i.e. the time between exciting slice 1 and 2, etc. In normal acquisitions, it is the time between exciting a particular slice, going off and exciting all the other slices in the stack sequentially, and then returning to that slice again to excite it and fill another line of K space with data. In other words, it is the time between filling one line of K space for a particular slice and filling the next line down in the same area of K space (Figure 3.33). This is why the TR is one of the parameters that governs scan time.

The *phase matrix* determines the number of lines that must be filled to complete the scan. As one line is filled per TR (in a typical pulse sequence) then if:

- a phase matrix of 128 is selected, 128 lines are filled and 128 TRs must be completed to finish the scan
- phase matrix of 256 is selected, 256 lines are filled and 256 TRs must be completed to finish the scan.

The *number of excitations* or NEX (also known as number of signal averages or acquisitions depending on manufacturer) is the number of times each line is filled with data. The signal can be sampled more than once by maintaining the same slope of phase gradient over several TRs instead of changing it every TR. In this way the same line of K space is filled several times, so that each line of K space contains more data. As there are more data in each line, the resultant image has a higher signal to noise ratio (*see* Chapter 4) but the scan time is proportionally longer.
For example:

- TR 1000 ms, phase matrix 256, 1 NEX scan time = 256 s
- TR 1000 ms, phase matrix 256, 2 NEX scan time = 512 s

Usually to fill each line more than once, the same slope of phase encoding gradient is used over two or more successive TRs, rather than filling all the lines once and then returning to repeat the process again.

Learning point: K space and scan time

Using the chest of drawers analogy:

- The TR is the time between filling the top drawer of chest of drawers 1 and filling the next drawer down in chest of drawers 1. During that time the top drawer in chest of drawers, 2, 3, 4, etc are filled sequentially.
- The phase matrix is the number of drawers in each of chest of drawers.
- The NEX is the number of times each drawer is filled, e.g. once, twice, three times, etc.
- The scan is over when all the drawers in all the chest of drawers are full with the required amount of data.

K space traversal and gradients

The way in which K space is traversed and filled depends on a combination of the polarity and amplitude of both the frequency and phase encoding gradients.

- The amplitude of the *frequency* encoding gradient determines how far to the *left and right* K space is traversed and this in turn determines the *size of the FOV in the frequency direction* of the image.
- The amplitude of the *phase* encoding gradient determines how far *up and down* a line of K space is filled. The steepest phase gradient slope in the acquisition determines the *phase matrix* of the image.

The polarity of each gradient defines the direction traveled through K space as follows:

- *frequency* encoding gradient *positive*, K space traversed from *left to right*
- *frequency* encoding gradient *negative*, K space traversed from *right to left*
- *phase* encoding gradient *positive*, fills *top* half of K space
- *phase* encoding gradient *negative*, fills *bottom* half of K space.

In addition, the RF pulse portion of a pulse sequence also defines movement through K space. For example, an excitation pulse always takes us to the center of K space.

K space filling and gradients are best described using an illustration of a typical gradient echo sequence (Figure 3.34). In a gradient echo sequence the frequency encoding gradient switches negatively to forcibly dephase the FID and then positively to rephase and produce a gradient echo (*see* Figure 5.22). When the frequency encoding gradient is negative, K space is traversed from

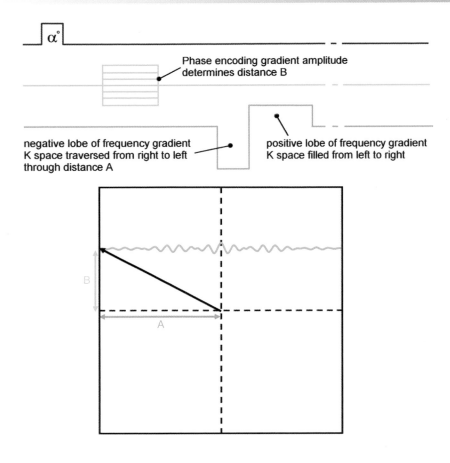

Figure 3.34   How gradients traverse K space.

right to left. The starting point of K space filling is at the center because the pulse sequence begins with an excitation pulse.

K space is initially traversed from the center to the left, to a distance (A) that depends on the amplitude of the negative lobe of the frequency encoding gradient. The phase encode in this example is positive and therefore a line in the top half of K space is filled. The amplitude of this gradient determines the distance traveled (B). The larger the amplitude of the phase gradient, the higher up in K space is the line that is filled with data from the echo. Therefore the combination of the phase gradient and the negative lobe of the frequency gradient determine at what point in K space data storage begins.

The frequency encoding gradient is then switched positively and during its application data are read from the echo. As the frequency encoding gradient is positive, data are placed in a line of K space from left to right. The distance traveled depends on the amplitude of the positive lobe of the gradient and determines the size of the FOV in the frequency direction of the image. This is only one example of how K space may be filled. If the phase gradient is negative then a line in the bottom half of K space is filled in exactly the same manner as above. K space traversal in spin echo sequences is more complex as the 180° RF pulse moves us through K space to the opposite side in both directions.

Options that fill K space

The way in which K space is filled depends on how the data are acquired and can be manipulated to suit the circumstances of the scan. This is especially true when reducing scan times. K space filling is manipulated in many imaging options, sequences and types of acquisition. These include the following:

- rectangular field of view (Chapter 4)
- anti-aliasing (Chapter 7)
- fast spin echo sequences (Chapter 5)
- keyhole imaging (Chapter 5)
- respiratory compensation (Chapter 7)
- parallel imaging (Chapter 5)
- single shot and echo planar imaging (Chapter 5).

The K space filling associated with the above options is discussed in the relevant chapters and are summarized in Table 3.4. However, it is appropriate here to describe two other options that use altered K space filling. These are:

- partial echo imaging
- partial or fractional averaging or half Fourier.

Table 3.4   K space filling options.

Option	Resolution	SNR	Scan time	Purpose
Partial averaging	same	less	less	reduce time when SNR is good
Partial echo	same	same	same	automatic for a short TE
Rectangular FOV	same	less	less	reduce time when anatomy is rectangular
Anti-aliasing (GE Philips)	same	same	same	to eliminate aliasing
Anti-aliasing (Siemens)	same	more	more	to eliminate aliasing
Fast spin echo	same	same	less	reduce scan time
Keyhole imaging	same	same	less	for temporal resolution and SNR
Respiratory compensation	same	same	slightly more	reduce respiratory artefact
Parallel imaging	same	same	less	reduce scan time
	more	less	same	increase resolution

Partial echo imaging

Partial echo imaging is performed when only part of the signal or echo is read during application of the frequency encoding gradient. As previously described, the peak of the echo or signal is usually centered in the middle of the acquisition window. For example, if the frequency encoding gradient is switched on for 8 ms, frequencies are digitized during 4 ms of rephasing and 4 ms of dephasing. This signal is mapped relative to the frequency axis of K space and the left half of the frequency area of K space is the mirror image of the right half.

When a very short TE is required, it is necessary to rephase the echo sooner than when using a longer TE. However, due to gradient limitations it may not be possible to switch the frequency encoding gradient on sooner than normal. By selecting partial or fractional echo it is possible to switch the frequency encoding gradient on at the normal time but have the peak of the echo occur sooner rather than centered in the middle of the acquisition window. This means that only the peak and the dephasing part of the echo are sampled and therefore initially only half of the frequency area of K space is filled (the right hand side of K space). However, due to the right to left symmetry of K space, the system can extrapolate the data in the right hand side of K space and place it also in the left hand side. Therefore although initially only the right hand side of K space is filled with data, after extrapolation, both sides contain data and overall signal is not lost from the image. Partial echo imaging is routinely used when very short TEs are selected. The use of a very short TE allows for maximum T1 and proton density weighting and slice number for a given TR (Figure 3.35).

Partial, fractional averaging or half Fourier

The negative and positive halves of K space on each side of the phase axis are symmetrical and a mirror image of each other. As long as at least half of the lines of K space that have been selected are filled during the acquisition, the system has enough data to produce an image. For example, if only 75% of K space is filled, only 75% of the phase encodings selected needs to be performed to complete the scan (Figure 3.36). The scan time is therefore reduced.

If 256 phase encodings, 1 NEX and TR of 1 s are selected:

$$\text{scan time} = 256 \times 1 \times 1$$
$$= 256\,\text{s}$$

If 256 phase encodings, 0.75 NEX and TR of 1 s are selected, only 75% of K space is filled with data during the scan. The rest is filled with zeros:

$$\text{scan time} = 256 \times 0.75 \times 1$$
$$= 192\,\text{s}$$

The scan time is reduced but fewer data are acquired so the image has less signal. It is not possible to extrapolate the missing data as in partial echo because the vertical phase axis of K space is the axis in which motion artefacts are seen, i.e. because of patient motion it is not possible to say that data in line +128 is exactly the same as line −128 because 256 TRs would elapse between filling these two lines and during this time it is likely the patient has moved. This is why zeroes are placed in the empty lines of K space and why signal is less than when all the lines are filled.

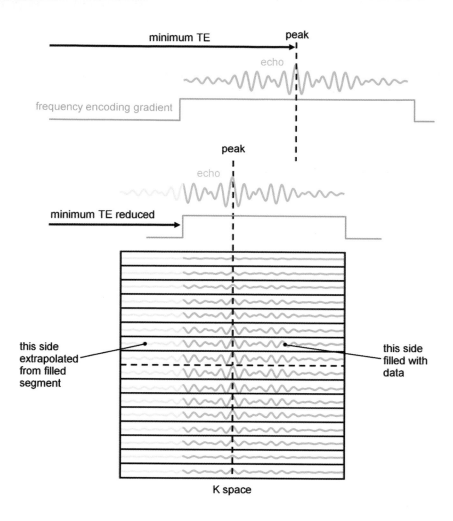

Figure 3.35 Partial echo.

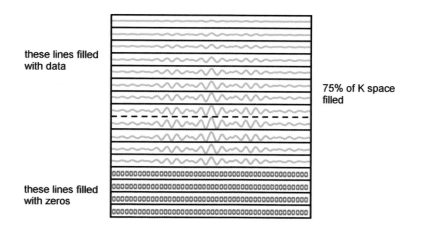

Figure 3.36 Partial Fourier.

Partial averaging can be used where a reduction in scan time is necessary, and where the resultant signal loss is not of paramount importance.

Types of acquisition

There are basically three ways of acquiring data:

- sequential
- two-dimensional volumetric
- three-dimensional volumetric.

Sequential acquisitions acquire all the data from slice 1 and then go on to acquire all the data from slice 2 (all the lines in K space are filled for slice 1 and then all the lines of K space are filled for slice 2, etc.). The slices are therefore displayed as they are acquired (not unlike computerized tomography scanning).

   Two-dimensional (2D) volumetric acquisitions fill one line of K space for slice 1, and then go on to fill the same line of K space for slice 2, etc. When this line has been filled for all the slices, the next line of K space is filled for slice 1, 2, 3, etc. This is the most common type of data acquisition.

Learning point: acquisition type and the chest of drawers

Let us go back to the chest of drawers analogy to explain the different types of acquisition. Imagine three chest drawers representing three slices in our acquisition.

- Sequential acquisition is one in which we would fill all the drawers for chest of drawers 1 before going onto chest of drawers 2. This is a type of acquisition that might be used for breath-holding techniques.
- Two-dimensional volumetric acquisition is one where we would fill the top drawer in each of the three chests of drawers in one TR and then in the next TR fill the next drawer down in each of the three chests of drawers. This is the most typical type of acquisition and the one we have assumed for many explanations in this chapter (Figure 3.37).

Refer to animation 3.3 on the supporting companion website for this book: www.wiley.com/go/mriinpractice

Three-dimensional (3D) volumetric acquisition (volume imaging) acquires data from an entire volume of tissue, rather than in separate slices. The excitation pulse is not slice selective, and the

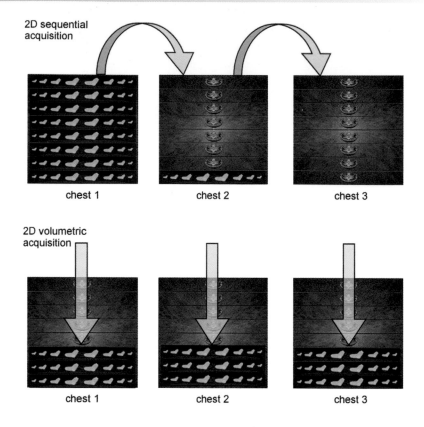

Figure 3.37   Data acquisition methods.

whole prescribed imaging volume is excited. At the end of the acquisition the volume or slab is divided into discrete locations or partitions by the slice select gradient that, when switched on, separates the slices according to their phase value along the gradient. This process is now called slice encoding. Many slices can be obtained (typically 128 to 256) without a slice gap. In other words, the slices are contiguous. The advantages of volume imaging are discussed in more detail in Chapter 4.

This chapter has introduced the basic mechanisms of gradients. A more detailed discussion, including high-speed gradient systems and their applications, is to be found in Chapter 9.

 For questions and answers on this topic please visit the supporting companion website for this book: www.wiley.com/go/ mriinpractice

As data acquisition and image formation have now been explored, the parameters available to the operator and how they interact with each other are described in the next chapter.

4

Parameters and trade-offs

Introduction

There are many parameters available to the operator when setting up a protocol. Although it is common to view a protocol as a way of examining a certain area or pathology, e.g. brain protocol, tumour protocol, it is important that protocols are considered in a much broader sense than this. A protocol is defined as a 'set of rules' and in MRI these rules are a variety of parameters that are selected by the operator. They include extrinsic contrast parameters, geometry parameters and a variety of imaging options.

The choice of pulse sequence determines the weighting and the quality of the images, and their sensitivity to pathology. The timing parameters selected specifically determine the weighting of the images. As previously discussed:

- TR determines the amount of T1 and proton density weighting
- flip angle controls the amount of T1 and proton density weighting
- TE controls the amount of T2 weighting.

The quality of the images is controlled by many factors, which also make up the parameters that are selected within a protocol. It is very important that the operator is aware of these factors and how they interrelate, so that the optimal image quality can always be obtained. The four main considerations determining image quality are:

MRI in Practice, Fourth Edition. Catherine Westbrook, Carolyn Kaut Roth, John Talbot.
© 2011 Blackwell Publishing Ltd. Published 2011 by Blackwell Publishing Ltd.

- signal to noise ratio (SNR)
- contrast to noise ratio (CNR)
- spatial resolution
- scan time.

Signal to noise ratio (SNR)

The **signal to noise ratio** is the ratio of the amplitude of the signal received to the average amplitude of the noise.

- The **signal** is the voltage induced in the receiver coil by the precession of the NMV in the transverse plane.
- The **noise** represents frequencies that exist randomly in space and time. It is equivalent to the hiss on a radio when the station is not tuned in properly, and some of it is energy left over from the 'Big Bang'. In the MR context, noise is generated by the presence of the patient in the magnet and the background electrical noise of the system. The noise is constant for every patient and depends on the build of the patient, the area under examination and the inherent noise of the system.

Noise occurs at all frequencies and is also random in time and space. The signal, however, is cumulative, occurs at time TE, depends on many factors and can be altered. The signal is therefore increased or decreased relative to the noise. Increasing the signal increases the SNR, while decreasing the signal decreases the SNR. Therefore, any factor that affects the signal amplitude in turn affects the SNR. The factors that affect the SNR include:

- magnetic field strength of the system
- proton density of the area under examination
- voxel volume
- TR, TE and flip angle
- NEX
- receive bandwidth
- coil type.

Magnetic field strength

The magnetic field strength plays an important part in determining SNR. As described in Chapter 1, as the field strength increases so does the energy gap between high- and low-energy nuclei. As the energy gap increases, fewer nuclei have enough energy to align their magnetic moments in opposition to B_0. Therefore the number of spin-up nuclei increases relative to the number of spin-down nuclei. The NMV therefore increases in size at higher field strengths and as a result there is more available magnetization to image the patient. SNR therefore increases. Although the magnetic field strength cannot be altered, when imaging with low field systems, SNR may be compromised and steps may have to be taken to boost the SNR that are not necessary when using high field systems. This usually manifests itself in longer scan times.

Proton density

The number of protons in the area under examination determines the amplitude of signal received. Areas of low proton density (such as the lungs) have low signal and therefore low SNR, while areas with a high proton density (such as the pelvis) have high signal and therefore high SNR. The proton density of a tissue is inherent to that tissue and cannot be changed (that is why it is an intrinsic contrast parameter, as discussed in Chapter 2). However, as the SNR is likely to be compromised when imaging areas of low proton density, steps may have to be taken to boost the SNR that are not necessary when scanning areas with a high proton density.

105

Voxel volume

The building unit of a digital image is a pixel. The brightness of the pixel represents the strength of the MRI signal generated by a unit volume of patient tissue (**voxel**). The voxel represents a volume of tissue within the patient, and is determined by the pixel area and the slice thickness (Figure 4.1). The pixel area is determined by the size of the FOV and the number of pixels in the FOV or matrix. Therefore:

$$\text{pixel area} = \text{FOV dimensions} \div \text{matrix size}$$

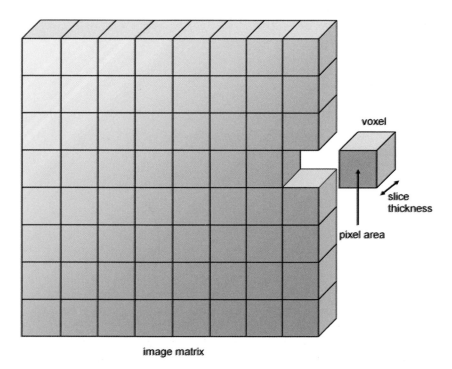

Figure 4.1   The voxel. The large green square is the FOV.

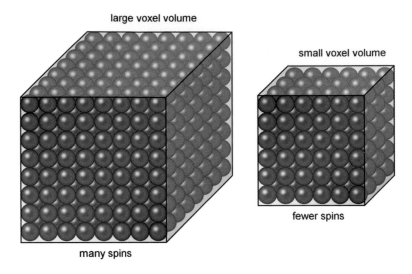

large voxel volume

small voxel volume

fewer spins

many spins

Figure 4.2   Voxel volume and SNR (spin numbers are not representative).

A **coarse matrix** is one with a low number of frequency encodings and/or phase encodings and results in a low number of pixels in the FOV. For a given FOV a coarse matrix results in large pixels and voxels. A **fine matrix** is one with a high number of frequency encodings and/or phase encodings, and results in a large number of pixels in the FOV. For a given FOV a fine matrix results in small pixels and voxels.

Large voxels contain more spins or nuclei than small voxels, and therefore have more nuclei within them to contribute towards the signal. Large voxels have a higher SNR than small voxels (Figure 4.2).

The SNR is therefore proportional to the voxel volume and any parameter that alters the size of the voxel changes the SNR. Any selection that decreases the size of the voxel decreases the SNR, and vice versa. This is achieved in three ways:

- *Changing the slice thickness*. Look at Figures 4.3, 4.4 and 4.5. In this example the voxel size is altered by halving the slice thickness from 10 mm to 5 mm. Doing this halves the voxel volume from 1000 mm^3 to 500 mm^3 and hence the SNR. Comparing Figure 4.4 with 4.5, it is clear that the thicker slice has a better SNR than the thin slice.
- *Changing the image matrix*. The image matrix is the number of pixels in the image. It is identified by two numbers: one denotes the number of pixels there are in the frequency direction (usually the long axis of the image), the other the number of phase pixels (usually the short axis of the image) (Figure 4.6). Look at Figures 4.7 and 4.8 where the phase matrix has been increased from 128 (Figure 4.7) to 256 (Figure 4.8). As the FOV has remained unchanged, there are smaller pixels and therefore voxels in Figure 4.8 than Figure 4.7. Therefore as the voxel volume has been halved in this example, the SNR is also halved.
- *Changing the FOV*. Look at Figures 4.9, 4.10 and 4.11. The FOV has been halved, which has halved the pixel dimension along both axes. Therefore the voxel volume and SNR are reduced to one quarter of the original value (from 1000 mm^3 to 250 mm^3). When comparing Figure 4.10 with 4.11 it is evident that the SNR is significantly reduced in Figure 4.11 but the resolu-

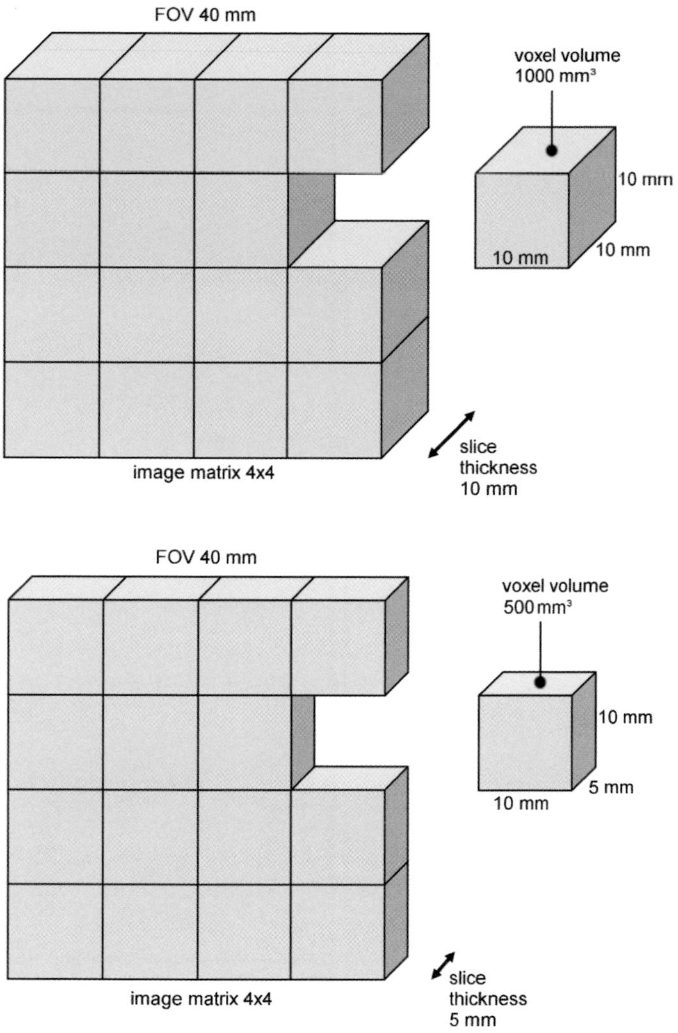

FOV 40 mm

voxel volume
1000 mm³

10 mm

10 mm

10 mm

image matrix 4x4

slice
thickness
10 mm

FOV 40 mm

voxel volume
500 mm³

10 mm

5 mm

10 mm

image matrix 4x4

slice
thickness
5 mm

Figure 4.3   Slice thickness vs SNR.

tion is increased. Depending on the area being imaged and the receiver coil used, it is sometimes necessary to take steps to increase the SNR when using a small FOV.

TR, TE and flip angle

Although TR, TE and flip angle are usually considered parameters that influence image contrast,
they also influence the SNR and therefore overall image quality. Spin echo pulse sequences generally have more signal than gradient echo sequences, as all the longitudinal magnetization is
converted into transverse magnetization by the 90° flip angle. Gradient echo pulse sequences only
convert a proportion of the longitudinal magnetization into transverse magnetization, as they use

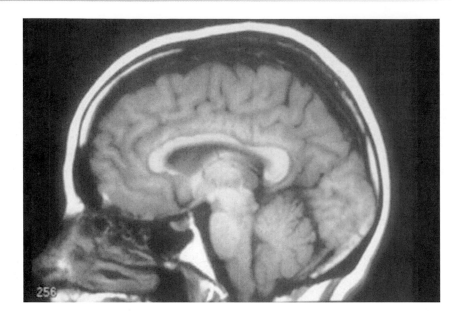

Figure 4.4   Sagittal T1 weighted image of the brain acquired with a slice thickness of 10 mm.

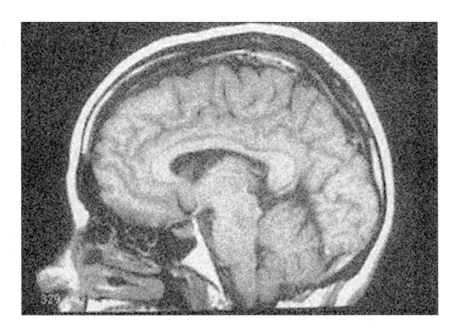

Figure 4.5   Sagittal T1 weighted image of the brain acquired with a slice thickness of 5 mm.

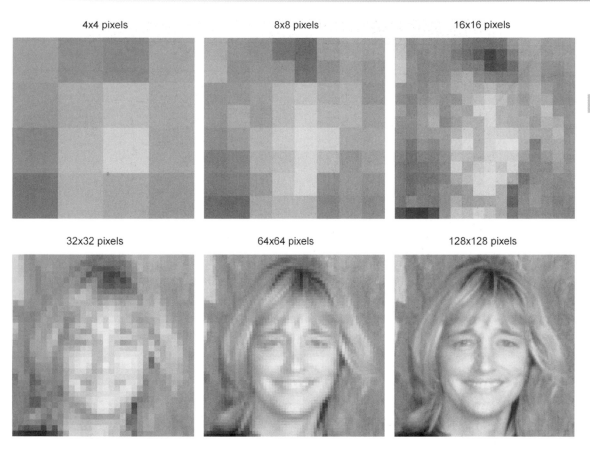

Figure 4.6   Changing the image matrix. Note how resolution changes.

flip angles other than 90°. In addition, the 180° rephasing pulse is more efficient at rephasing than the rephasing gradient of gradient echo sequences, and so the resultant echo has greater signal amplitude.

- The flip angle controls the amount of transverse magnetization that is created which induces a signal in the coil (Figures. 4.12, 4.13 and 4.14). The maximum signal amplitude is created with flip angles of 90°. Look at Figures 4.13 and 4.14 in which the flip angle has been altered from 90° to 10°. The resultant SNR is significantly reduced so that steps are necessary to increase it to improve image quality.
- The TR controls the amount of longitudinal magnetization that is allowed to recover before the next excitation pulse is applied. A long TR allows full recovery of the longitudinal magnetization so that more is available to be flipped in the next repetition. A short TR does not allow full recovery of longitudinal magnetization, so less is available to be flipped (*see* Figure 2.8). Look at Figures 4.15, 4.16, 4.17 and 4.18, where the TR has been increased from 140 ms to 700 ms. It is easy to see how the SNR has improved as the TR increases. This is because as the TR increases more longitudinal magnetization is available to create transverse magnetization

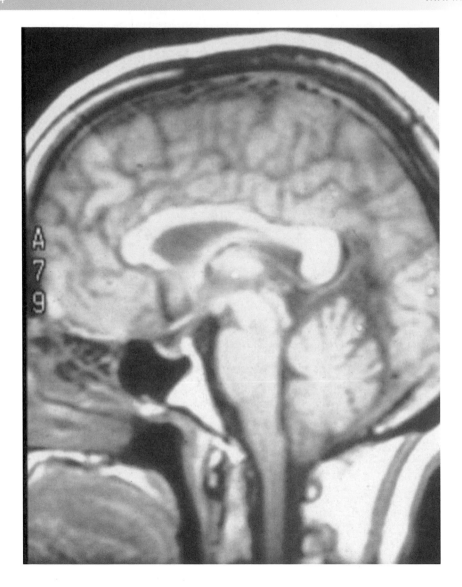

Figure 4.7   Sagittal T1 weighted image of the brain acquired with a 128 phase matrix.

after excitation. However, as the TR is one of factors that affects scan time (*see* Chapter 3), increasing the TR also increases scan time and the chance of patient movement.

- The TE controls the amount of transverse magnetization that is allowed to decay before an echo is collected. A long TE allows considerable decay of the transverse magnetization to occur before the echo is collected, while a short TE does not (Figure 4.19). Look at Figures 4.20, 4.21, 4.22 and 4.23 where the TE has been increased from 11 ms to 80 ms. The SNR dramatically decreases as the TE increases, because there is less transverse magnetization available to be rephased and produce an echo. This is why T2 weighted sequences that use a long TE usually have a lower SNR than T1 or PD weighted sequences that use a short TE.

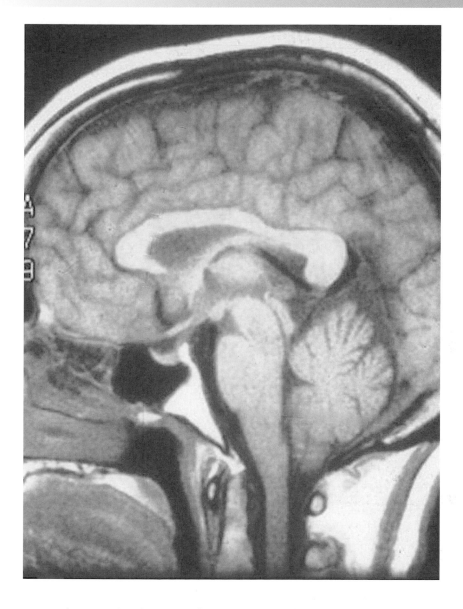

Figure 4.8   Sagittal T1 weighted image of the brain acquired with a 256 phase matrix.

Summary

- A long TR increases SNR and a short TR reduces SNR
- A long TE reduces SNR and a short TE increases SNR
- The lower the flip angle, the lower the SNR

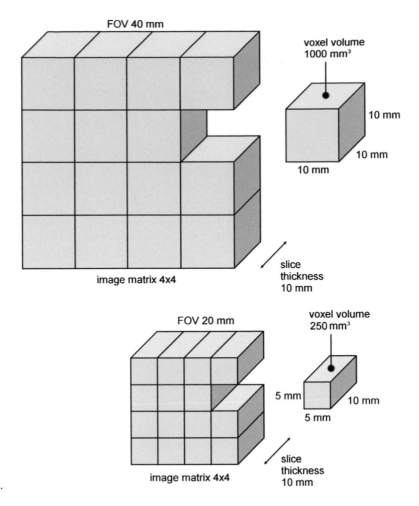

Figure 4.9   FOV vs SNR.

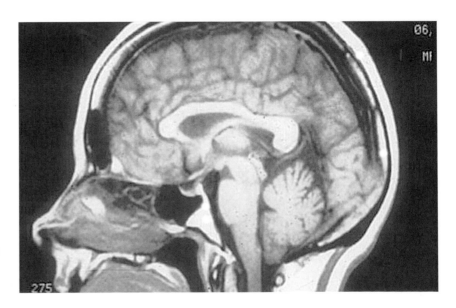

Figure 4.10   Sagittal T1 weighted image of the brain acquired with a FOV of 24 cm.

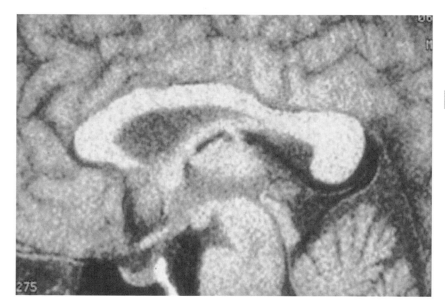

Figure 4.11 Sagittal T1 weighted image of the brain acquired with a FOV of 12 cm.

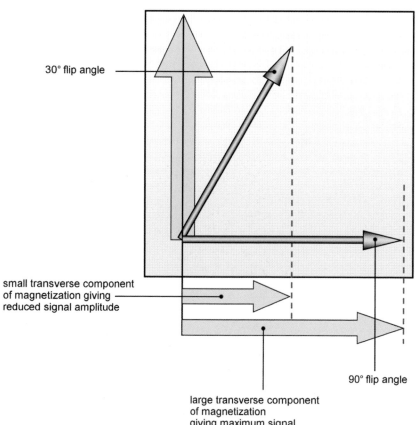

30° flip angle

small transverse component of magnetization giving reduced signal amplitude

90° flip angle

large transverse component of magnetization giving maximum signal

Figure 4.12 Flip angle vs SNR.

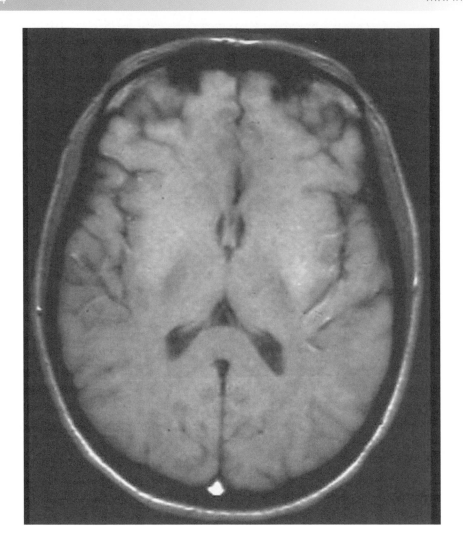

Figure 4.13   Axial gradient echo image through the brain using a flip angle of 90°.

Number of signal averages (NEX, NSA, Naq)

This is the number of times data are collected with the same amplitude of phase encoding slope. The NEX controls the amount of data stored in each line of K space (*see* Chapter 3). Referring to the chest of drawers analogy, the NEX is the number of times each drawer is filled with data. Doubling the NEX therefore doubles the amount of data that is stored in each line of K space, while halving the NEX halves the amount of data stored.

The data contain both signal and noise. Noise is random, as it is in a different position each time data are stored. Signal, however, is not random, as it always occurs at the same place when it is collected. The presence of random noise means that doubling the NEX only increases the SNR by $\sqrt{2}\,(=1.4)$. Therefore increasing the NEX is not necessarily the best way of increasing SNR. This is demonstrated in Figure 4.24.

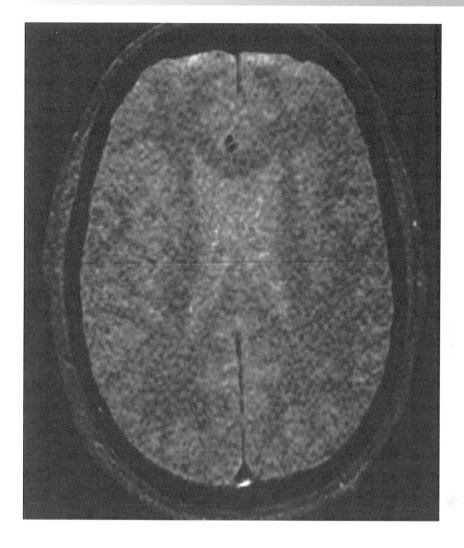

Figure 4.14   Axial gradient echo image through the brain using a flip angle of 10°.

To double the SNR we need to increase the NEX and the scan time by a factor of four. To triple it requires a ninefold increase in NEX and scan time. Increasing the scan time increases the chances of patient movement. Look at Figures 4.25 and 4.26 where the NEX has been increased from 1 to 4. The SNR is undoubtedly greater in Figure 4.26 but took four times longer to acquire than Figure 4.25. Increasing the NEX also reduces motion artefact. This is discussed later in Chapter 7.

Receive bandwidth

This is the range of frequencies that are sampled during the application of the readout gradient. Reducing the receive bandwidth results in less noise being sampled relative to signal. By applying

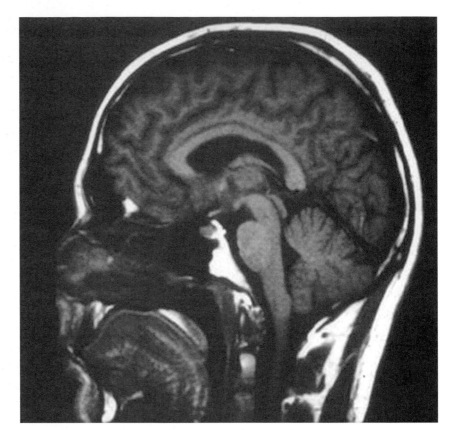

Figure 4.19 Sagittal T1 weighted image through the brain using a TE of 11 ms.

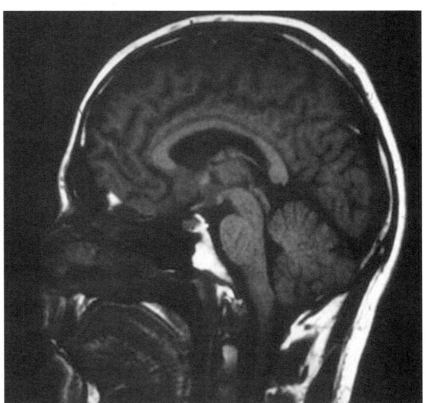

Figure 4.20 Sagittal T1 weighted image through the brain using a TE of 20 ms.

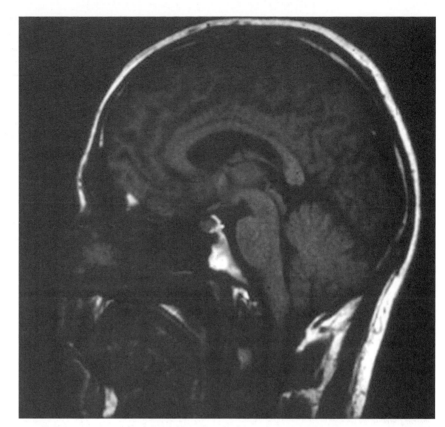

Figure 4.21 Sagittal T1 weighted image through the brain using a TE of 40 ms.

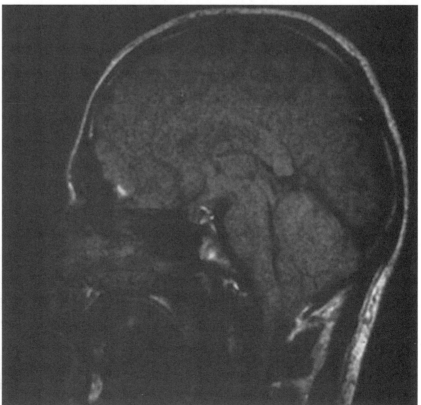

Figure 4.22 Sagittal T1 weighted image through the brain using a TE of 80 ms.

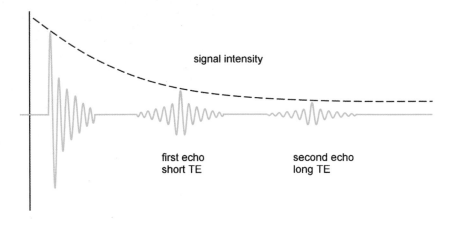

Figure 4.23   TE vs SNR.

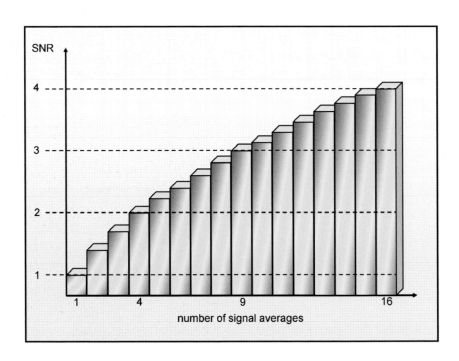

Figure 4.24   NEX vs SNR.

a filter to the frequency encoding gradient, noise frequencies much higher and lower than signal frequencies are filtered out.

Look at Figure 4.27. The areas shaded in green and red represent the ratio of signal to noise respectively (where signal frequencies are the same as noise frequencies the squares are shaded orange). In the left-hand diagram (that represents a broad receive bandwidth), there are 15 green

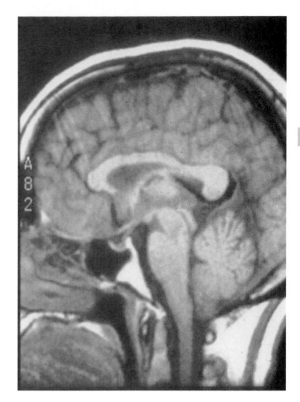

Figure 4.25 Sagittal T1 weighted image through the brain using a NEX of 1.

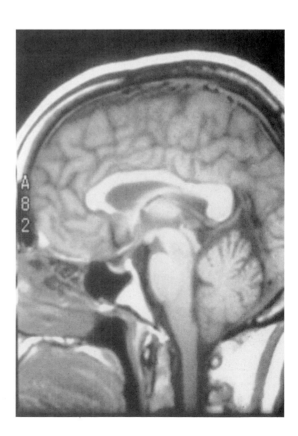

Figure 4.26 Sagittal T1 weighted image through the brain using a NEX of 4.

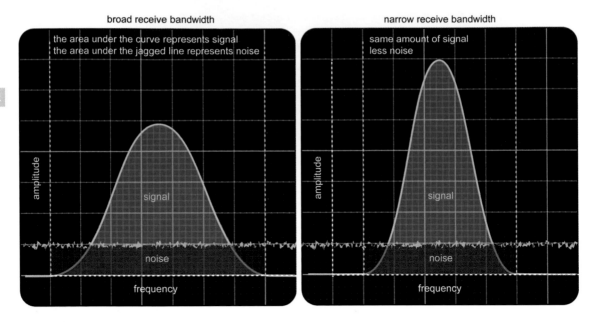

Figure 4.27   Bandwidth vs SNR.

signal squares and seven red noise squares. Therefore the SNR is approximately 2:1. In the right-hand diagram (that represents a narrow receive bandwidth), there are still 15 green signal squares but only five red noise squares. Therefore the SNR has increased to 3:1. Although the height of the signal curve is lower in the left-hand diagram than the right-hand diagram, the area under each curve is the same (i.e. 15 green squares). The height of the signal curve in the left-hand diagram is lower because frequencies are spread over a wider frequency range than in the right-hand diagram. Therefore as the receive bandwidth decreases, the SNR increases as less noise is sampled as a proportion of signal. Halving the bandwidth increases the SNR by about 40%, but increases the sampling time or acquisition window. As a result, reducing the bandwidth increases the minimum TE available (*see* Chapter 3). Reducing the bandwidth also increases chemical shift artefact (*see* Chapter 7).

Learning point: when to use a reduced receive bandwidth

Although these restrictions apply, there are some clinical situations where reducing the receive bandwidth is advantageous. Lengthening TEs are not important when a long TE is required for T2 weighting. In addition, chemical shift artefact only occurs when water and fat co-exist in the same voxel. Therefore reducing the receive bandwidth is a useful way of significantly improving SNR when performing T2 weighted images in conjunction with chemical saturation techniques (*see* Chapter 6) which remove signal from either fat or water and eliminate chemical shift artefact (*see* Chapter 7). Alternatively, broadening the receive bandwidth is often necessary when very short TEs are required. Although this decreases SNR because more noise frequencies are sampled, to achieve very short TEs the sampling time or acquisition window must be significantly reduced. This is especially relevant in fast gradient echo imaging (*see* Chapter 5).

Type of coil

The type of coil used affects the amount of signal received and therefore the SNR. Coil types are discussed in Chapter 9. Quadrature coils increase SNR because two coils are used to receive signal. Phased array coils increase SNR even more as the data from several coils are added together. Surface coils placed close to the area under examination also increase the SNR. The use of the appropriate receiver coil plays an extremely important role in optimizing SNR. In general, the size of the receiver coil should be chosen such that the volume of tissue imaged optimally fills the sensitive volume of the coil. Large coils, however, increase the likelihood of aliasing, because tissue outside the FOV is more likely to produce signal. The position of the coil is also very important for maximizing SNR. To induce maximum signal, the coil must be positioned in the transverse plane perpendicular to B_0. Angling the coil, as sometimes happens when using surface coils, results in a reduction of SNR (Figure 4.28).

Summary

To optimize image quality the SNR must be the highest possible. To achieve this:

- use spin echo pulse sequences where possible
- try not to use a very short TR and a very long TE
- use the correct coil and ensure that it is well tuned and positioned, and immobilized correctly
- use a coarse matrix
- use a large FOV
- select thick slices
- use as many NEX as possible.

Contrast to noise ratio (CNR)

The contrast to noise ratio is defined as the difference in the SNR between two adjacent areas. It is controlled by the same factors that affect SNR. The CNR is probably the most critical factor affecting image quality as it directly determines the eyes' ability to distinguish areas of high signal from areas of low signal. Image contrast depends on both intrinsic and extrinsic parameters as discussed in Chapter 2 and therefore these factors also affect CNR. From a practical point of view the CNR is increased in the following ways.

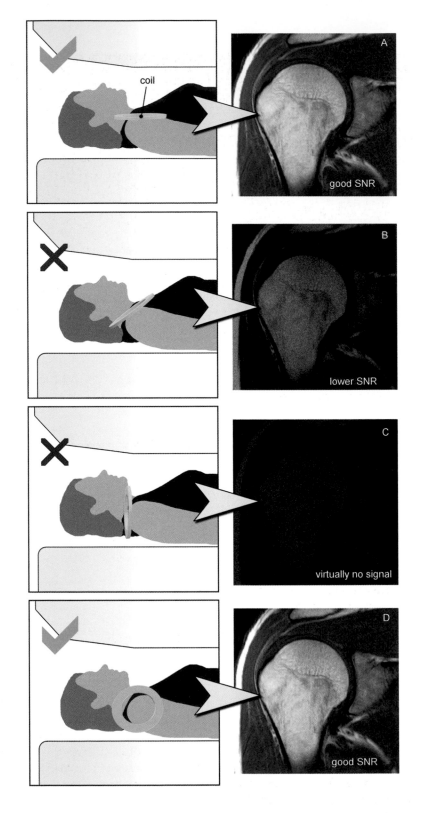

Figure 4.28 Coil position vs SNR.

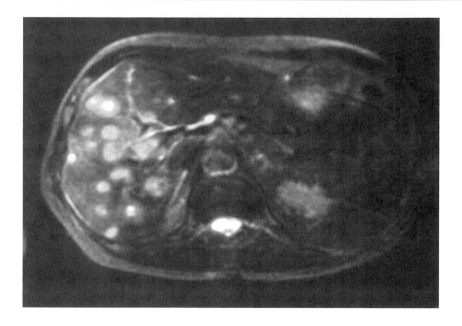

Figure 4.29   Axial T2 weighted image with through the liver. Lesions within the liver have a much greater signal than normal liver. Hence the CNR is high and they are well seen.

Using a T2 weighted image. Although a T2 weighted image often has a lower SNR than a T1 weighted image (due to the longer TE), the ability to distinguish tumor from normal tissue is often much greater because of the high signal of the tumor compared with the low signal of surrounding anatomy, i.e. the CNR is higher. This is shown in Figure 4.29 where, although overall image quality is poor, liver lesions are seen well because their signal intensity is very different from normal liver.

Using contrast agents. The purpose of administering contrast agents is to increase the CNR between pathology (which enhances) and normal anatomy (which does not) (*see* Chapter 11).

Using chemical pre-saturation technique. By saturating out normal anatomy, pathology is often seen more clearly (*see* Chapter 6 and Figure 6.19).

Using magnetization transfer contrast (MTC). In MRI, only protons that have a sufficiently long T2 time can be imaged. Other protons whose transverse components decay before the signal can be collected cannot be visualized adequately. These protons, mainly bound to large proteins, membranes and other macromolecules are called bound protons. The protons that have longer T2 times can be visualized and are termed free protons. There is always a transfer of magnetization between the bound and the free protons, which causes a change in the T1 values of the free protons. This can be exploited by selectively saturating the bound protons, which reduces the intensity of the signal from the free protons due to **magnetization transfer contrast (MTC)**. The MTC saturation band is applied before the excitation pulse at a bandwidth that selectively destroys the transverse components of magnetization of the bound protons. The use of MTC increases the CNR between pathological and normal tissues and is useful in many areas, including angiography and joint imaging.

Spatial resolution

The **spatial resolution** is the ability to distinguish between two points as separate and distinct, and is controlled by the voxel size. The voxel size is affected by:

- slice thickness
- FOV
- number of pixels or matrix (*see* Figure 4.1).

Small voxels result in good spatial resolution, as small structures can be easily differentiated (Figure 4.30). Large voxels, on the other hand, result in low spatial resolution, as small structures are not resolved so well. In large voxels, individual signal intensities are averaged together and not represented as distinct within the voxel. This results in **partial voluming.**

- The thinner the slice, the greater the ability to resolve small structures in the slice select plane. Reducing the slice thickness therefore increases spatial resolution, while increasing the

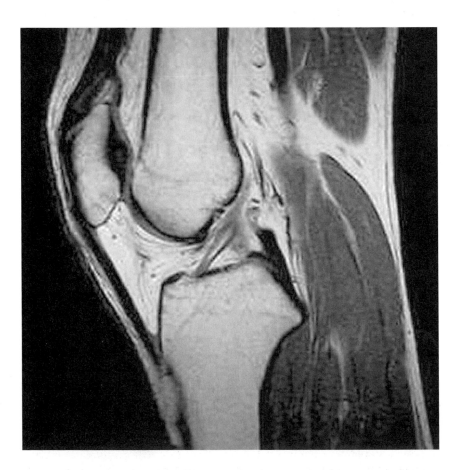

Figure 4.30   High resolution sagittal image of the knee.

slice thickness reduces spatial resolution and increases partial voluming. However, thinner slices result in smaller voxels and reduced SNR (Figures 4.4 and 4.5).

- The matrix determines the number of pixels in the FOV. Small pixels increase spatial resolution as they increase the ability to distinguish between two structures close together in the patient. Increasing the matrix therefore increases the spatial resolution. However, fine matrices result in smaller voxels and therefore reduced SNR (Figures 4.7 and 4.8).
- The size of the FOV also determines the pixel dimensions. For a given matrix a large FOV results in large pixels, while a small FOV produces small pixels. Increasing the FOV size therefore decreases the spatial resolution. However, a small FOV results in smaller voxels and therefore reduced SNR (Figures 4.10 and 4.11).

Spatial resolution and pixel dimension

Systems employ a variety of different methods to allow operator control of the geometry of the voxel. Square pixels always provide better spatial resolution than rectangular pixels as the image is equally resolved along both the frequency and phase axis. If the FOV is square, the pixels are also square if an even matrix is selected, e.g. 256×256 and this optimizes spatial resolution. If the FOV is square and an uneven matrix is selected, for example, 256×128, the pixels are rectangular (Figure 4.31) and this results in decreased spatial resolution.

Typically, the operator controls the geometry of a voxel by selecting the FOV dimensions, the image matrix and the slice thickness. Usually, the frequency matrix is the highest number and the phase matrix is altered to change the scan time and the resolution. If the FOV is square and the phase matrix is less than the frequency matrix, the pixels are longer in the phase direction than in the frequency direction. The spatial resolution is therefore reduced along the phase axis. If the FOV is rectangular, the pixels will be square if the matrix selected produces a pixel with the same dimensions along phase as well as frequency. Some systems automatically keep the pixels square regardless of the matrix and FOV selected. For example:

> Square FOV 256×256 mm
> Image matrix 256×256
> Pixel dimension is 1 mm $\times 1$ mm (square)

> Rectangular FOV 256×128 mm
> Image matrix 256×128
> Pixel dimension is 1 mm $\times 1$ mm (square) (Figure 4.32).

Rectangular FOV

When scanning anatomy that has a smaller dimension in the phase axis then frequency, a **rectangular FOV** may be desired. To acquire a square FOV, high-resolution image is costly in time, and rectangular FOV maintains spatial resolution but reduces the scan time as only a portion of the total number of phase encodings that are normally required are performed.

The dimension of the FOV in the phase direction is reduced compared to that in the frequency direction and so should be used when imaging anatomy that fits into a rectangle, for example a sagittal lumbar spine image. In the example shown in Figures 4.33 and 4.34 that compares a square FOV (256×256 mm) with a rectangular FOV (256 mm $\times 128$ mm), the pixel dimension and

even matrix square field of view

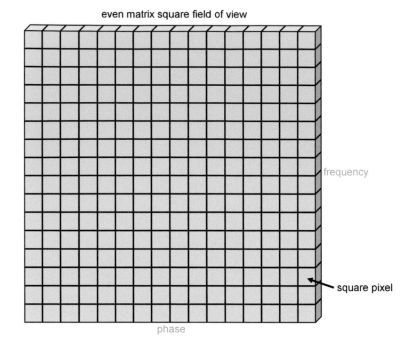

frequency

square pixel

phase

uneven matrix square field of view

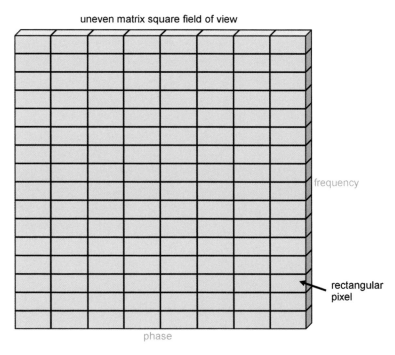

frequency

rectangular
pixel

phase

Figure 4.31   Pixel size vs matrix size.

even matrix square field of view

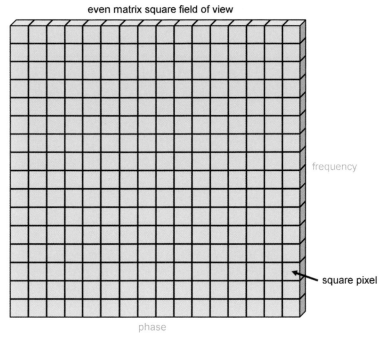

frequency

square pixel

phase

uneven matrix rectangular field of view

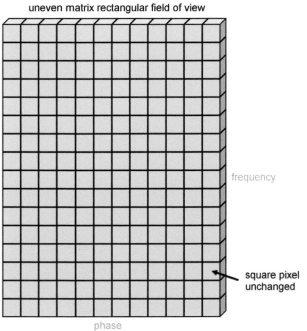

frequency

square pixel
unchanged

phase

Figure 4.32   Square pixels.

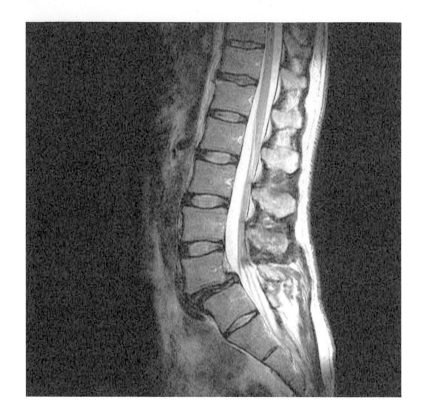

Figure 4.33 Sagittal T2 weighted image of the lumbar spine using a square FOV of 24 cm and image matrix of 256 × 256.

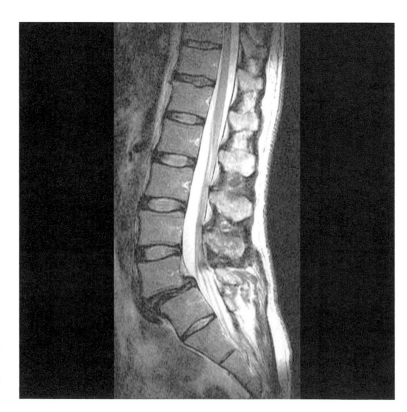

Figure 4.34 Sagittal T2 weighted image of the lumbar spine using a rectangular FOV of 12 cm in the phase direction. The scan time is half that of Figure 4.33 but the phase resolution remains unchanged.

therefore spatial resolution are the same for both FOVs. However as only 128 pixels exist in the phase axis in the rectangular FOV, only 128 phase encodes are required (128 lines of K space filled). Therefore the scan time is half that of a square FOV (Figures 4.33 and 4.34).

Learning point: rectangular FOV and K space filling using the chest of drawers analogy

In rectangular FOV, the FOV in the phase direction is smaller than that in the frequency direction and the scan time is reduced, but the resolution of the image remains unchanged because the pixel dimensions remain unchanged. Using the chest of drawers analogy for K space described in Chapter 3, the height of the chest of drawers determines the top and bottom-most drawer that is filled with data. This in turn determines the number of phase encodes required to complete the scan. For example, if a 256 × 256 matrix is selected lines +/−128 must be filled with data (Figure 4.35).

To reduce the scan time, fewer phase encodes must be performed between these outer lines, or fewer drawers filled. To achieve this, the increment between each phase encoding step is increased. The phase increments are the difference in angle between successive phase encoding slopes and correspond to the depth of each drawer in the chest of drawers analogy. The size of the phase increment or the depth of the drawer is inversely proportional to the size of the FOV in the phase direction when compared to frequency. Therefore deep drawers result in smaller dimension FOVs in the phase direction compared with frequency and shallow drawers, larger dimension FOVs in the phase direction when compared with frequency. For example, if the phase increment is halved, the FOV in the phase direction is double that of the FOV in the frequency direction and vice versa. In rectangular FOV, the phase increment is increased so that fewer phase encodes are performed between lines +/−128. This reduces the scan time and at the same time reduces the size of the FOV in the phase direction compared to frequency producing a rectangular FOV. Using this analogy it is easy to see that some signal may be lost because fewer data are being acquired (fewer lines or drawers are filled with data).

Scan time

The scan time is the time to complete data acquisition or the time to fill K space (*see* Chapter 3). Scan times are important in maintaining image quality, as long scan times give the patient more chance to move during the acquisition. Any movement of the patient will probably degrade the images. As multiple slices are selected during a 2D and 3D volumetric acquisition, movement

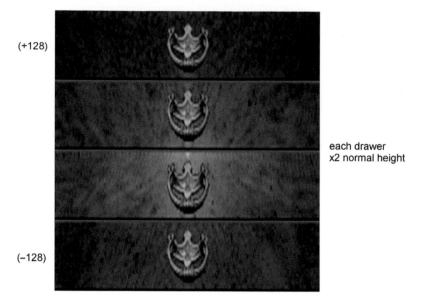

(+128)

each drawer
x2 normal height

(−128)

Figure 4.35   Rectangular FOV and the chest of drawers.

Summary

To improve image quality the spatial resolution must be optimized. The spatial resolution can be maintained by:

- selecting as thin a slice as possible
- selecting a fine matrix
- selecting a small FOV
- selecting rectangular FOV where possible.

during these types of acquisition affects all the slices. During a sequential acquisition, movement of the patient only affects those slices that are acquired while the patient is moving. As discussed in Chapter 3, the factors that affect scan time are:

- *TR* – the time of each repetition or MR experiment or the times between filling consecutive drawers. Doubling the TR doubles the scan time and vice versa
- *phase matrix* – the number of phase encodings determines the number of lines of K space or the number of drawers that are filled with data to complete the scan. If the number of phase encodings is doubled, the scan time also doubles
- *NEX* – the number of times data are collected with the same slope of phase encoding gradient or the number of times each drawer is filled with data. Doubling the NEX doubles the scan time and vice versa.

Learning point: how resolution affects the minimum TE

Resolution is controlled by the size of the voxel. To achieve a small voxel and therefore good resolution, we need to use thin slices, a small FOV and a fine matrix.

- The slice thickness is determined by the slope of the slice select gradient. Therefore to achieve *thin slices* the slice select gradient slope is *steep*.
- The size of the frequency FOV is determined by the slope of the frequency encoding gradient. To achieve a *small FOV*, the frequency encoding gradient slope is *steep*.
- The matrix size in the phase direction is determined by the number of phase encodings performed. To achieve a *fine matrix* a high proportion of the phase encoding gradient slopes are *steep*.

If gradient slopes have to be steep during a pulse sequence because thin slices, fine matrices or a small FOV have been selected, their rise times are greater. The **rise time** of a gradient is the time required for it to achieve the correct slope (*see* Chapter 9). Steep gradient slopes result in a higher rise time for the gradient than shallow gradient slopes. Steep gradient slopes therefore stress the gradient coils more than shallow gradient slopes. This therefore increases the minimum TE as the system cannot collect the signal until all the gradient functions have been completed. A small FOV, thin slices and fine matrices increase the minimum TE and may result in fewer slices being available. If the TE increases, the selection and encoding of each slice takes longer, and therefore fewer slices can be excited in a given TR.

Summary

To reduce the likelihood of patient movement, the scan time should always be as short as possible. To achieve the shortest scan time:

- use the shortest TR possible
- select the coarsest matrix possible
- reduce the NEX to a minimum.

Summary

SNR is proportional to:

- pixel area/FOV^2
- slice thickness
- proton density
- $\sqrt{NEX}$

- $1/\sqrt{}$(number of phase encodings)
- $1/$(number of frequency encodings)
- $1/\sqrt{}$(receive bandwidth)
- TR, TE and flip angle.

Spatial resolution is determined by:

- FOV
- matrix size
- slice thickness.

Scan time is proportional to:

- TR
- number of phase encodings
- NEX.

Trade-offs

It is probably now obvious that there are many trade-offs when selecting parameters within a pulse sequence. Ideally an image has high SNR, good spatial resolution and is acquired in a very short scan time. However, this is rarely achievable as increasing one factor inevitably reduces one or both of the other two. It is vital that the user has a full understanding of all the parameters that affect each image quality parameter and the trade-offs involved. Table 4.1 gives the result of optimizing image quality. Table 4.2 gives the parameters and their associated trade-offs.

Decision making

The decisions made when setting up a protocol depend on the area to be examined, the condition and co-operation of the patient, and the clinical throughput required. There are really no rules in MRI. This can be very frustrating when trying to learn, but also makes the subject interesting and challenging. Every facility has protocols established with the co-operation of the manufacturer and the radiologist. However, here are a few tips for optimizing image quality.

- Always choose the correct coil and position it correctly. This often makes the difference between a good or bad quality examination.
- Make sure that the patient is comfortable. This is very important as a patient is more likely to move if they are uncomfortable. Immobilize the patient as much as possible to reduce the likelihood of movement.
- Try to ascertain from the radiologist exactly what protocols are required before the scan. This saves a lot of time, as radiologists can be difficult to track down.
- The scan plane, pulse sequence type and weighting required are usually (but not always) decided by the radiologist. In our view, SNR is the most important image quality factor. There is no point in having an image with good spatial resolution if the SNR is poor. Sometimes, however, good spatial resolution is vital but if the SNR is low, the images will be of poor quality and the benefit of good spatial resolution is lost.

Table 4.1   The results of optimizing image quality.

To optimize image	Adjusted parameter	Consequence
Maximize SNR	↑ NEX	↑ scan time
	↓ matrix	↓ scan time (p/matrix)
	–	↓ resolution
	↑ slice thickness	↓ resolution
	↓ receive bandwidth	↑ minimum TE
	–	↑ chemical shift
	↑ FOV	↓ resolution
	↑ TR	↓ T1 weighting
	–	↑ number of slices
	↓ TE	↓ T2 weighting
Maximize resolution (assuming a square FOV)	↓ slice thickness	↓ SNR
	↑ matrix	↓ SNR
	–	↑ scan time (p/matrix)
	↓ FOV	↓ SNR
Minimize scan time	↓ TR	↑ T1 weighting
	–	↓ SNR
	–	↓ number of slices
	↓ phase matrix	↓ resolution
	–	↑ SNR
	↓ NEX	↓ SNR
	–	↑ movement artefact
	↓ slice number in volume imaging	↓ SNR

It is very important to keep the scan time as short as possible. Again, there is no point having an image with great SNR and spatial resolution if it took so long to acquire that the patient has moved during the scan. Remember, any patient can move – not just a restless one. The longer the patient is expected to lie on the table, the more likely it is that they will move.

As each system varies considerably, the following are only guidelines. The parameters given are not etched in stone but are only meant as indicators and are appropriate at most common clinical field strengths, i.e. 0.5 T to 1.5 T. It is inadvisable to select:

Table 4.2   Parameters and their associated trade-offs.

Parameter	Benefit	Limitation
TR ↑	↑ SNR	↑ scan time
	↑ number of slices	↓ T1 weighting
TR ↓	↓ scan time	↓ SNR
	↑ T1 weighting	↓ number of slices
TE ↑	↑ T2 weighting	↓ SNR
TE ↓	↑ SNR	↓ T2 weighting
NEX ↑	↑ SNR	↑ scan time
	↑ signal averaging	
NEX ↓	↓ scan time	↓ SNR
		↓ signal averaging
Slice thickness ↑	↑ SNR	↓ resolution
	↑ coverage	↑ partial voluming
Slice thickness ↓	↑ resolution	↓ SNR
	↓ partial voluming	↓ coverage
FOV ↑	↑ SNR	↓ resolution
	↑ coverage	
	↓ aliasing (pFOV)	
FOV ↓	↑ resolution	↓ SNR
		↓ coverage
		↑ aliasing (pFOV)
(p)Matrix ↑	↑ resolution	↑ scan time
		↓ SNR if pixel small
(p)Matrix ↓	↓ scan time	↓ resolution
	↑ SNR if pixel large	
Receive bandwidth ↑	↓ chemical shift	↓ SNR
	↓ minimum TE	

Table 4.2   *Continued*

Parameter	Benefit	Limitation
Receive bandwidth ↓	↑ SNR	↑ chemical shift
		↑ minimum TE
Large coil	↑ area of received signal	↓ SNR
		sensitive to artefacts
		aliasing with small FOV
Small coil	↑ SNR	↓ area of received signal
	less sensitive to artefacts	
	less prone to aliasing with small FOV	

- a very short TR in spin echo sequences (choose 400 ms not 200 ms)
- a very long TE (choose 100 ms not 200 ms)
- very low flip angles (choose 20° not 5°)
- very thin slices (choose 4 mm not 3 mm)
- a very small FOV (choose 120 mm not 80 mm), unless you are using a good local coil.

In most centers, the protocols selected work well and the radiologists are happy with the parameters set. However, it is worth remembering that, for example, a 1 mm difference in slice thickness can make all the difference in improving SNR without noticeably reducing the spatial resolution. Also remember that as the FOV size decreases, the dimensions of the pixel along both axes are reduced (assuming that the system operates with a square FOV). Under these circumstances, the FOV is the most potent controller of SNR. Using a 160 mm FOV instead of an 80 mm FOV can be important in maintaining SNR.

If the area under examination has inherently good signal (for example the brain), and the correct coil has been selected, it is usually possible for a fine matrix and fewer NEX to be used to achieve good quality images in terms of SNR and spatial resolution. However, when examining an area with inherently low signal (for example the lungs), selection of more NEX and a coarser matrix may be necessary. Try to do all this and keep the scan time as low as possible. It is usually not practical to have sequences that last 30 minutes each.

Volume imaging

Volume imaging is advantageous in that very small lesions can be demonstrated because the slice thickness can be drastically reduced compared with conventional imaging, and there is no slice gap. In conventional imaging the slice thickness affects the SNR. In volume imaging the entire volume of tissue is excited and the volume contains no gap, the SNR is superior and so fewer NEX can be used. The other main advantage of volumes is that as data are collected from a slab, the slab can be manipulated to look at the anatomy within the volume in any plane and at any angle of obliquity.

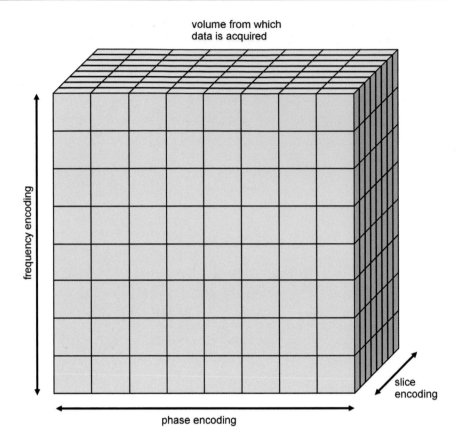

**volume from which
data is acquired**

frequency encoding

*slice
encoding*

phase encoding

Figure 4.36   Encoding in a volume acquisition.

The disadvantages of volume imaging are that in general, the scan times associated with them are relatively long. For this reason, they are usually used in conjunction with faster pulse sequences. In volume imaging, slices are sectioned out by a technique known as slice encoding (Figure 4.36). This is another series of phase encoding steps along the slice select axis. Therefore, just as the number of phase encoding steps increases the scan time in conventional spin echo, the number of slices also affects the scan time in volume imaging. Therefore:

$$\text{scan time} = \text{TR} \times \text{NEX} \times \text{number of phase encodings} \times \text{number of slice encodings}.$$

The greater the number of slices prescribed, the longer the scan time. However, this is offset somewhat by the fact that the greater the slice number the greater the SNR, and so the NEX can be reduced.

Volume imaging and resolution

To obtain equal resolution in every plane and at every angle of obliquity, each voxel should be symmetrical (**isotropic**). That is to say, the voxel should have equal dimensions in every plane. If this is not true, the volume has poorer resolution in the planes other than the one in which it was acquired. For example, if a FOV of 240 mm and matrix of 256 × 256 is used, each pixel has a dimension of 0.9 mm (FOV/matrix). If the slice thickness selected is 3 mm, resolution is worse when the voxel is viewed from the side. Under these conditions, the voxel is **anisotropic**.

Sometimes volumes are acquired purely because the slices are contiguous and not because they are to be viewed in another plane, for example coronal volumes of the brain can be very useful in detecting small temporal lobe lesions. However, they are not generally used to look at the brain axially or coronally. In this instance, 3 mm slices at 64 locations will cover the head adequately. In volume imaging of a joint, on the other hand, reformatting in other planes may be paramount. Under these circumstances it is important to obtain isotropic voxels, so thinner slices (1 mm or less) are required, although the number of slice locations may have to be increased to cover the anatomy.

The uses of volume imaging

Volume imaging has many potential applications, but it is widely used for imaging of joints, especially the knee, where anatomy is often confusing and not strictly in plane. Volumes can be very useful for following ligaments or other structures that cross over the imaging plane. Volumes should also be used when looking for very small lesions. The slice thickness can be lowered to less than 1 mm in most systems, and so extremely good resolution can be achieved. Lesions in the temporal lobes or posterior fossa especially lend themselves to volume imaging.

Summary

- Volume imaging allows reformatting in any plane
- Isotropic voxels give equal resolution in every plane
- The scan time depends on the slice number and the TR, phase encoding number and the NEX
- Increasing the slice number increases the SNR, but also increases the scan time
- Volume imaging increases the SNR as a whole volume of tissue is excited

Manipulating SNR, image contrast, spatial resolution and scan time is a real art and takes some time and experience. Even after many years the operator will probably get things wrong occasionally. However, perseverance is important, and eventually results in good image quality.

 For questions and answers on this topic please visit the supporting companion website for this book: www.wiley.com/go/ mriinpractice

As image quality factors and trade-offs have been explored, it is now important to understand pulse sequences and their individual uses. These are discussed in Chapter 5.

5

Pulse sequences

Introduction

Understanding pulse sequences forms an integral part of learning MRI. Pulse sequences enable us to control the way in which the system applies pulses and gradients. In this way, image weighting and quality is determined. There are many different pulse sequences available, and each is designed for a specific purpose. This chapter discusses the mechanisms, uses and parameters for each of the common pulse sequences, and their advantages and disadvantages. Each manufacturer uses different acronyms to distinguish between individual pulse sequences, which can be very confusing to the user. A table comparing the common acronyms for each of the main manufacturers is included (Table 5.2). This is provided as a guide only; it is not in any way meant to compare the performance or specification of each system. The parameters given are general as they depend on field strength. However, the parameters given should be suitable for most current clinical field strengths.

MRI in Practice, Fourth Edition. Catherine Westbrook, Carolyn Kaut Roth, John Talbot.
© 2011 Blackwell Publishing Ltd. Published 2011 by Blackwell Publishing Ltd.

Learning point: what is a pulse sequence?

The definition of a pulse sequence is a series of RF pulses, gradient applications and intervening time periods. The RF pulses are applied for excitation purposes and, in the case of spin echo, for rephasing purposes. The gradients are applied to spatially encode signal (*see* Chapter 3) and to rephase and dephase spins depending on the type of pulse sequence and imaging option selected. The intervening time periods refer to the time intervals between these various functions, some of which are extrinsic contrast parameters that are selected at the console (*see* Chapter 2). Therefore a pulse sequence is a carefully co-ordinated and timed sequence of events to generate a particular type of image contrast. They can be thought of like dances. All dances involve movement of the feet as a series of steps, just as all pulse sequences involve RF pulses and gradients. However, just as the timing and the co-ordination of steps determines the type of dance, e.g. tango, foxtrot, etc., so the timing and co-ordination of elements within a pulse sequence determines the resultant image contrast.

Pulse sequences can generally be categorized as follows.

Spin echo pulse sequences (spins are rephased by a 180° rephasing pulse):

- conventional spin echo
- fast or turbo spin echo
- inversion recovery.

Gradient echo pulse sequences (spins are rephased by a gradient):

- coherent gradient echo
- incoherent gradient echo
- steady state free precession
- balanced gradient echo
- fast gradient echo
- echo planar imaging.

SPIN ECHO PULSE SEQUENCES

Conventional spin echo

Mechanism

This pulse sequence has previously been discussed in Chapter 2. To recap, spin echo uses a 90° excitation pulse followed by one or more 180° rephasing pulses to generate a spin echo.

If only one echo is generated, a T1 weighted image can be obtained using a short TE and a short TR. For proton density and T2 weighting, two RF rephasing pulses, generating two spin echoes, are applied. The first echo has a short TE and a long TR to achieve proton density weighting, and the second has a long TE and a long TR to achieve T2 weighting (*see* Figures 2.23, 2.24 and 2.25).

Uses

Spin echo pulse sequences are the gold standard for most imaging. They may be used for almost every examination. T1 weighted images are useful for demonstrating anatomy because they have a high SNR. In conjunction with contrast enhancement, however, they can show pathology. T2 weighted images also demonstrate pathology. Tissues that are diseased are generally more edematous and/or vascular. They have increased water content and consequently have a high signal on T2 weighted images and can therefore be easily identified (*see* Figures 2.23 to 2.26).

Parameters

T1 weighting

- Short TE 10–30 ms
- Short TR 300–700 ms
- Typical scan time 4–6 min

Proton density/T2 weighting

- Short TE 20 ms/long TE 80 ms+
- Long TR 2000 ms+
- Typical scan time 7–15 min

Advantages

- good image quality
- very versatile
- what you set is what you get (i.e. the contrast is truly based on the T1 and T2 relaxation times of tissues)
- true T2 weighting sensitive to pathology

Disadvantages

- scan times relatively long

Fast or turbo spin echo

Mechanism

As the name suggests, fast or turbo spin echo is a spin echo pulse sequence, but with scan times that are much shorter than conventional spin echo. To understand how fast spin echo achieves this, it is important to recap on data acquisition in conventional spin echo (*see* Chapter 3). A 90° excitation pulse is followed by a 180° rephasing pulse. Only one phase encoding step is applied per TR on each slice and therefore only one line of K space is filled per TR (Figure 5.1).

As the scan time is a function of the TR, NEX and number of phase encodings, to reduce the scan time one or more of these factors should be reduced. Decreasing the TR and the NEX affects image weighting and SNR, which is undesirable. Reducing the number of phase encodings reduces the spatial resolution, which is also a disadvantage (*see* Chapter 4). In fast spin echo, the scan time is reduced by performing more than one phase encoding step and subsequently filling more than one line of K space per TR. This is achieved by using several 180° rephasing pulses to produce a train of echoes or echo train (Figure 5.2). At each rephasing, an echo is produced and a different phase encoding step is performed.

In conventional spin echo, raw image data from each echo are stored in K space, and the number of 180° rephasing pulses applied corresponds to the number of echoes produced per TR. Each echo is used to produce a separate image (usually proton density and T2). In fast spin echo,

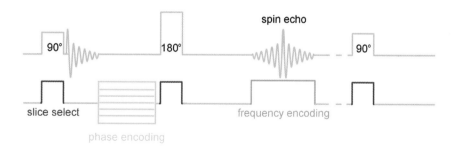

Figure 5.1   Spatial encoding in conventional spin echo.

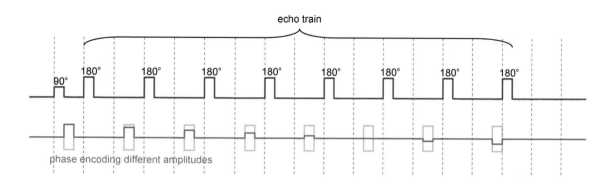

Figure 5.2   The echo train.

data from each echo are placed into *one* image. The number of 180° rephasing pulses performed per TR corresponds to the number of echoes produced and the number of lines of K space filled. This number is called the **turbo factor** or the **echo train length**. The higher the turbo factor, the shorter the scan time as more phase encoding steps are performed per TR.

For example:

- In conventional spin echo, 256 phase matrix selected, 256 phase encodings must be applied. Assuming 1 NEX has been selected: 256 TR times elapse to complete the scan.
- In fast spin echo, using the same parameters but selecting a turbo factor of 16, 16 phase encoding steps are performed every TR. Therefore 256 ÷ 16 (16) TR times elapse to complete the scan. The scan time is therefore reduced to 1/16 of the original.

At each 180°/phase encoding combination, a different amplitude of phase encoding gradient slope is applied to fill out a different line of K space. In conventional spin echo only one line is filled per TR, while in fast spin echo several lines corresponding to the turbo factor are filled (Figure 5.2). Therefore K space is filled more rapidly and the scan time is reduced.

Learning point: the chest of drawers and fast spin echo

Using the chest of drawers analogy from Chapter 3, in conventional spin echo one drawer is opened per TR to fill one line of K space with data points. In fast spin echo, to decrease the scan time but maintain resolution, all the drawers must be filled (phase resolution) but more than one drawer must be opened per TR to fill K space more quickly, reducing the scan time. This is achieved by performing more than one application of the phase encoding gradient per TR, each one to a different slope to open a different drawer.

For example, if 10 drawers are to be opened per TR, then the phase encoding gradient must be applied 10 different times to 10 different amplitudes per TR to open 10 different drawers. Once the drawers are opened, there must be data to put into them. This requires producing 10 echoes, one for each drawer. To do this, 10 different 180° pulses must be applied. The number of RF pulses corresponds to the number of echoes and the number of drawers opened per TR. This is called the echo train length or turbo factor and indicates how much faster the scan is compared with conventional spin echo, i.e. a turbo factor of 16 indicates 16 drawers are opened per TR and the scan time is 16 times faster than conventional spin echo.

Weighting in fast spin echo

The echoes are generated at different TE times and therefore data collected from them have variable weighting. All these data are stored and placed into one image. So how is a fast spin echo sequence weighted correctly? The TE selected is only an **effective TE**. In other words, it is the TE

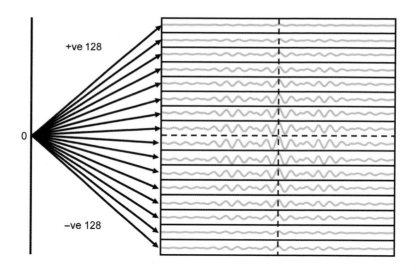

Figure 5.3   Phase encoding gradient slopes.

at which the operator wishes to weight the resultant image. To achieve this weighting, the system orders the phase encoding steps so that steep or shallow slopes are applied to the various echoes produced. As described in Chapter 3, each phase encoding step applies a different slope of gradient to phase shift the signal by a different amount. If 256 phase encodings are performed, the phase encoding gradient is switched on to varying degrees from +128 to −128 (or +128 to −127 if the 0 line is included) (Figure 5.3).

Very steep phase encoding slopes reduce the amplitude of the resultant echo. Shallow phase encoding slopes result in an echo that has maximum signal amplitude (Figure 5.4) (*see* Chapter 3). The system orders the phase encodings so that the shallow slopes that produce maximum signal are centered on the effective TE selected. The steep slopes that produce much smaller signal amplitude are placed away from the effective TE. The resultant image contains data from all the echoes in the echo train, but data from echoes collected around the effective TE have more impact on image contrast as they fill the central lines of K space, which produce the greatest signal amplitude. Data from echoes collected at the wrong weighting (other TEs) have much less of an effect on the contrast, as they fill the outer lines of K space and therefore have a smaller signal amplitude and a greater spatial resolution (Figure 5.5).

If a TE of 100 ms is selected, with a TR 4000 ms and a turbo factor of 16, T2 weighting is required. The shallowest phase encodings are performed on echoes occurring around 100 ms. Data acquired from these phase encodings have a TE at or close to 100 ms. Phase encodings performed at the very beginning and end of the echo train are steep, and the signal amplitude of these echoes is small. They contain either proton density or very heavily T2 weighted data, which are present in the image but whose impact is less predominant.

Uses

Generally speaking, the contrast seen in fast spin echo images is similar to spin echo and, therefore, these sequences are useful in most clinical applications. In the central nervous system, pelvis

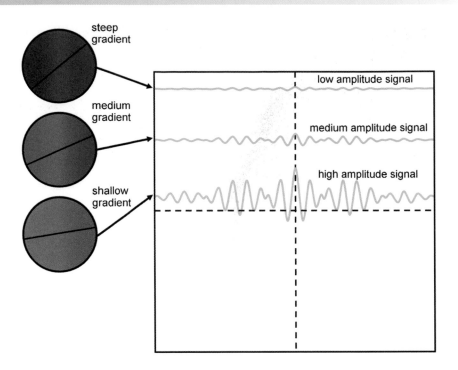

Figure 5.4 Phase encoding vs signal amplitude.

and musculoskeletal regions, fast spin echo has largely replaced spin echo especially for T2 weighting. In the chest and abdomen, respiratory artefact is sometimes troublesome if respiratory compensation techniques are not compatible with fast spin echo software. This is offset by the fact that the shorter scan times of fast spin echo enable images to be produced while the patient holds their breath.

There are, however, two contrast differences between spin echo and fast spin echo, both of which are due to the repeated, closely spaced 180° pulses of the echo train. First, fat remains bright on T2 weighted images due to the multiple RF pulses, which reduce the effects of spin–spin interactions in fat (**J coupling**) (Figure 5.6). However, fat saturation techniques can be used to compensate for this (*see* Chapter 6). Second, the repeated 180° pulses can increase magnetization transfer effects so that muscle, for example, appears darker on fast spin echo images than in conventional spin echo. In addition, the multiple 180° pulses reduce magnetic susceptibility effects, which can be detrimental when looking for small hemorrhages.

Image blurring may occur in fast spin echo images at the edges of tissues with different T2 decay values. This is because each line of K space filled during an echo train contains data from echoes with a different TE. When using long echo trains, late echoes that have a low signal amplitude contribute to the resolution of K space. If these echoes are negligible, then resolution is lost from the image and blurring occurs. This, however, may be reduced by decreasing the spacing between echoes and/or the turbo factor. In addition, artefact from metal implants is significantly reduced when using fast spin echo because the repeated 180° RF pulses compensate for field inhomogeneity (*see* Chapter 7).

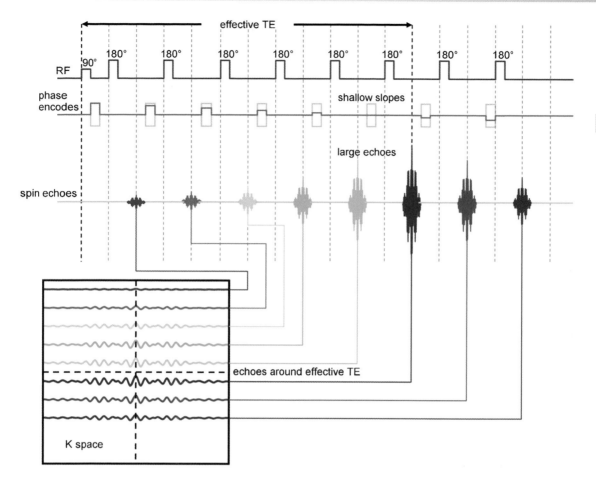

Figure 5.5   K space filling and phase re-ordering.

Parameters

These are similar to conventional spin echo. However, the turbo factor now plays an important role in image weighting. The higher the turbo factor, the shorter the scan time, but the result-ant image has more of a mixture of weighting because there are more data collected at the wrong TE. This is not as important in T2 weighted scans, as the proton density data are offset somewhat by the heavily T2 weighted data. In T1 and proton density weighting, on the other hand, larger turbo factors place too much T2 weighting in the image and hence shorter turbo factors must be used. The scan time savings in T1 weighted imaging are therefore not as great as with T2 weighting.

For T1 weighting (Figure 5.7):

- TR   300–700 ms
- effective TE   minimum
- turbo factor   2–8.

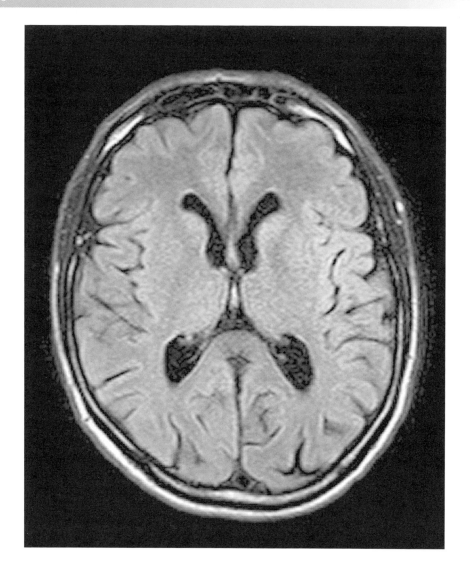

Figure 5.20   Axial FLAIR image through the brain.

Parameters

- long TI   1700–2200 ms (to suppress CSF depending on field strength)
- long TE   70 ms+ (to enhance signal from pathology)
- long TR   6000 ms+ (to allow full recovery)
- long turbo factor   16–20 (to enhance signal from pathology)
- average scan time   13–20 min

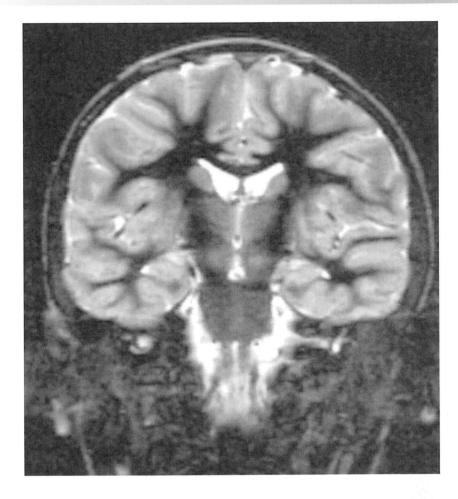

Figure 5.21   Coronal IR sequence using a TI that nulls white matter.

IR prep sequences

There are two further modifications of fast IR that were specifically developed to null blood in cardiac imaging (*see* Chapter 8). Double IR prep begins with two 180° pulses. One is non-slice selective and inverts all spins in the imaging volume, and the other is slice selective and re-inverts spins within a slice. A TI corresponding to the null point of blood (about 800 ms) completely nulls the signal from blood in the slice so that black blood imaging results. This is useful when looking at the morphology of the heart and great vessels. Triple IR prep adds a further inverting pulse at the TI of fat (about 150 ms) to null fat and blood together. This is useful when determining fatty infiltration of the heart walls (*see* Figure 8.3).

GRADIENT ECHO PULSE SEQUENCES
Conventional gradient echo

Mechanism

Gradient echo pulse sequences have been discussed in Chapter 2. To recap, gradient echo sequences use variable flip angles so that the TR and therefore the scan time can be reduced without producing saturation. T2* and proton density weighting, which are normally associated with long TRs and scan times, can therefore be acquired using short TRs because the sequence begins with a flip angle less than 90°. A gradient rather than a 180° rephasing RF pulse is used to rephase the FID. The frequency encoding gradient is used for this purpose because it is quicker to apply than a 180° pulse and therefore the minimum TE can be reduced. The frequency encoding gradient is initially applied negatively to increase dephasing of the FID, and then its polarity is reversed producing rephasing of the gradient echo. However, the gradient does not compensate for magnetic field inhomogeneities, so the resultant echo displays a great deal of T2* information (Figure 5.22).

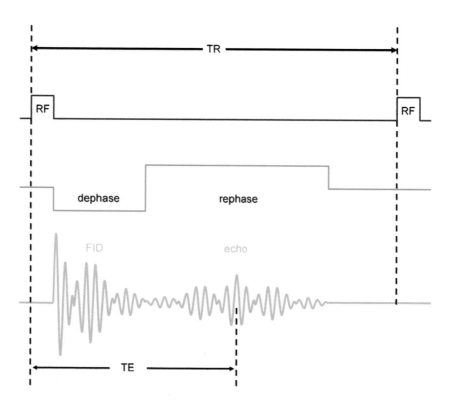

Figure 5.22   A basic gradient echo sequence showing how a bipolar application of the frequency encoding gradient produces a gradient echo.

Uses

Gradient echo pulse sequences can be used to acquire T2*, T1 and proton density weighting. However, there is always some degree of T2* weighting due to the absence of a 180° rephasing pulse. Gradient echo sequences allow for a reduction in the scan time as the TR is greatly reduced. They can be used for single-slice or volume breath-hold acquisitions in the abdomen, and for dynamic contrast enhancement. They are very sensitive to flow as gradient rephasing is not slice selective, so flowing nuclei always give a signal, as long as they have been previously excited (*see* Chapter 6). Because of this, gradient echo sequences may be used to produce angiographic-type images.

165

Parameters

The flip angle, in conjunction with the TR, determines the degree of saturation and therefore T1 weighting. To prevent saturation (necessary for T2* and proton density weighting) the flip angle should be small and the TR long enough to permit full recovery (although if the flip angle is small full recovery occurs using a much shorter TR than in spin echo imaging). If saturation and therefore T1 weighting is required, the flip angle should be large and the TR short, so that full recovery cannot occur. The TE controls the amount of T2* dephasing. To minimize T2* the TE should be short. To maximize it, the TE should be long (*see* heat analogy in Chapter 2 and Figures 2.36 and 2.37).

T1 weighting

- large flip angle   70–110° (to maximize saturation)
- short TR   less than 50 ms (to maximize saturation)
- short TE   1–5 ms (to minimize T2*)
- average scan time   several seconds to minutes.

T2* weighting

- small flip angle   5–20° (to minimize saturation)
- long TR   200 ms+ (to minimize saturation)
- long TE   15–25 ms (to maximize T2*)
- average scan time   several seconds to minutes.

Proton density weighting

- small flip angle   5–20° (to minimize saturation)
- long TR   200 ms+ (to minimize saturation)
- short TE   5–10 ms (to maximize T2*)
- average scan time   several seconds to minutes.

In conventional gradient echo the TR does not always affect image contrast. Once a certain value of TR has been exceeded, the NMV recovers fully, regardless of the flip angle selected. Under these circumstances the flip angle and TE control the degree of saturation and dephasing respectively.

The steady state and echo formation

The **steady state** is a term used in many scientific contexts. It is defined as the stable condition that does not change over time. For example, if a pot of water is placed on a stove, the stove will gradually heat up the pot and the water. In addition heat energy is lost from the pot and the water through processes such and conduction, convection and evaporation. If the amount of heat energy from the stove equals the amount of heat energy lost by convection, conduction and evaporation, then the temperature of the pot and water will remain constant and stable. This is an example of the steady state because the energy 'in' equals the energy 'out'.

In MRI, energy is given to hydrogen during excitation and, as described by the classical theory, the amount of energy applied is indicated by the flip angle. Energy is lost by hydrogen through spin lattice energy transfer and the amount of energy lost is determined by the TR. Therefore by selecting a certain combination of TR and flip angle, we can insure that the overall energy of hydrogen remains constant as the energy 'in' as determined by the flip angle equals the energy 'out' as determined by the TR. There are, therefore, critical values of flip angle and TR to maintain the steady state (Figure 5.23).

As RF has a low frequency and hence low energy, for most values of flip angle very short TRs are required to achieve the steady state. In fact the TRs required are shorter than the T1 and T2 relaxation times of the tissues. There is therefore no time for transverse magnetization to decay before the pulse sequence is repeated. Generally, flip angles of 30° to 45° in conjunction with a TR less than 50 ms achieve the steady state.

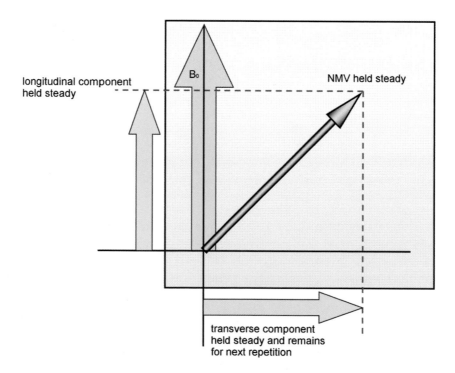

Figure 5.23   The steady state.

Table 5.1   T1 and T2 relaxation times and signal intensity of brain tissue in the steady state at 1 T.

Tissue	T1 time (ms)	T2 time (ms)	T1/T2	Signal intensity
Water	2500	2500	1	↑
Fat	200	100	0.5	↑
Cerebrospinal fluid	2000	300	0.15	↓
White matter	500	100	0.2	↓

In the steady state, there is co-existence of both longitudinal and transverse magnetization. In particular, the transverse component of magnetization does not have time to decay during the pulse sequence and builds up over successive TRs. This transverse magnetization is produced as a result of previous excitations, but remains over several TR periods in the transverse plane. It is called the **residual transverse magnetization** and it affects image contrast as it induces a voltage in the receiver coil. It affects image contrast as it results in tissues with long T2 times (such as water), appearing bright on the image. Generally speaking, as the TR is so short, magnetization in tissues does not have time to reach its T1 or T2 times before the next excitation pulse is applied. Therefore in the steady state image contrast is not due to differences in T1 and T2 times of tissues but rather to the ratio of T1 to T2, i.e. in tissues where T1 and T2 times are similar, the signal intensity is high.

In the human body, fat and water have this parity (fat, very short T1 and T2 times; water, very long T1 and T2 times) and therefore return high signal intensity in steady state sequences (Table 5.1). Other tissues such as muscle return a lower signal intensity because they do not have a similar T1 and T2 decay time. Most gradient echo sequences use the steady state as the shortest TR and scan time is achieved. Gradient echo sequences are classified according to whether the residual transverse magnetization is in phase (coherent) or out of phase (incoherent).

Learning point: echo formation

The steady state involves repeatedly applying RF pulses at time intervals less than the T2 and T1 times of all the tissues. There is therefore a build-up of residual transverse magnetization and in the steady state, this is rephased by RF pulses to produce a spin echo.

This happens because every RF pulse (regardless of its net amplitude as determined by the flip angle) contains energies that are sufficient to rephase transverse magnetization (they also contain energies that cause resonance but this is not relevant for this explanation). These energies rephase the residual transverse magnetization left over from previous RF excitation pulses to form a spin echo. This occurs at exactly the same time as the next RF pulse because the residual transverse magnetization takes the same time to rephase as it took to dephase in the first place. Therefore, when utilizing the steady state, the TR equals the tau of the spin echo.

Look at Figures 5.24 and 5.25. You will see from these diagrams that a train of RF pulses generates two signals:

- a *FID*, which occurs as a result of the withdrawal of the previous RF pulse and, once rephased, contains either T2* or T1 information depending on the TE
- a *stimulated echo* whose peak occurs at the same time as a subsequent RF pulse and contains T2* and T2 information.

The first RF pulse (RF pulse 1, shown in red) produces a FID (also shown in red). The second RF pulse (RF pulse 2, shown in orange) also produces a FID (also shown in orange). However, because the TR between RF pulse 1 and 2 is shorter than the relaxation times of the tissues, transverse magnetization is still present when the RF pulse 2 is applied. RF pulse 2 produces a FID and rephases the residual transverse magnetization still present from the first RF pulse. A spin or stimulated echo is therefore produced. This occurs at the same time as the third RF pulse (RF pulse 3, shown in blue) because the time for rephasing this transverse magnetization is the same time it took to dephase. Therefore at RF pulse 3 there are two signals: a FID (shown in blue) produced as a result of the excitation properties of RF pulse 3, and a spin echo (shown in red) that was produced by RF pulse 1 and rephased by RF pulse 2.

Any two RF pulses produce a spin echo. The first RF pulse excites the nuclei regardless of its net amplitude; the second RF pulse rephases the FID and any residual magnetization present to produce a spin echo (Figures 5.24 and 5.25). These echoes are termed **Hahn** or **stimulated echoes** depending on the amplitude of the RF pulses involved. Any two 90° RF pulses produce a Hahn echo (after Erwin Hahn who discovered them). Any two RF pulses with varying amplitude, i.e. with flip angles other than 90°, are called stimulated echoes. This type of echo is used in steady state gradient echo sequences. Most gradient echo sequences contain data from FIDs and stimulated echoes. Their contrast is determined by which of these are digitized and used in the resultant image. In practice, echo production is so rapid that the tails of FID signals merge with stimulated echoes, resulting in a continuous signal of varying amplitude. However, in the interests of simplicity, the diagrams in this chapter show them separately.

Summary

- The steady state is created when the TR is shorter than the relaxation times of tissues and the energy 'in' as determined by the flip angle equals the energy 'out' during the TR period
- Residual magnetization therefore builds up in the transverse plane
- The residual transverse magnetization is rephased by subsequent RF pulses to produce stimulated echoes
- The resultant image contrast is due to the ratio of T1 to T2 in a particular tissue and whether the FID and or the stimulated echo are sampled

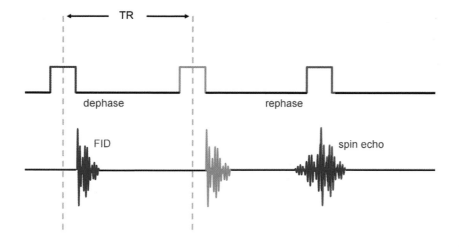

Figure 5.24   Echo formation in the steady state I.

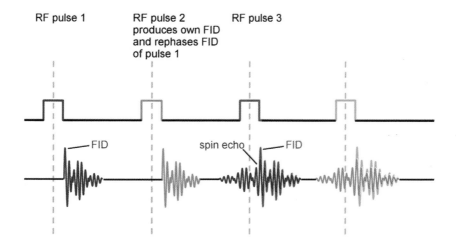

Figure 5.25   Echo formation in the steady state II.

Coherent gradient echo

Mechanism

Coherent gradient echo pulse sequences use a variable flip angle excitation pulse followed by gradient rephasing to produce a gradient echo. The steady state is maintained by selecting a TR shorter than the T1 and T2 times of the tissues. There is therefore residual transverse magnetization left over when the next excitation pulse is delivered. These sequences keep this residual magnetization coherent by a process known as rewinding. Rewinding is achieved by reversing the slope of the phase encoding gradient after readout (Figure 5.26). This results in the residual magnetization rephasing, so that it is in phase at the beginning of the next repetition.

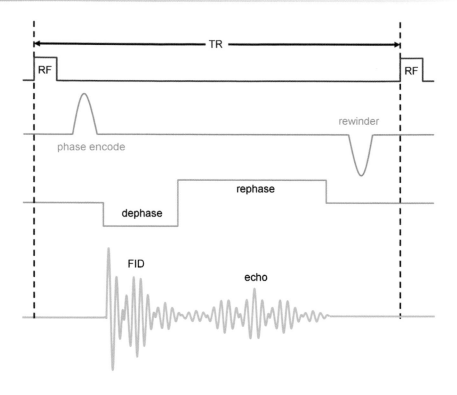

Figure 5.26   The coherent gradient echo sequence.

The rewinder gradient rephases all transverse magnetization regardless of when it was created. Therefore the resultant echo contains information from the FID and the stimulated echo. These sequences can therefore be used to achieve T1 or T2* weighted images, although traditionally they are used in conjunction with a long TE to produce T2* weighting.

Uses

Coherent gradient echo pulse sequences usually produce rapid images that are T2* weighted (Figures 5.27 and 5.28). As water is bright they are often said to give an angiographic, myelographic or arthrographic effect. They can be used to determine whether a vessel is patent, or whether an area contains fluid. They can be acquired slice by slice, or in a 3D volume acquisition. As the TR is short, slices can be acquired in a single breath hold.

Parameters

To maintain the steady state:

- flip angles   30–45°
- TR   20–50 ms.

To maximize T2*:

- long TE   15–25 ms
- use gradient moment rephasing to accentuate T2* and reduce flow artefact (*see* Chapter 6)
- average scan time: seconds for single slice, minutes for volumes.

Advantages

- very fast scans, breath-holding possible
- very sensitive to flow so good for angiography
- can be acquired in a volume acquisition

Disadvantages

- reduced SNR in 2D acquisitions
- magnetic susceptibility increases (*see* Chapter 7)
- loud gradient noise

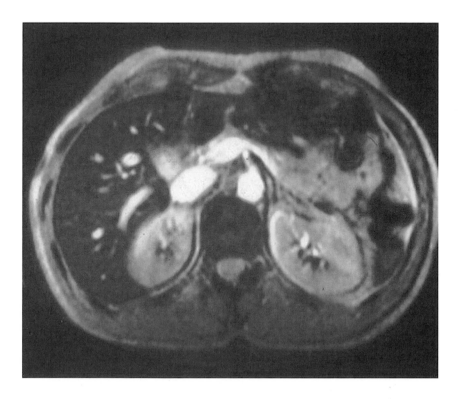

Figure 5.27   Axial breath-hold coherent gradient echo sequence through the abdomen showing vessel patency in the aorta and inferior vena cava.

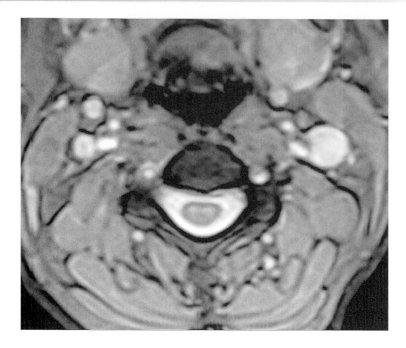

Figure 5.28   Axial coherent gradient echo sequence through the cervical spine. Note the high signal in the carotid arteries and jugular veins.

Incoherent gradient echo (spoiled)

Mechanism

Incoherent gradient echo pulse sequences begin with a variable flip angle excitation pulse and use gradient rephasing to produce a gradient echo. The steady state is maintained so that residual transverse magnetization is left over from previous repetitions. These sequences dephase or spoil this magnetization so that its effect on image contrast is minimal. Only transverse magnetization from the previous excitation is used, enabling T1 contrast to dominate. There are two ways to achieve spoiling, as follows.

RF spoiling. In this sequence RF is transmitted at a particular frequency to excite a slice and at a specific phase. The receiver coil digitally communicates with the transmit coil and only frequencies from echoes that have just been created by the excitation pulse are digitized. Using the watch analogy from Chapter 1, disregard the precessional rotation of transverse magnetization for the purposes of this explanation and look at Figure 5.29. The first RF excitation pulse applied to a particular slice has a phase of 3 o'clock. This means that the resultant transverse magnetization is created at 3 o'clock in the transverse plane. Spins dephase and are rephased by a gradient to produce a gradient echo. The receiver coil, which is situated in the transverse plane, samples frequencies within this echo and data from them are sent to K space to produce the resultant image.

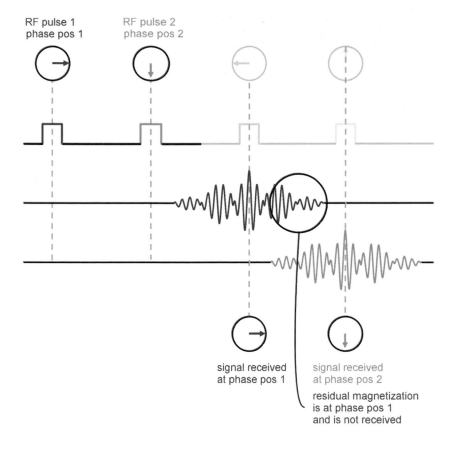

RF pulse 1
phase pos 1

RF pulse 2
phase pos 2

signal received
at phase pos 1

signal received
at phase pos 2

residual magnetization
is at phase pos 1
and is not received

Figure 5.29   RF spoiling in the incoherent gradient echo sequence.

A short TR period later the process is repeated, but this time the RF excitation pulse creates transverse magnetization at a different phase, such as 6 o'clock. Spins dephase and are rephased by a gradient to produce a second gradient echo. The receiver coil samples frequencies within this echo and data from them are sent to K space to produce the resultant image. However, as the TR was so short, magnetization created at 3 o'clock is still present as it has not had time to decay. This is the residual transverse magnetization, but because it has a different phase to the transverse magnetization just created, it is not sampled and therefore does not impact image contrast. This is RF spoiling and enables only information from the most recently created magnetization to affect image contrast.

Gradient spoiling. Gradients can be used to dephase and rephase the residual magnetization. Gradient spoiling is the opposite of rewinding. In gradient spoiling, the slice select, phase encoding and frequency encoding gradients can be used to dephase the residual magnetization, so that it is incoherent at the beginning of the next repetition. In this way, T2* or T2 effects are reduced. Generally, the uses and parameters involved in these sequences are similar to those used in RF spoiling. However, most manufacturers use RF spoiling in incoherent gradient echo sequences.

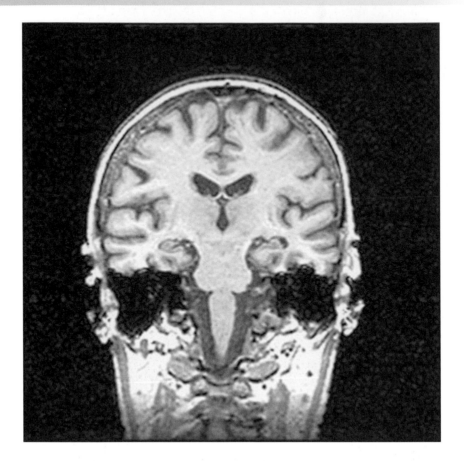

Figure 5.30   Coronal incoherent gradient echo sequence through the brain. This was acquired as part of a volume acquisition enabling T1 weighted high-resolution imaging.

Uses

As the stimulated echo that contains mainly T2* and T2 information is spoiled, RF spoiled pulse sequences produce T1 or proton density weighted images, although fluid may have a rather high signal due to gradient rephasing (Figure 5.30). They can be used for 2D and volume acquisitions, and as the TR is short, 2D acquisitions can be used to acquire T1 weighted breath-hold images. RF spoiled sequences demonstrate good T1 anatomy and pathology after gadolinium.

Parameters

To maintain the steady state:

- flip angle   30–45°
- TR   20–50 ms.

To maximize T1:

- short TE   5–10 ms
- average scan time   several seconds for single slice, minutes for volumes.

Advantages

- can be acquired in a volume or 2D
- breath holding possible
- good SNR and anatomical detail in volume
- can be used after gadolinium contrast injection

Disadvantages

- SNR poor in 2D
- loud gradient noise

Steady state free precession (SSFP)

Mechanism

In gradient echo sequences the TE is not long enough to measure the T2 time of tissues as a TE of at least 70 ms is required for this. In addition, gradient rephasing is so inefficient that any echo is dominated by T2* effects and therefore true T2 weighting cannot be achieved. The SSFP sequence overcomes this problem to obtain images that have a sufficiently long TE and less T2* than in other steady state sequences. This is achieved in the following manner.

As previously described, every RF pulse, regardless of its net magnitude, contains energies that have sufficient magnitude to rephase spins and produce a stimulated echo. However, in SSFP we need to digitize frequencies only from this stimulated echo and not from the FID. To do this, the stimulated echo must be repositioned so that it does not occur at the same time as the subsequent excitation pulse. This is achieved by applying a rewinder gradient, which speeds up the rephasing so that the stimulated echo occurs sooner (Figure 5.31).

The resultant echo demonstrates more true T2 weighting than conventional gradient echo sequences. This is because:

- *The TE is now longer than the TR.* In SSFP, there are usually two TEs.
- The actual TE is the time between the echo and the next excitation pulse.
- The effective TE is the time from the echo to the excitation pulse that created its FID. Therefore:

$$\text{effective TE} = (2 \times \text{TR}) - \text{TE}.$$

If the TR is 50 ms and the TE is 10 ms, then:

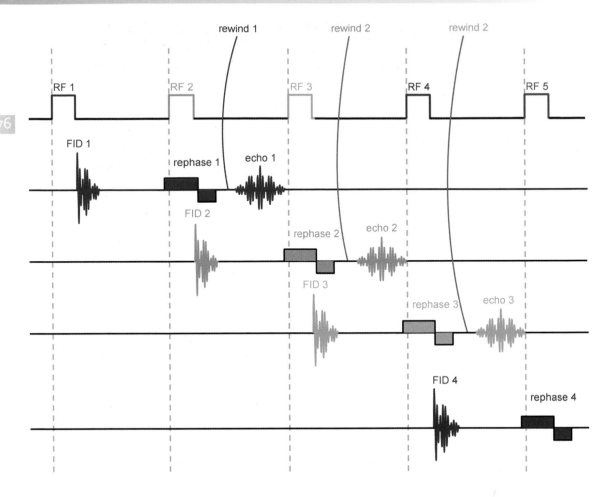

Figure 5.31 The SSFP sequence. Note how a rewinder gradient repositions each spin echo so that it no longer occurs at the same time as an excitation pulse but just before it. It can therefore be sampled on its own and the effects of the FID are eliminated.

$$\text{effective TE} = (2 \times 50) - 10 = 90 \, \text{ms}.$$

This means that spins within the echo have had 90 ms to dephase between their excitation pulse and the regeneration of the echo. T2 weighting results.

Rephasing has been initiated by an RF pulse rather than a gradient so that more T2 information is present. The rewinder gradient merely repositions the stimulated echo at a time when it can be received.

Uses

SSFP sequences were used to acquire images that demonstrate true T2 weighting (Figure 5.32). They were especially useful in the brain and joints with both 2D and 3D volumetric acquisitions.

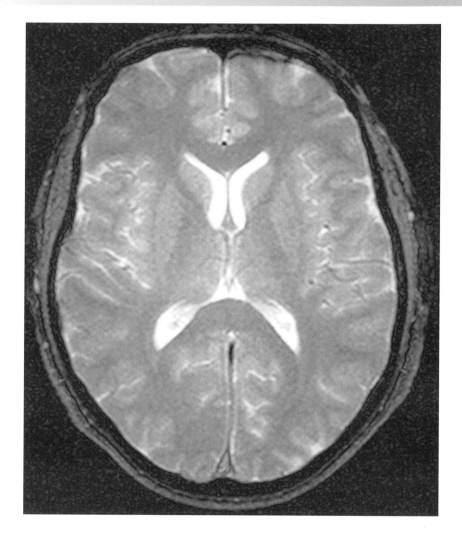

Figure 5.32   Axial SSFP image through the brain.

FSE has now largely replaced this sequence as it produces better T2 weighting in short scan times. However, the process of shifting the stimulated echo is used in sequences where rapid data acquisition and long TEs are required. An example of this is in perfusion imaging (*see* Chapter 12).

Learning point: T2* vs true T2

It is important to understand the difference between the terms true T2 and T2*. This is best demonstrated in imaging of the cervical spine. If the suspected pathology is a herniated disc, then using a T2* gradient echo sequence such as coherent gradient echo is appropriate. The disc will be demonstrated as low signal intensity disc bulge into a high signal intensity CSF-filled thecal sac and will produce a change in morphology (Figure 5.33). If, however, the pathology is more subtle, for example a small MS plaque within the cord, then we need to use a true T2 weighted sequence where the contrast seen depends on differences between the T2 times of the pathology and surrounding cord (Figure 5.34). In these circumstances it is better to use spin echo type sequences such as CSE, FSE or SSFP that use TEs long enough to measure the T2 decay times of tissues present.

Parameters

To maintain the steady state:

- flip angle   30–45°
- TR   20–50 ms.

The actual TE affects the effective TE. The longer the actual TE, the lower the effective TE. Actual TE should therefore be as short as possible.

- Average scan time – seconds for slice-by-slice acquisitions to several minutes for volumes. Some manufacturers suggest decreasing the effective TE to reduce magnetic susceptibility, and increasing the flip angle to create more transverse magnetization, which results in higher SNR.

Advantages

- can be acquired in a volume and in 2D
- truer T2 weighting achieved than in conventional GE

Disadvantages

- susceptible to artefacts
- image quality can be poor
- loud gradient noise

Learning point: differentiating common steady state sequences

As previously explained, the steady state produces two signals:

- a *FID* made up of transverse magnetization that has just been created
- a *stimulated echo* made up of the residual transverse magnetization component.

Coherent gradient echo, incoherent gradient echo and SSFP pulse sequences can be differentiated according to whether they use one or both of these signals.

- Coherent gradient echo samples both the FID and the stimulated echo to produce either T1 or T2* weighted images depending on the TE used (Figure 5.35).
- Incoherent pulse sequences samples the FID only to produces mainly T1 weighted images (Figure 5.36).
- SSFP samples the stimulated echo only to produce images that are more T2 weighted (Figure 5.37).

Balanced gradient echo

Mechanism

This sequence is a modification of the coherent gradient echo sequence that uses a balanced gradient system to correct for phase errors in flowing blood and CSF, and an alternating RF excitation scheme to enhance steady state effects. In addition, both the FID and the spin echo are collected within a single readout. This results in images where fat and water produce a higher signal, greater SNR and fewer flow artefacts than coherent gradient echo in shorter scan times.

The balanced gradient system is shown in Figure 5.38. As the area of the gradient under the line equals that above the line, moving spins accumulate a zero phase change as they pass along the gradients. As a result, spins in blood and CSF are coherent and have a high signal intensity. This gradient formation is the same as flow compensation or gradient moment rephasing (*see* Chapter 6). In balanced gradient echo this gradient is applied in the slice and frequency axes.

In addition, higher flip angles and shorter TRs are used than in coherent gradient echo, producing a higher SNR and shorter scan times. Normally this combination of flip angle and TR would result in saturation and therefore enhanced T1 contrast. However, saturation is avoided by changing the phase of the excitation pulse every TR. This is achieved by selecting a flip angle of 90°, for example, but in the first TR period only applying half of this, i.e. 45°. In successive TRs the full flip angle is applied but with alternating polarity so that the resultant transverse magnetization is created at a different phase every TR (i.e. 180° apart) (Figure 5.39). In this way, saturation is avoided and fat and water, which have T1/T2 values approaching parity, return much higher signal than tissues that do not. The resultant images display high SNR, good CNR between fat, water and surrounding tissues, fewer flow voids and in very short scan times.

Uses

Balanced gradient echo was developed initially for imaging the heart and great vessels but is now also used in spinal imaging, especially the cervical spine and internal auditory meatus as CSF flow is reduced. It is also sometimes used in joint and abdominal imaging (Figures 5.40 and 5.41).

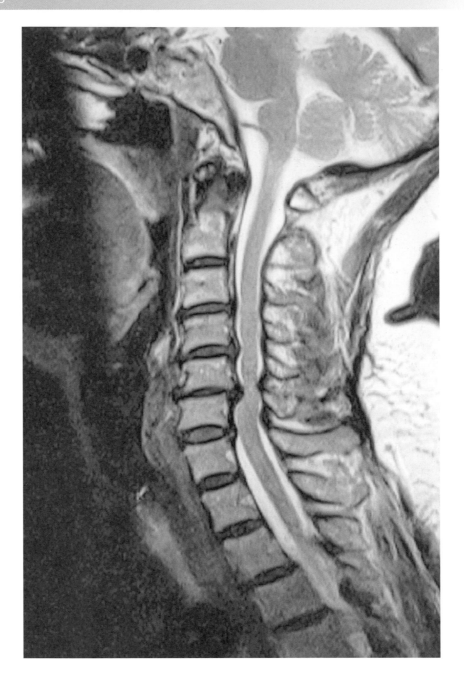

Figure 5.33   Sagittal T2* weighted coherent gradient echo sequence through the cervical cord. The prolapsed discs are well seen as they indent the thecal sac.

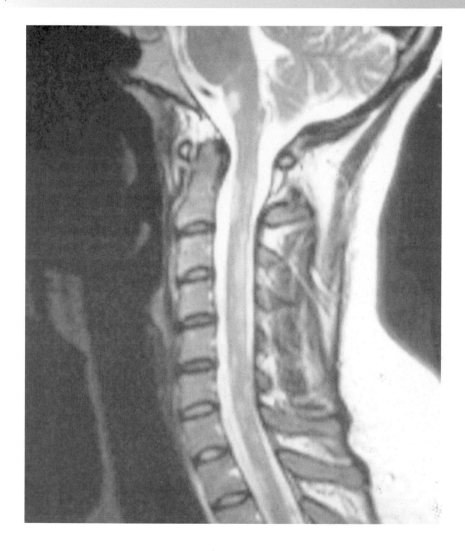

Figure 5.34   Sagittal T2 weighted FSE sequence through the cervical spine showing MS plaques within the cord. It is possible that these may have been missed in a T2* weighted sequence where the TE is not long enough to measure the T2 decay times of the pathology and the surrounding cord.

Parameters

- large flip angle   90° (enhances SNR)
- short TR   10 ms (reduces scan time and flow artefact)
- long TE   15 ms (to enhance T2*)

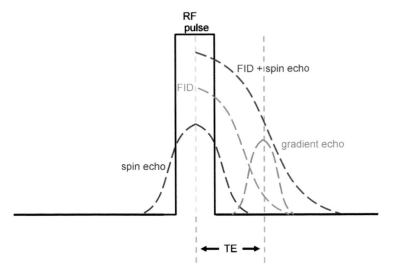

Figure 5.35 Echo formation in coherent gradient echo.

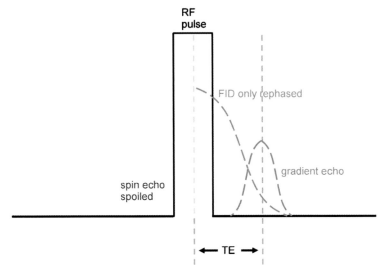

Figure 5.36 Echo formation in incoherent gradient echo.

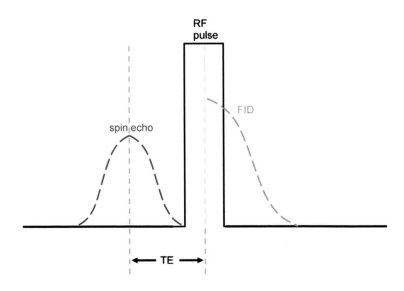

Figure 5.37 Echo formation in SSFP.

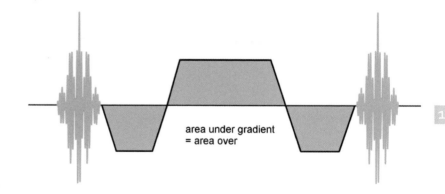

Figure 5.38   Balanced gradient system in balanced gradient echo.

area under gradient = area over

183

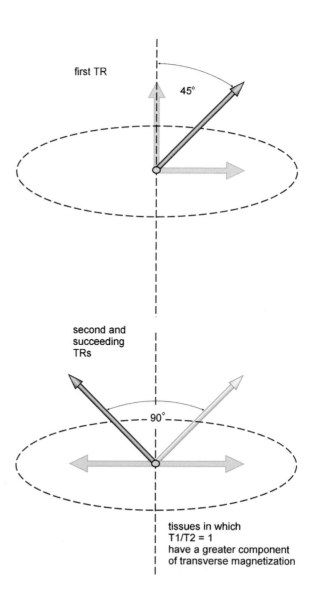

first TR

45°

second and succeeding TRs

90°

tissues in which T1/T2 = 1 have a greater component of transverse magnetization

Figure 5.39   Maintenance of the steady state in balanced gradient echo.

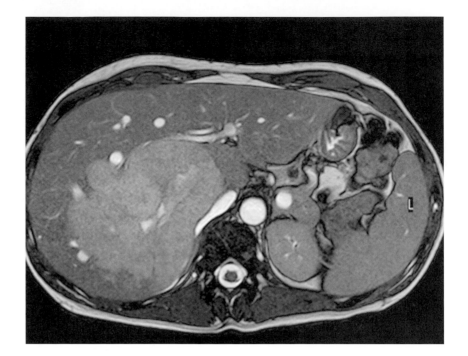

Figure 5.40 Axial balanced gradient echo image through the abdomen.

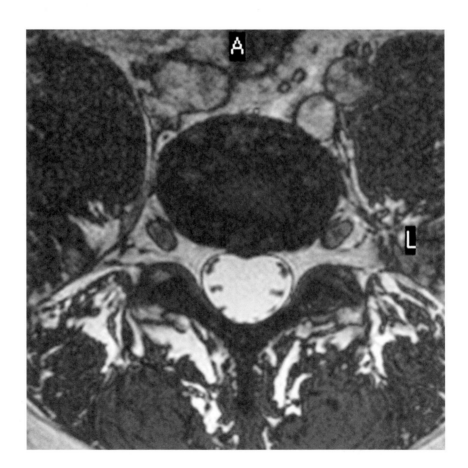

Figure 5.41 Axial balanced gradient echo image through the lumbar spine.

Fast gradient echo

Very fast pulse sequences have been developed that can acquire a volume in a single breath hold. These usually employ coherent or incoherent gradient echo sequences but the TE is significantly reduced. This is achieved by applying only a portion of the RF excitation pulse, so that it takes much less time to apply and switch off. Only a proportion of the echo is read (partial echo). These measures ensure that the TE is kept to a minimum, so that the TR and therefore the scan time can be reduced accordingly. In addition, many fast sequences use extra pulses, applied before the pulse sequence begins, to pre-magnetize the tissue. In this way, certain contrast can be obtained. This pre-magnetization is achieved in the following two ways.

- A 180° pulse is applied before the pulse sequence begins. This inverts the NMV into full satu- ration, and at a specified delay time the pulse sequence itself begins. This can be used to enhance T1 contrast or to null signal from certain organs and tissues, and is similar to inver- sion recovery.
- A 90°/180°/90° combination is applied before the pulse sequence begins. The first 90° pulse produces transverse magnetization. The 180° pulse rephases this, and at a specified time later the second 90° pulse is applied. This drives the coherent transverse magnetization into the longitudinal plane, so that it is available to be flipped when the pulse sequence begins. This is used to produce T2 contrast and is sometimes known as **driven equilibrium** (*see* also DRIVE which uses a similar principle).

Fast gradient systems permit multi-slice gradient echo sequences with TEs as short as 0.7 ms. Multiple images can therefore be acquired in a single breath hold and are free from respira- tory motion artefacts. In addition, fast gradient echo acquisitions are useful when temporal reso- lution is required. This is especially important after the administration of contrast when the selection of fast gradient echo permits dynamic imaging of an enhancing lesion (*see* Chapter 8). This important technique has applications in many areas, including the abdominal viscera and the breast.

K space filling in fast gradient echo sequences

To scan rapidly, it is usually necessary to fill K space in a different way to normal acquisitions. There are several permutations, most of which enhance signal and contrast and achieve rapid scan times.

Centric K space filling

This fills K space linearly (line by line), but instead of starting at an outer edge and working either upwards or downwards, fills the central lines first. This is achieved by applying all the shallowest phase encoding gradients first, leaving the steep ones until the end of the pulse sequence. In this way, signal and contrast are maximized as the central lines are filled when echoes have their highest amplitude, as they have not yet decayed. This type of K space filling is important when using fast gradient echo techniques in which SNR and contrast is compromised (Figure 5.42).

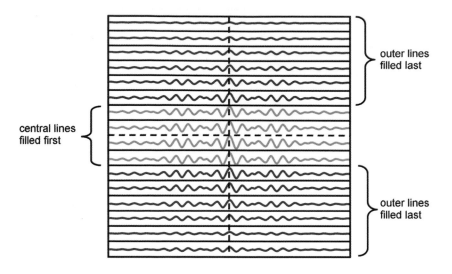

Figure 5.42   Centric K space filling.

Keyhole filling

This fills K space linearly and similarly to centric K space filling except that the central lines are only filled during a certain part of the sequence. This type of filling is used mainly in contrast enhanced angiography where we need to have a high temporal resolution for data acquired when gadolinium is present in the imaging volume (*see* Chapter 8). Before gadolinium arrives in the imaging volume, the system fills the outer resolution lines of K space. When gadolinium is in the imaging volume only a percentage of the central lines are filled. This means that acquisition times are short in this part of the sequence. At the end of the scan, the system 'stitches' the outer and central lines together to produce an image that has resolution and contrast. The contrast portion is acquired only when the gadolinium is present (Figure 5.43).

In addition to the main sequences discussed here, each manufacturer has their own modifications of the steady state sequences. These modifications include adding algorithms to correct for artefacts and altering how data from the FID and stimulated echoes are acquired. They result in mainly T2 or T2* weighted imaging, but have unique contrast and artefact characteristics. We advise you to consult manufacturers information for details about these sequences.

Single shot imaging techniques

As shown in fast spin echo, the scan time is significantly reduced by filling more than one line of K space at once. Taking this concept to the limits, the fastest scan time possible would be one where all the lines are filled during one repetition. This is termed **single shot (SS)** imaging and this method collects all the data required to fill all the lines of K space from a single echo train. The echo train may consist of spin echoes (generated by a train of 180° RF pulses) termed single shot fast/turbo spin echo (SS–FSE or SS–TSE) or a train of gradient echoes termed **echo planar imaging (EPI)**. To achieve this, multiple echoes are generated and each is phase encoded by a different slope of gradient to fill all the required lines of K space in a single TR period. For example, if a phase matrix of 128 is required then an echo train of 128 echoes is produced and individually

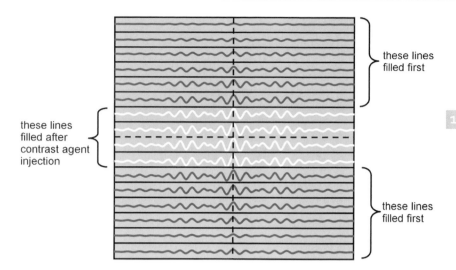

these lines
filled after
contrast agent
injection

these lines
filled first

these lines
filled first

Figure 5.43   Keyhole
imaging.

187

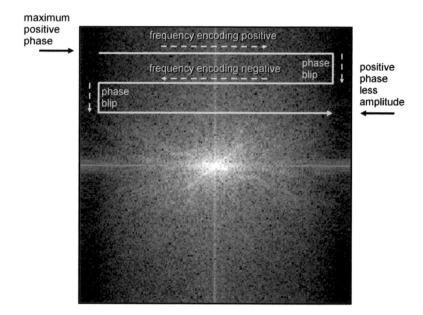

maximum
positive
phase

frequency encoding positive

frequency encoding negative

phase
blip

phase
blip

positive
phase
less
amplitude

Figure 5.44   K space
filling in EPI.

phase encoded to fill 128 lines of K space in a single TR period. To fill all K space in one repetition, the readout and phase encode gradients must rapidly switch on and off and change direction (*see* Chapter 3).

The readout gradient must switch from positive to negative; positively to fill a line of K space from left to right and negatively to fill a line from right to left. This rapid change in gradient polarity also rephases the FID produced after the excitation pulse to generate the gradient echoes used in EPI. As the readout gradient switches its polarity so rapidly it is said to oscillate.

The phase gradient also has to switch on and off rapidly but its polarity does not need to change in this type of K space traversal. Look at Figure 5.44. The first application of the phase gradient is maximum positive to fill the top line. The next application (to encode the next echo in the echo

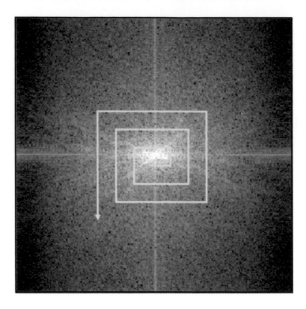

Figure 5.45   Spiral K space filling.

train) is still positive but its amplitude is slightly less so that the next line down is filled. This process is repeated until the center of K space is reached when the phase gradient switches negatively to fill the bottom lines. The amplitude is gradually increased until maximum negative polarity is achieved, filling the bottom line of K space. This type of gradient switching is called **blipping** (Figure 5.44). This type of single shot imaging is the simplest form in that although all lines are filled in one TR, lines are filled linearly.

Spiral K space filling

A more complex type of K space traversal is shown in Figure 5.45. In this example both the readout and the phase gradient switch their polarity rapidly and oscillate. In this spiral form of K space traversal, the readout gradient oscillates to fill lines from left to right and then right to left, and K space filling begins at the center; the phase gradient must also oscillate to fill a line in the top half followed by a line in the bottom half. To understand this more clearly, place a pen at the center of K space on the diagram and work out the amplitude and polarity of each gradient as you move your pen along. In this example, the pen is never removed from the paper, indicating that there is no TR; all K space is filled in one go. Other modifications of spiral or radial K space filling ensure rapid filling of K space with enhanced filling of the central lines. These currently include:

- *elliptical K space filling*, where the central ellipse portion of K space is acquired as a volume acquisition during a contrast enhanced MR angiogram. As the central portion of K space is filled, the volume, acquired in a relatively long scan time, can show arterial flow only. Venous flow is suppressed
- *propeller K space filling*, where lines are acquired as a block, thereby reducing the scan time, but the blocks are rotated about the central axis of K space. In this way the central portion

of K space is acquired every TR and therefore the SNR and CNR are increased. In addition, because the central portion of K space is sampled every TR, this is equivalent to using multiple NEX and results in a reduction in motion artefact due to motion averaging (*see* Chapter 4).

As all the echoes must be encoded before the transverse magnetization has decayed to zero, images contain a significant amount of T2* decay and SNR is relatively poor. To compensate for this, K space may be acquired in segments. This is called multi-shot where data are acquired in several TR passes. In multi-shot EPI the effective time between echoes is dramatically reduced. As chemical shift, distortion and blurring are all proportional to echo spacing, artefacts in multi-shot are reduced relative to single shot. There are two multi-shot methods.

- *K space segmentation by acquisition* acquires a section of K space at a time (e.g. four quarters) so that there are four excitations and TR periods. If a 128 phase matrix is required then 32 lines, repeated four times, fills K space.
- *K space segmentation by echo* uses a turbo factor that is repeated several times (e.g. turbo factor of 4 repeated 32 times). Data from the first echoes are placed in the top quarter of K space, data from the second echoes in the next quarter, and so on.

Both methods increase the scan time compared to single shot imaging methods but produce images with improved quality.

Single shot sequences place exceptional strains on the gradients and therefore gradient modifications are required at significant cost. The slew rates of the gradients must be about four times that of conventional gradients (*see* Chapter 9). Two types of gradient power supply modifications can be used.

- *Resonant power supplies* allow the readout and phase gradients to oscillate at the same frequency, reducing gradient requirements. The disadvantage is that they are only able to operate at a fixed frequency and amplitude. In practical terms this means that the gradients could only be used for EPI sequences so that the system would require two power supplies: one for EPI and one for conventional imaging.
- *Non-resonant power supplies* produce any gradient waveform so that both EPI and conventional sequences may be run off the same supply. This significantly reduces the cost but also the specifications of the gradients as they have to be able to cope with both types of sequence.

EPI contrast and parameters

In EPI, gradient echoes are typically generated by oscillation of the readout gradient. However, different contrasts are achieved by either beginning the sequence variable RF excitation pulse termed **gradient echo EPI (GE–EPI)** or with 90° and 180° RF pulses termed **spin echo EPI (SE–EPI)**. GE–EPI begins with an excitation pulse of any flip angle and is followed by EPI readout of gradient echoes (Figure 5.46). In this scenario, images are acquired in one TR pass in milliseconds.

In SE–EPI the sequence begins with a 90° excitation pulse followed by a 180° rephasing pulse followed by an EPI readout of gradient echoes (Figure 5.47). The application of the refocusing pulse helps to clean up some of the artefacts caused by magnetic field inhomogeneities and chemical shift. SE–EPI has longer scan times but generally better image quality than GE–EPI, but the extra RF pulses increase RF deposition to the patient. EPI sequences may be preceded

189

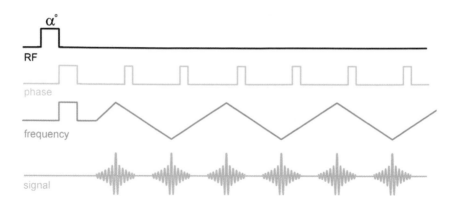

Figure 5.46   GE–EPI sequence.

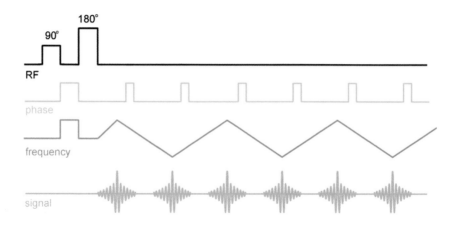

Figure 5.47   SE–EPI sequence.

with any type of RF pulse. An example is EPI–FLAIR (180°/90°/180° followed by EPI readout) where CSF is nulled but the sequence is significantly faster than in conventional FLAIR sequencing (Figure 5.49)

In all single shot techniques, because all K space is filled at once the recovery rates of individual tissues are not critical. For this reason the TR is said to equal infinity (because it is infinitely long). Either proton density or T2 weighting is achieved by selecting either a short or long effective TE, which corresponds to the time interval between the excitation pulse and when the center of K space is filled. T1 weighting is possible by applying an inverting pulse before the excitation pulse to produce saturation.

Hybrid sequences, which combine gradient and spin echoes, such as **GRASE (gradient and spin echo)** are an effective compromise. Typically, a series of gradient rephasings are followed by an RF rephasing pulse (Figure 5.48). The hybrid sequence uses the benefits of both types of rephasing methods: the speed of the gradient and the ability of the RF pulse to compensate for T2* effects.

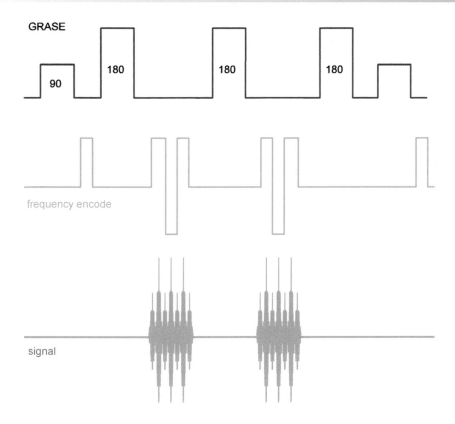

Figure 5.48   GRASE sequence.

These sequences increase the scan time to more than 100 ms per image but the benefits in terms of image quality are significant.

Uses and limitations

Some typical EPI and GRASE images are shown in Figures 5.49, 5.50 and 5.51, and in Chapter 12. EPI and single shot techniques have increased the use of functional MRI (*see* Chapter 12). Scanning rapidly enables freezing of physiological motion, which is advantageous when imaging the heart and coronary vessels (*see* Chapter 8) and when performing interventional techniques (*see* Chapter 12). Rapid imaging also enables visualization of physiology such as perfusion and blood oxygenation (*see* Chapter 12). Concerns over safety have, however, been expressed. The rapid switching of gradients causes nerve stimulation and gradient noise is severe, so acoustic insulation and ear protection are essential. In addition, many artefacts are seen in EPI including distortion and chemical shift.

As each echo is acquired rapidly, chemical shift in the frequency direction is relatively small. However, there is a larger chemical shift along the phase axis. This phase directional chemical shift artefact does not appear in standard spin or gradient echo acquisitions since echoes with different phase encodes are acquired at exactly the same time after excitation. In single shot imaging,

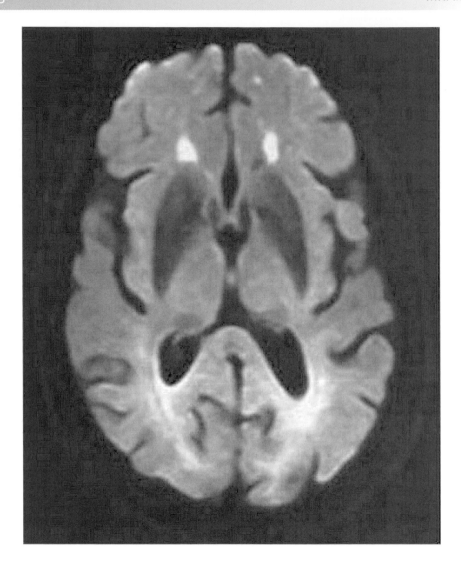

Figure 5.49   Axial EPI–FLAIR sequence through the brain. Note how the CSF signal is nulled.

however, the length of time required to perform a train of phase encodes means that phase encodes are applied at different times after excitation. This results in chemical shifts for fat of typically 10–20 pixels compared with the 1–2 pixel misregistration in spin echo imaging.

Other artefacts seen in single shot imaging include blurring and ghosting. Blurring occurs as the result of T2* decay during the course of the acquisition. If the train of echoes takes a similar time to decay, the signal from the end of the acquisition is reduced, resulting in a loss of resolution and blurring. In EPI acquisitions, half FOV ghosts occur as the result of small errors in the timing and shape of readout gradients. This causes differences between echoes acquired with positive and negative readout gradients. These errors cause a ghost of the real image that appears shifted in the phase direction by one half of the FOV. Since it is difficult to eliminate these errors, a cor-

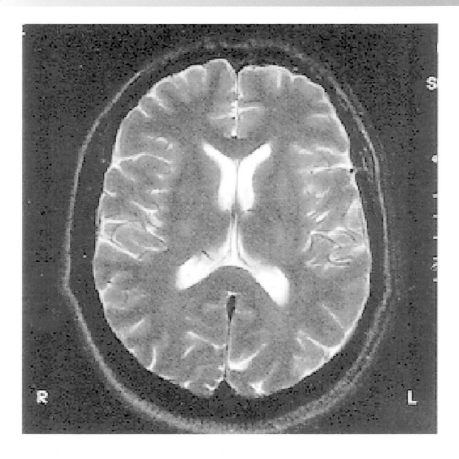

Figure 5.50   Axial GRASE image through the brain.

rection is usually performed during image reconstruction using information acquired during the reference scan. Despite these problems these sequences have a significant place in clinical MRI.

PARALLEL IMAGING TECHNIQUES

Parallel imaging or sensitivity encoding is a technique that fills K space more efficiently than conventional imaging by filling multiple lines of K space per TR (as in FSE). Unlike FSE, however, these lines are acquired by assigning them to certain coils that are coupled together to enable them to acquire data simultaneously. Therefore we need to have coils specifically designed for this purpose and software to link them electronically. Typically two, four, six or eight coils are used and arranged around the area to be imaged, although coils are also constructed with multiple coils or channels built in. The number of coils or channels may exceed 32. In this example let us assume a four-coil configuration (Figure 5.52):

- coil 1 acquires line 1 and every fourth line thereafter
- coil 2 acquires line 2 and every fourth line thereafter
- coil 3 acquires line 3 and every fourth line thereafter
- coil 4 acquires line 4 and every fourth line thereafter.

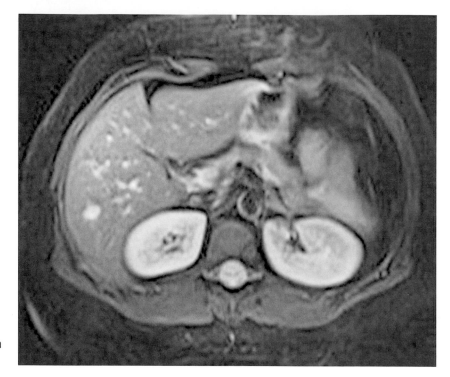

Figure 5.51 Axial
SE–EPI image through
the abdomen.

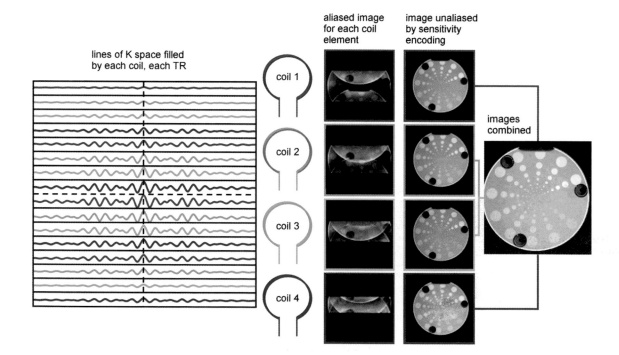

Figure 5.52 Parallel imaging.

Hence every TR, four lines of K space are acquired. In the first TR period:

- coil 1 acquires line 1
- coil 2 acquires line 2
- coil 3 acquires line 3
- coil 4 acquires line 4.

In TR period 2:

- coil 1 acquires line 5
- coil 3 acquires line 6
- coil 3 acquires line 7
- coil 4 acquires line 8, and so on.

The process is repeated until all the lines are filled. As four lines are acquired per TR, the scan time is decreased by a factor of 4. This is sometimes called the **reduction** or **acceleration factor** and is similar to the turbo factor in FSE. The reduction factor equals the number of coils or channels in the configuration. The coil configuration can also be used to increase the resolution, e.g. achieve a phase matrix of 512 in the time of a 128 or a combination of both scan time reduction and improved resolution. For example two coils or channels are used to halve the scan time and two are used to double the phase resolution.

Now let's look at the lines acquired by each coil. You can see from Figure 5.52 that each coil has acquired every fourth line and that as a result the gap between each line is four times greater than if K space had been filled normally. Using the chest of drawers analogy in Chapter 3, this means that the depth of each drawer has quadrupled and, as this dimension is inversely proportional to the size of the FOV in the phase direction, the size of the FOV in the phase direction is reduced to a quarter of its original size as in rectangular FOV (*see* Chapter 4). As a result, aliasing of tissue outside the FOV in the phase direction occurs and therefore each coil produces a wrapped image (*see* Chapter 7). To rectify this, the system uses the sensitivity profile of each coil to calculate where signal is coming from relative to the coil so that it can map it correctly onto the image. This profile determines the position of signal relative to the coil based on its amplitude. Signal coming from near to the coil has a higher amplitude than that furthest away. As a result of this process, the image is unwrapped, and using algorithms,the unwrapped data from each coil are combined to produce a single image (*see* Figure 9.21).

Uses

Parallel imaging is an important development and can be used to either reduce scan times or improve resolution. It can be used with most pulse sequences with the appropriate software and coil configurations. Although it has obvious benefits in terms of scan time and/or resolution, it results in a slight loss of SNR. In addition, chemical shift may increase due to different resonant frequencies being mapped across each coil. Patient movement also causes misalignment between under-sampled data and reference scans.

The choice of each pulse sequence is often a quite difficult one. There are now so many that we are really spoilt for choice. However, generally speaking every pulse sequence is designed to produce a certain contrast, image quality and data acquisition. These factors should be taken into account when selecting a particular pulse sequence. Table 5.2 should help most readers apply the terms used in this and other chapters to their type of system. Table 5.3 compares the various rapid imaging techniques.

Table 5.2   A comparison of acronyms used by manufacturers.

	GE	Philips	Siemens
Spin echo	SE	SE	SE
Fast spin echo	FSE	TSE	TSE
Inversion recovery	IR	IR	IR
Short tau inversion recovery	STIR	STIR	STIR
Fluid attenuated inversion recovery	FLAIR	FLAIR	FLAIR
Coherent gradient echo	GRASS	FFE	FISP
Incoherent gradient echo	SPGR	T1FFE	FLASH
Balanced gradient echo	FIESTA	BFFE	True FISP
Steady state free precession	SSFP	T2 FFE	PSIF
Fast gradient echo	Fast GRASS/SPGR	TFE	Turbo FLASH
Echo planar	EPI	EPI	EPI
Parallel imaging	ASSET	SENSE	iPAT
Spatial pre-saturation	SAT	REST	SAT
Gradient moment rephasing	Flow comp	Flow comp	GMR
Signal averaging	NEX	NSA	AC
Anti-aliasing	No phase wrap	Foldover suppression	Oversampling
Rectangular FOV	Rect FOV	Rect FOV	Half Fourier imaging
Respiratory compensation	Resp comp	PEAR	Resp trigger
Driven equilibrium	FR-FSE	DRIVE	RESTORE

Abbreviations used in Table 5.2

AC	number of acquisitions	iPAT	integrated parallel acquisition technique
ASSET	array spatial and sensitivity encoding technique	MP RAGE	magnetization prepared rapid gradient echo
		NEX	number of excitations
DRIVE	driven equilibrium	NSA	number of signal averages
FFE	fast field echo	PEAR	phase encoding artefact reduction
FIESTA	free induction echo stimulated acquisition	PSIF	mirrored FISP
FISP	free induction steady precession	REST	regional saturation technique
FLAIR	fluid attenuated inversion recovery	RESTORE	restore turbo spin echo
FLASH	fast low angled shot	SENSE	sensitivity encoding
Flow comp	flow compensation	SPGR	spoiled GRASS
FR-FSE	fast recovery fast spin echo	SSFP	steady state free precession
FSE	fast spin echo	STIR	short tau inversion recovery
GMR	gradient moment rephasing	TFE	turbo field echo
GRASS	gradient recalled acquisition in the steady state	TSE	turbo spin echo
		Turbo FLASH	magnetization prepared sub second imaging

Table 5.3 Single and multi-shot methods.

	Sequence	Readout	Time
FSE	90/180	multiple SE	min/sec
GRASE	90/180	GE	min/sec
SE-EPI	90/180	GE	sec/sub sec
GE-EPI	variable flip	GE	sec/sub sec
IR-EPI	180/90/180	GE	sec/sub sec

 For questions and answers on this topic please visit the supporting companion website for this book: www.wiley.com/go/ mriinpractice

6

Flow phenomena

Introduction

This chapter specifically explores artefacts produced from nuclei that move during the acquisition of data. Flowing nuclei exhibit different contrast characteristics from their neighboring stationary nuclei, and originate primarily from nuclei in blood and CSF. The motion of flowing nuclei causes mismapping of signals and results in artefacts known as phase ghosting. The causes of flow artefact are collectively known as **flow phenomena**. The principal phenomena are:

- time of flight
- entry slice phenomenon
- intra-voxel dephasing.

First, however, the common mechanisms and types of flow are analyzed.

THE MECHANISMS OF FLOW

There are four principal types of flow (Figure 6.1).

- Laminar flow is flow that is at different but consistent velocities across a vessel. The flow at the center of the lumen of the vessel is faster than at the vessel wall, where resistance slows down the flow. However, the velocity difference across the vessel is constant.

MRI in Practice, Fourth Edition. Catherine Westbrook, Carolyn Kaut Roth, John Talbot.
© 2011 Blackwell Publishing Ltd. Published 2011 by Blackwell Publishing Ltd.

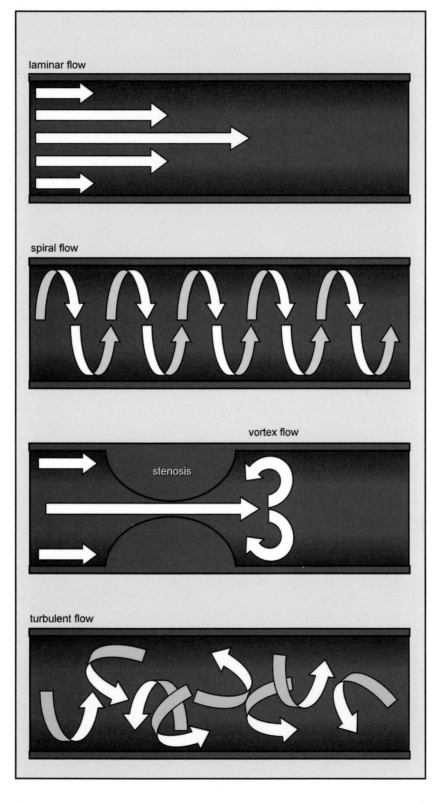

Figure 6.1 The different types of flow.

- Spiral flow is where the direction of flow is spiral.
- Vortex flow is flow that is initially laminar but then passes through a stricture or stenosis in the vessel. Flow in the center of the lumen has a high velocity but near the walls, the flow spirals.
- Turbulent flow is flow at different velocities that fluctuates randomly. The velocity difference across the vessel changes erratically.

200

Learning point: flow mechanisms

Flow mechanisms are often termed as follows:

- first order motion laminar flow (constant velocity)
- second order motion acceleration
- third order motion jerk.

Only first order flow can be compensated for as the system can only correct for flow that is at a constant velocity and direction during data acquisition.

FLOW PHENOMENA

Time of flight phenomenon

To produce a signal, a nucleus must receive an excitation pulse and a rephasing pulse. If a nucleus receives the excitation pulse only and is not rephased, it does not produce a signal. Similarly, if a nucleus is rephased but has not previously been excited, it does not produce a signal. Stationary nuclei always receive both excitation and rephasing pulses, but flowing nuclei present in the slice for the excitation may have exited the slice before rephasing. This is called **time of flight phenomenon** (Figure 6.2). The effects of the time of flight phenomenon depend on the type of pulse sequence used.

 Refer to animation 6.1 on the supporting companion website for this book: www.wiley.com/go/mriinpractice

Time of flight in spin echo pulse sequences

In a spin echo pulse sequence, a 90° excitation pulse and a 180° rephasing pulse are applied to each slice. Every slice is therefore selectively excited and rephased. Stationary nuclei within the slice receive both the 90° and the 180° RF pulses and produce a signal.

Nuclei flowing perpendicular to the slices may be present within the slice during the 90° pulse, but may have exited the slice before the 180° pulse can be delivered. These nuclei are excited but

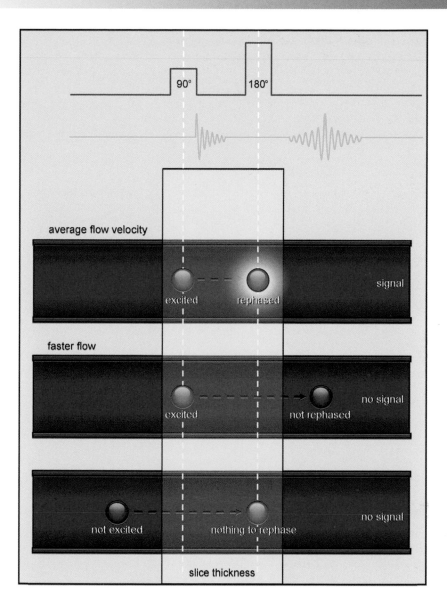

Figure 6.2   The time of flight phenomenon.

not rephased and do not therefore give a signal. Alternatively, nuclei not present in the slice during excitation may be present during rephasing. These nuclei have not previously been excited and do not therefore give a signal. Time of flight phenomena result in a signal void from the nuclei; and so the vessel appears dark. Time of flight effects depend on the following.

- *Velocity of flow.* As the velocity of flow increases, a smaller proportion of flowing nuclei are present in the slice for both the 90° and the 180° RF pulses. As the velocity of flow increases,

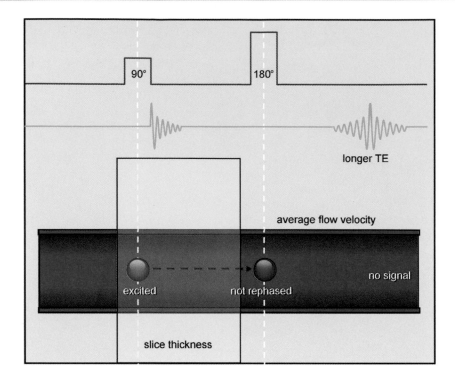

Figure 6.3 Time of flight vs TE.

the time of flight effect increases. This is called **high velocity signal loss**. As the velocity of flow decreases, a higher proportion of flowing nuclei are present in the slice for both the 90° and the 180° RF pulses. Therefore as the velocity of flow decreases, the time of flight effect decreases. This is called **flow-related enhancement.**

- *TE.* As the TE increases, a higher proportion of flowing nuclei have exited the slice between the excitation pulse and the 180° rephasing pulse. Therefore at a longer TE, more nuclei have received only one pulse and the signal void increases (Figure 6.3).
- *Slice thickness.* For a given constant velocity, nuclei take longer to travel through a thick slice compared with a thin slice. Therefore, nuclei are more likely to receive both the 90° and 180° pulse in thick slices. As the thickness of the slice decreases, the nuclei are more likely to receive only one pulse and the signal void increases.

Time of flight in gradient echo pulse sequences

In gradient echo pulse sequences, a variable excitation pulse is followed by gradient rephasing. Each slice is selectively excited by the RF pulse, but the rephasing gradient is applied to the whole body. In other words, the excitation pulse is slice selective, but the gradient rephasing is not. Therefore, a flowing nucleus that receives an excitation pulse is rephased regardless of its slice position and produces a signal. In addition, the very short TR usually associated with gradient echo sequences tends to saturate stationary nuclei, which receive repeated RF pulses so that flowing nuclei appear to have a higher signal. This is explored later. In gradient echo pulse sequences therefore, flow signal enhancement is increased and these pulse sequences are often said to be flow-sensitive.

Summary

- Time of flight phenomena produce flow related enhancement or high velocity signal loss
- Flow-related enhancement increases as the:
  - velocity of flow decreases
  - TE decreases
  - slice thickness increases
- High velocity signal void increases as the:
  - velocity of flow increases
  - TE increases
  - slice thickness decreases

Entry slice phenomenon

Entry slice phenomenon is related to the excitation history of the nuclei. Nuclei that receive repeated RF pulses during an acquisition with a short TR are said to be **saturated** because their magnetic moments are more likely to be orientated in the spin-down direction (*see* Chapter 1). This is because the TR is not long enough for longitudinal recovery of magnetization in the tissues in which the nuclei reside. Nuclei that have not received these repeated RF pulses are said to be **fresh**, as their magnetic moments are mainly orientated in the spin-up direction. The signal that they produce is different from that of the saturated nuclei (Figure 6.4).

Stationary nuclei within a slice become saturated after repeated RF pulses, especially when the TR is short. Nuclei flowing perpendicular to the slice enter the slice fresh, as they were not present during repeated excitations. They therefore produce a different signal from the stationary nuclei. This is called **entry slice phenomenon** or **inflow effect** as it is most prominent in the first slice of a 'stack' of slices.

The slices in the middle of the stack exhibit less entry slice phenomenon, as flowing nuclei have received more excitation pulses by the time they reach these slices. In other words, they become less fresh and more saturated and their signal intensity depends mostly on the TE, TR, flip angle and the contrast characteristics of the tissue in which they are situated.

Entry slice phenomenon only decreases if nuclei receive repeated excitations. The rate at which the nuclei receive the excitation pulses determines the magnitude of the phenomenon. Any factor that affects the rate at which a nucleus receives repeated excitations affects the magnitude of the phenomenon. The magnitude of entry slice phenomenon therefore depends on the following.

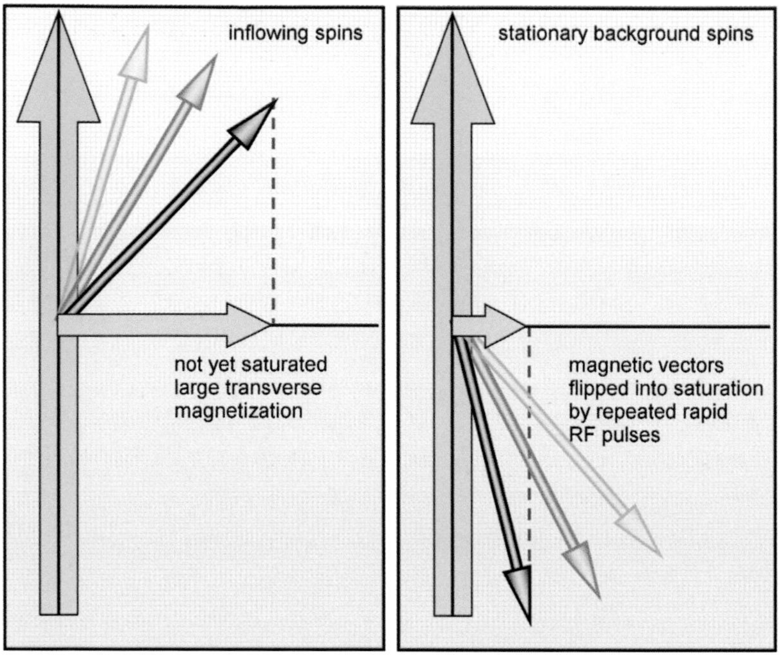

Figure 6.4   Contrast differences between saturated and fresh spins.

- *TR.* The TR is the time between each excitation pulse. A short TR results in an increase in the rate at which the RF is delivered. In other words, a short TR decreases the time between successive RF pulses. A short TR therefore reduces the magnitude of entry slice phenomenon.
- *Slice thickness.* Flowing nuclei with a constant velocity take longer to travel through thick slices than thin slices. Nuclei traveling through thick slices are likely to receive more RF pulses than nuclei traveling through thin slices. Entry slice phenomenon therefore decreases in thick slices compared with thin slices.
- *Velocity of flow.* The velocity of flow also affects the rate at which a flowing nucleus receives RF. Fast-flowing nuclei are more likely to have traveled to the next slice when RF is delivered than slow nuclei. Entry slice phenomenon is therefore decreased as the velocity of flow decreases.
- *Direction of flow.* The direction of flow is probably the most important factor in determining the magnitude of entry slice phenomenon. Flow that is in the same direction as slice selection is called **co-current.** Flow that is in the opposite direction to slice selection is called **counter-current** flow.
  - *Co-current flow.* Flowing nuclei travel in the same direction as slice selection. The flowing nuclei are more likely to receive repeated RF excitations as they move from one slice to the next. They therefore become saturated relatively quickly, and so entry slice phenomenon decreases rapidly.

Refer to animation 6.2 on the supporting companion website for this book: www.wiley.com/go/mriinpractice

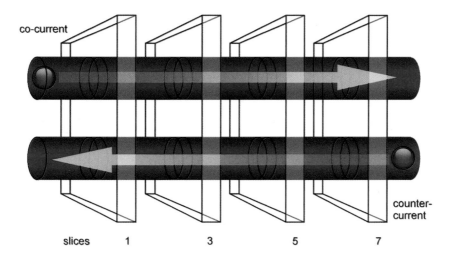

Figure 6.5   Co- and counter-current flow.

— *Counter-current flow.* Flowing nuclei travel in the opposite direction to slice excitation. Flowing nuclei stay fresh as when they enter a slice they are less likely to have received previous excitation pulses. Entry slice phenomenon does not therefore decrease rapidly and may still be present deep within the slice stack (Figure 6.5).

Learning point: entry slice phenomenon in clinical imaging

Look at Figures 6.6 to 6.9. These are four axial slices through the abdomen prescribed and excited from the most inferior position to the most superior position, i.e. Figure 6.6 is slice 1, Figure 6.7 is slice 2, Figure 6.8 is slice 3 and Figure 6.9 is slice 4 in the stack of slices. Slice 1 was acquired first; slice 4 last, in the acquisition.

Look at the signal intensity of the aorta and inferior vena cava (IVC) in these images. Although they both contain blood and should be the same signal intensity on all slices, it is clear that this is not the case. In slice 1 the IVC has high signal intensity and the aorta low signal intensity. In slice 4 the contrast is opposite, i.e. the IVC is dark and the aorta is bright. In addition the IVC is darker on slice 4 than the aorta is on slice 1.

These appearances are due to entry slice phenomena. In slice 1, nuclei in the IVC are fresh because they have traveled up from the legs and have received no previous RF pulses because they are not positioned in the stack of slices. Therefore in slice 1 these nuclei receive their first RF pulse and return a high signal as their magnetic moments are mainly in the spin-up direction and are not saturated. Nuclei in the aorta, however, are saturated and return a low signal because they have been excited by RF pulses as they have traveled down through the stack of slices during acquisition and their magnetic moments are primarily orientated in the spin-down direction.

In slice 4, the effect is opposite to that in slice 1. Nuclei in the aorta are now fresh as they have been traveling from the head and arms and received no previous RF pulses. Therefore in slice 4 these nuclei receive their first RF pulse and return a high signal as their magnetic moments are mainly orientated in the spin-up direction. Nuclei in the IVC, however, are saturated by repeated RF pulses as they travel through the stack during the acquisition and their magnetic moments are primarily orientated in the spin-down direction. In slices 2 and 3, however, this inflow effect decreases as nuclei in both vessels have received RF pulses.

The IVC is darker on slice 4 than the aorta is on slice 1 because flow in the IVC is co-current to slice excitation while flow in the aorta is counter-current. Therefore nuclei in the IVC receive more RF pulses because they are traveling in the same direction as slice excitation than nuclei in the aorta that are traveling in the opposite direction to slice excitation. This effect is rarely seen in clinical imaging because flow compensation techniques such as spatial pre-saturation eliminate it. This is discussed later.

Summary

Entry slice phenomenon increases:

- at the first slice in the stack
- when using a long TR
- in thin slices
- with fast flow
- in counter-current flow

Intra-voxel dephasing

Gradients alter the magnetic field strength, precessional frequency and phase of nuclei. Nuclei flowing along a gradient rapidly accelerate or decelerate depending on the direction of flow and gradient application. Flowing nuclei therefore either gain phase (if they have been accelerated) or lose phase (if they have been decelerated) (*see* watch analogy in Chapter 1).

If a flowing nucleus is adjacent to a stationary nucleus in a voxel, there is a phase difference between the two nuclei. This is because the flowing nucleus has either lost or gained phase relative to the stationary nucleus due to its motion along the gradient. Therefore nuclei within the same voxel are out of phase with each other, which results in a reduction of total signal amplitude from the voxel. This is called **intra-voxel dephasing** (Figure 6.10). The magnitude of intra-voxel dephasing depends on the degree of turbulence. In turbulent flow, intra-voxel dephasing effects are irreversible. In laminar flow, the intra-voxel dephasing can be compensated for as long as the velocity and direction of flow are constant.

Summary

- Flow affects image quality
- Time of flight effects give signal void or enhancement
- Entry slice phenomenon effects give a different signal intensity to flowing nuclei
- The signal intensity of the lumen is also affected by the mechanism of flow

FLOW PHENOMENA COMPENSATION

Introduction

Flowing nuclei therefore produce a very confusing range of signal intensities. Ideally, these should be compensated for, so that their adverse effects on image quality and interpretation can be minimized. There are several methods available to help reduce flow artefacts and these are now discussed. These techniques also reduce phase mismapping in pulsed flow such as blood and CSF. This is discussed in more detail in Chapter 7. The methods for reducing flow phenomena are:

- even echo rephasing
- gradient moment nulling
- spatial pre-saturation.

Even echo rephasing

If two or more echoes are produced in a spin echo pulse sequence, intra-voxel dephasing may be reduced by acquiring the second and succeeding even echoes at a multiple of the first TE; for example, two echoes, first TE 40 ms and second TE 80 ms. This works on the principle that flowing nuclei that are out of phase at the first echo are in phase at the second echo as long as the nuclei are given exactly the same amount of time to rephase as they were given to dephase. In other words, if at the first TE of 40 ms they are out of phase, 40 ms later (at 80 ms) they will be in phase again. This is called **even echo rephasing** and can be used to reduce artefact in a T2 weighted image.

Gradient moment rephasing (nulling)

Gradient moment rephasing compensates for the altered phase values of the nuclei flowing along a gradient. It uses additional gradients to correct the altered phases back to their original values

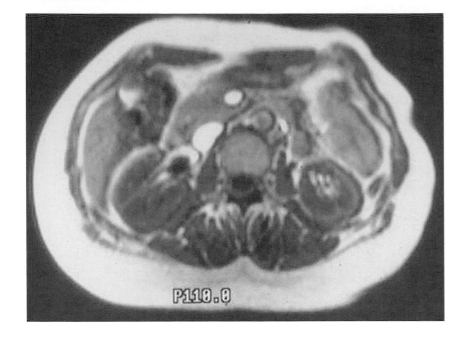

Figure 6.6 Axial T1 weighted image slice 1 (most inferior).

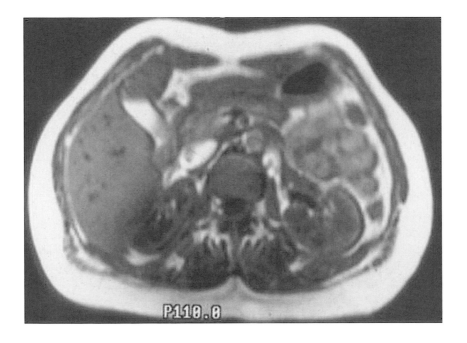

Figure 6.7 Axial T1 weighted image slice 2.

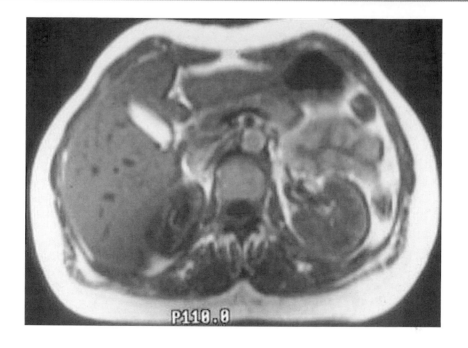

Figure 6.8   Axial T1 weighted image slice 3.

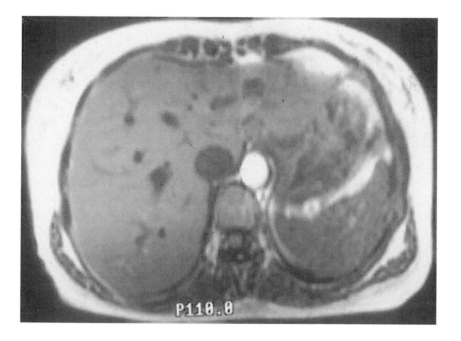

Figure 6.9   Axial T1 weighted image slice 4 (most superior).

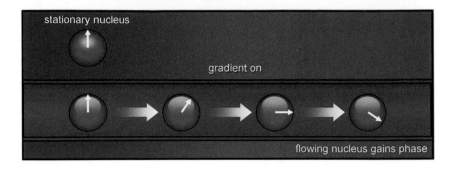

Figure 6.10   Intra-voxel dephasing.

and follows the same principles as the balanced gradient system used in balanced gradient echo sequences (*see* Chapter 5). Flowing nuclei do not gain or lose phase due to the presence of the main gradient.

Gradient moment rephasing is performed by the slice select gradient and/or the readout gradient. The gradient alters its polarity from positive to double negative and then back to positive again. A flowing nucleus traveling along these gradients experiences different magnetic field strengths, and its phase changes accordingly. This is shown in Figure 6.11, where a flowing spin gains 90° of phase as it passes along the first positive lobe of the gradient and then loses 180° of phase as it passes through the double negative lobe of the gradient. Its net phase change at this stage is that it has lost 90° of phase. As it then passes through the last positive lobe of the gradient this is corrected so that the net phase change is zero.

Gradient moment rephasing predominantly reduces intra-voxel dephasing. As the phase shifts of flowing nuclei are corrected, flow motion artefacts are reduced. In Figure 6.12 ghosting of the aorta is clearly seen. This is removed in Figure 6.13 where gradient moment rephasing has been applied.

Gradient moment rephasing assumes a constant velocity and direction across the gradients at all times. It is most effective on slow laminar flow and is therefore often termed **first order motion compensation**. Pulsatile flow is not strictly constant, so gradient moment rephasing is often more effective on venous rather than arterial flow. It is also less effective on turbulent fast flow perpendicular to the slice.

As gradient moment rephasing uses extra gradients, it increases the minimum TE. If the system has to perform extra gradient tasks, more time must elapse before it is ready to read an echo. As a result, fewer slices may be available for a given TR, or the TR and therefore the scan time may be automatically increased to scan the selected slices.

Spatial pre-saturation

Spatial pre-saturation pulses nullify the signal from flowing nuclei so that the effects of entry slice and time of flight phenomena are minimized. Spatial pre-saturation delivers a 90° RF pulse to a volume of tissue outside the FOV. A flowing nucleus within the volume receives this 90° pulse. When it then enters the slice stack, it receives an excitation pulse and is saturated. If it is fully

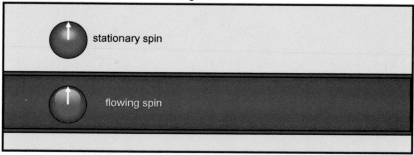

no gradient

stationary spin

flowing spin

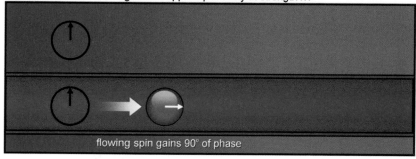

gradient applied positively at strength x1

flowing spin gains 90° of phase

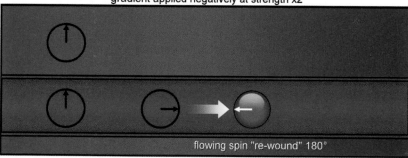

gradient applied negatively at strength x2

flowing spin "re-wound" 180°

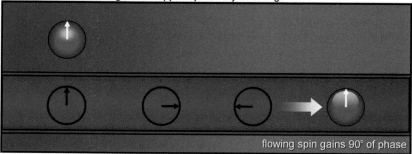

gradient applied positively at strength x1

flowing spin gains 90° of phase

211

Figure 6.11   Gradient moment rephasing (nulling).

Refer to animation 6.3 on the supporting companion website for this book: www.wiley.com/go/mriinpractice

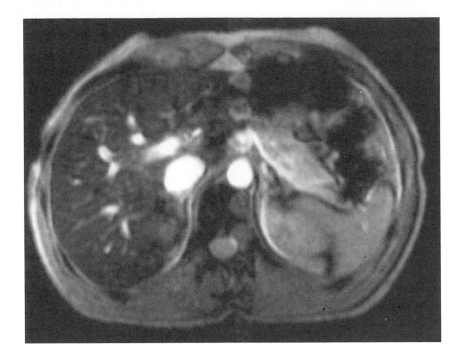

Figure 6.12 Axial T2* coherent gradient echo through the abdomen demonstrating flow artefact in the aorta. No gradient moment rephasing was used.

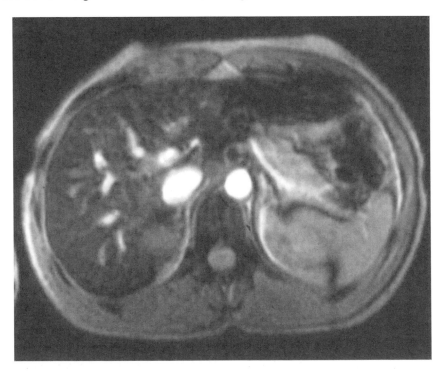

Figure 6.13 Axial T2* coherent gradient echo through the abdomen with gradient moment rephasing. The artefact has largely been largely eliminated.

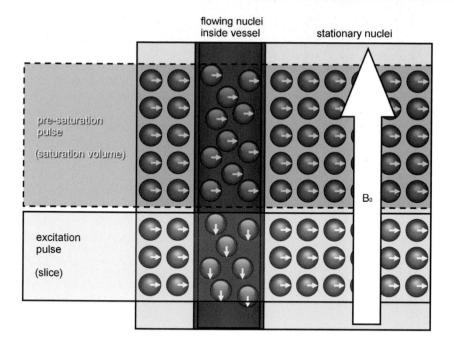

Figure 6.14   Spatial pre-saturation.

saturated to 180°, it has no transverse component of magnetization and produces a signal void (Figure 6.14).

To be effective, pre-saturation pulses should be placed between the flow and the imaging stack so that signal from flowing nuclei entering the FOV is nullified. In sagittal and axial imaging, pre-saturation pulses are usually placed above and below the FOV so that arterial flow from above and venous flow from below are saturated. Right and left pre-saturation pulses are sometimes useful in coronal imaging (especially in the chest), to saturate flow from the subclavian vessels.

Spatial pre-saturation pulses can be brought into the FOV itself. This permits artefact-producing areas (such as the aorta) to be pre-saturated so that phase mismapping can be reduced (*see* Chapter 7). Pre-saturation pulses are only useful if they are applied to tissue. If they are applied to air they are not effective. They increase the amount of RF that is delivered to the patient, which may increase heating effects (*see* Chapter 10). The use of pre-saturation pulses may also decrease the number of slices available and should therefore be used appropriately.

Pre-saturation pulses are also only effective if the flowing nucleus receives the 90° pre-saturation pulse. Pulses are applied around each slice just before the excitation pulse. The TR and the number of slices therefore govern the interval between the delivery of each pre-saturation pulse. To optimize pre-saturation, use all the slices permitted for a given TR. As pre-saturation produces a signal void, it is usually used in T1 and proton density weighted images where fluid (blood and CSF) is dark anyway. Figures 6.15 and 6.16 show axial T1 weighted gradient echo images of the abdomen with and without pre-saturation. Ghosting of the aorta seen on Figure 6.15 is largely eliminated by using spatial pre-saturation pulses in Figure 6.16. Note also that the signal intensity of the aorta is reduced by using pre-saturation.

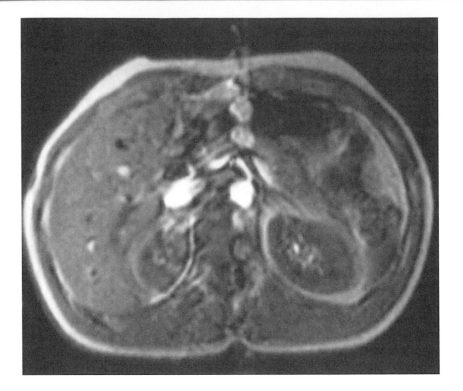

Figure 6.15   Axial T2* coherent gradient echo through the abdomen demonstrating flow artefact in the aorta. No spatial pre-saturation was used.

Pre-saturation nullifies signal and can therefore be used specifically to eliminate certain signals. The main uses of this are:

- chemical pre-saturation
- spatial inversion recovery (SPIR).

Chemical pre-saturation

Hydrogen exists in different chemical environments in the body, mainly fat and water (*see* Chapter 2). The precessional frequency of fat is slightly different from that of water. As the main magnetic field strength increases, this frequency difference also increases. For example at 1.5 T the precessional frequency between fat and water is approximately 220 Hz, so fat precesses 220 Hz lower than water. At 1.0 T this frequency difference is reduced to 147 Hz. The frequency difference between fat and water is called **chemical shift** and can be used to specifically null the signal from either fat or water. This technique is important to differentiate pathology (which is mainly water) and normal tissue (which often contains fat). To saturate or null either fat or water, the precessional difference between the two must be sufficiently large so that they can be isolated from each other. Fat or water saturation is therefore most effectively achieved on high field systems.

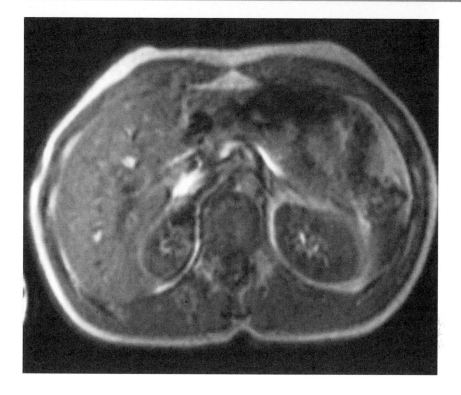

Figure 6.16 Axial T2* coherent gradient echo through the abdomen using spatial pre-saturation inferiorly and superiorly to the slice. The artefact has been largely eliminated and vessel signal has been nulled.

Fat saturation

To saturate fat signal, a 90° pre-saturation pulse must be applied at the precessional frequency of fat to the whole FOV (Figure 6.17). The excitation RF pulse is then applied to the slices and the magnetic moments of the fat nuclei are flipped into saturation. If they are flipped to 180°, they do not have a component of transverse magnetization and produce a signal void. The water nuclei, however, are excited, rephased and produce a signal. Figures 6.18 and 6.19 compare axial T2 weighted images of the parotid gland, with and without fat pre-saturation. Using fat saturation has increased the CNR between the lesion and normal tissue as fatty components in the base of the skull have been nulled.

Water saturation

To saturate water signal the pre-saturation pulse must be applied at the precessional frequency of water to the whole FOV (Figure 6.20). The RF excitation pulse is then applied to the slices, and the magnetic moments of nuclei in water are flipped into saturation. If they are flipped to 180° they do not have a transverse component of magnetization and produce a signal void. The fat

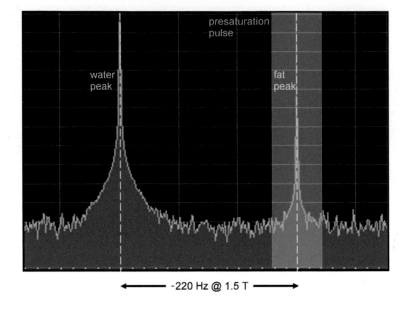

-220 Hz @ 1.5 T

Figure 6.17   Fat saturation.

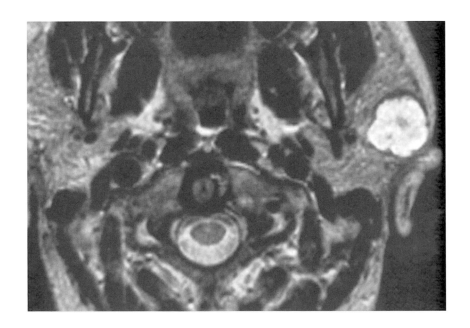

Figure 6.18   Axial FSE T2 weighted image without fat saturation.

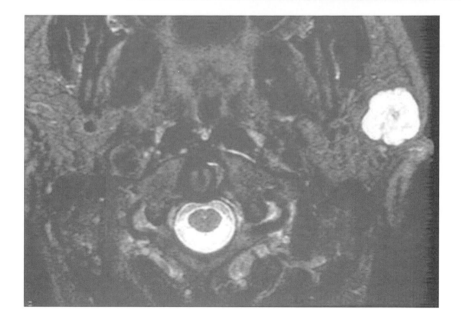

Figure 6.19 Axial T2 weighted image with fat saturation.

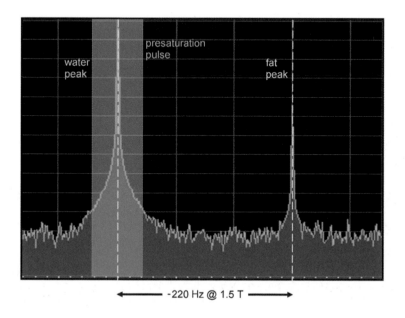

Figure 6.20 Water saturation.

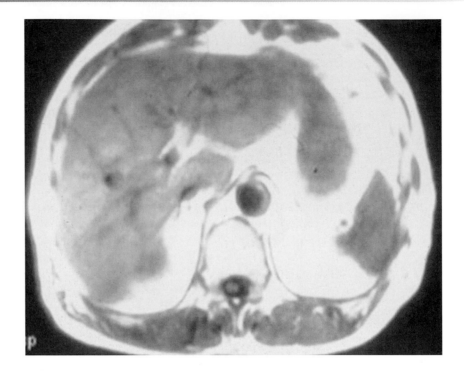

Figure 6.21   Axial T1 weighted image without water saturation.

nuclei, however, are excited, rephased and produce a signal. Figures 6.21 and 6.22 compare axial T1 weighted images of the liver, with and without water pre-saturation. Any fatty lesions in the liver are better demonstrated after water saturation as normal liver signal is nulled.

To be used effectively, there should be an even distribution of fat or water throughout the FOV. Pre-saturation RF is transmitted at the same frequency and evenly to the whole FOV, so that a particularly dense area of fat receives the same pre-saturation energy as an area with very little fat. Under these circumstances fat saturation is less effective. In addition, the gradients applied for spatial encoding vary the frequency across each slice. For this reason chemical pre-saturation often appears non-uniform across the slice or imaging volume. Therefore optimal saturation occurs at the center of a slice or in the central portion of the imaging volume. Fat and water pre-saturation delivers extra RF into the patient and therefore reduces the number of slices available for a given TR.

The pre-saturation pulses are delivered to the FOV before the excitation of each slice. The interval between the pre-saturation pulses is called the **SAT TR** and is equal to the scan TR divided by the number of slices. If the SAT TR is longer than the T1 times of fat or water, the magnetic moments of fat or water may not be saturated as they have had time to recover before each pre-saturation pulse is delivered. To prevent this, always prescribe the maximum number of slices available for a given TR so that the SAT TR is reduced to a minimum.

Any tissue can be nulled in this way as long as an RF pulse matching its precessional frequency is applied to the imaging volume before excitation. For example, silicone may be saturated to null its signal in breast imaging. This is a useful technique for ruptured implants. Spatial pre-saturation is also useful to reduce artefacts such as phase mismapping and aliasing (*see* Chapter 7).

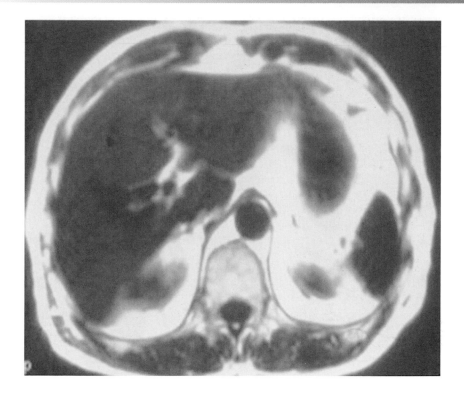

Figure 6.22   Axial T1 weighted image with water saturation.

Spatial inversion recovery (SPIR)

In this technique an RF pulse at the precessional frequency of fat is applied to the imaging volume, but unlike chemical pre-saturation this has a magnitude of 180°. The magnetic moments of fat are therefore totally inverted into the −Z direction. After a time TI, which corresponds to the null point of fat, the 90° excitation pulse is applied. As fat has no longitudinal magnetization at this point, the excitation pulse produces no transverse magnetization in fat. Therefore the fat signal is nulled (Figures 6.23 and 6.24).

This technique therefore combines fat saturation and inverting mechanisms similar to STIR (*see* Chapter 5) to eliminate fat signal. However, it has several advantages over both of these techniques. Chemical saturation is very dependent on homogeneity of the main magnetic field as it requires the precessional frequency of fat to be the same over the whole imaging volume. SPIR is much less susceptible to this because nulling also occurs by selecting an inversion time corresponding to the null point of fat. This depends on the T1 recovery time of fat rather than its precessional frequency and relaxation times are not affected by small changes in homogeneity. However, as STIR sequences totally rely on the T1 recovery times to null signal rather than precessional frequencies, they are less likely to be affected by inhomogeneity than fat saturated methods such as SPIR or fat saturation.

Figures 6.25 and 6.26 compare a STIR image with a SPIR image and clearly show more uniform nulling of fat in the STIR sequence. However, in STIR sequences, gadolinium may be nulled along

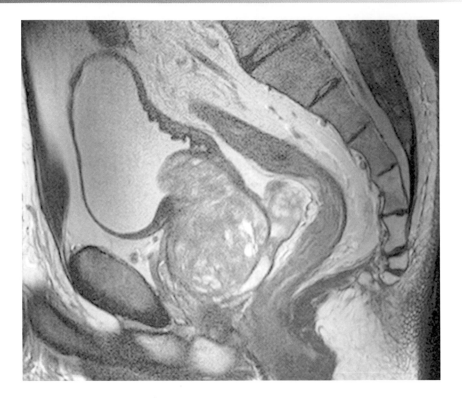

220

Figure 6.23   Sagittal T2 weighted FSE image of the pelvis.

with fat, as gadolinium shortens the T1 recovery time of tissues taking up contrast to that of fat (*see* Chapter 11). Therefore STIR sequences must never be used after giving gadolinium. However, in SPIR sequences this does not occur because fat is selectively inverted and nulled, leaving gadolinium untouched. Therefore SPIR may be used to null the signal from fat in sequences where gadolinium has been given.

Learning point: suppression techniques

We have discussed several ways of nulling fat signal. Unless a lipoma (a fatty tumor) is present, fat is usually considered normal tissue. In sequences where both fat and water or fat and gadolinium return a high signal it is often necessary to null the signal from fat to visualize water (which may indicate pathology) more clearly. Examples of this are in T2 weighted TSE sequences. Currently fat is nulled in the following ways:

- fat saturation
- STIR
- SPIR
- out of phase imaging (Dixon technique). This is used in gradient echo sequences to null the signal from voxels in which fat and water nuclei co-exist. This is achieved by selecting a TE when fat and water are out of phase with each other. As they are incoherent, no signal is received from the voxel (Figures 6.27 and 6.28) (*see* more on the phase difference between fat and water in Chapter 7).

It is possible to null the signal from many types of tissues, however. This can be achieved by applying a saturation pulse at the specific frequency of the tissue to be nulled into the FOV before the excitation pulse is applied. Tissue can also be nulled using an inverting pulse followed by an excitation pulse at a delay time equivalent to the null point of the tissue (*see* Chapter 5). Liver and spleen may be specifically nulled as can materials such as silicone.

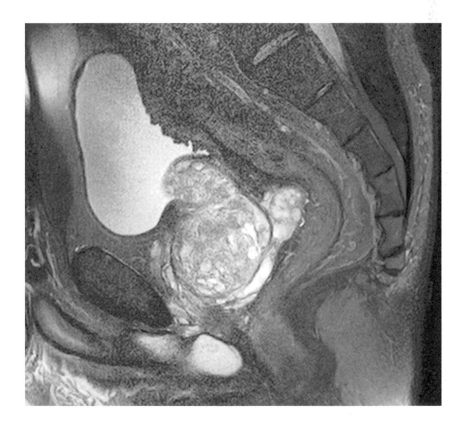

Figure 6.24   Sagittal T2 weighted FSE image of the pelvis with SPIR. Fat has been suppressed.

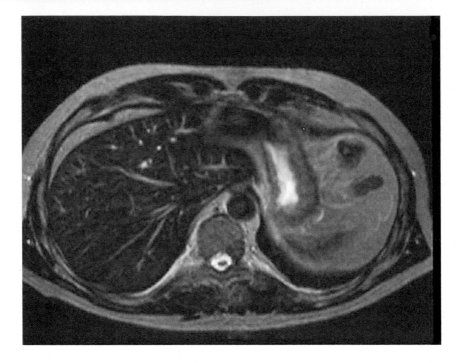

Figure 6.25   Axial STIR image. Fat is uniformly suppressed.

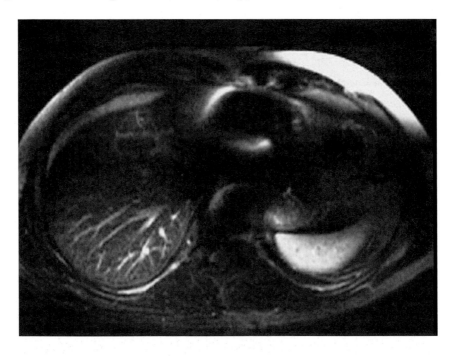

Figure 6.26   Axial SPIR image. Non-uniform suppression of fat is clearly seen due to field inhomogeneities.

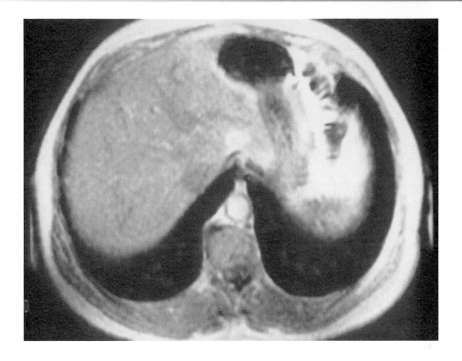

Figure 6.27 Axial gradient echo in phase image.

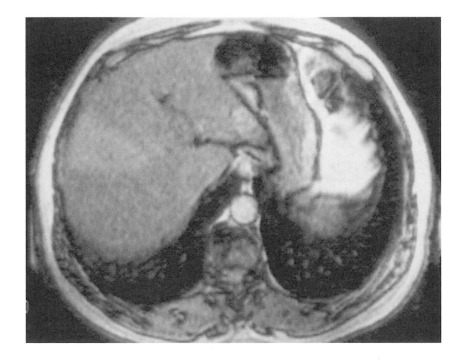

Figure 6.28 Axial gradient echo out of phase image.

Summary

Even echo rephasing:

- uses balanced echoes in which even echoes demonstrate less dephasing than odd echoes
- reduces intra-voxel dephasing
- is mainly used in T2 weighted sequences.

Gradient moment rephasing:

- uses additional gradients to correct altered phase values
- reduces artefact from intra-voxel dephasing
- is most effective on slow, laminar flow within the slice.

Pre-saturation:

- uses additional RF pulses to nullify signal from flowing nuclei
- reduces artefact due to time of flight and entry slice phenomenon (spatial pre-saturation)
- gives flowing nuclei a signal void (spatial pre-saturation)
- is mainly used in T1 weighted images (spatial pre-saturation)
- is effective on fast and slow flow (spatial pre-saturation)
- increases the RF deposition to the patient
- can be used inside the FOV to nullify signal from fat or water and to reduce aliasing (chemical pre-saturation).

For questions and answers on this topic please visit the supporting companion website for this book: www.wiley.com/go/mriinpractice

Now that flow phenomena have been discussed, it is appropriate to proceed to explore other artefacts that are commonly seen on MR images. These are described in the next chapter.

7

Artefacts and their compensation

Introduction

All MRI images have artefacts to some degree. It is therefore very important that the causes of these artefacts are understood and compensated for if possible. Some artefacts are irreversible and may only be reduced rather than eliminated. Others can be avoided altogether. This chapter discusses the appearances, causes and remedy of the most common artefacts encountered in MRI.

Phase mismapping

Appearance

Phase mismapping or ghosting produces replications of moving anatomy across the image in the phase encoding direction. It usually originates from anatomy that moves periodically throughout the scan, such as the chest wall during respiration (Figure 7.1), pulsatile movement of vessels and CSF, swallowing and eye movement. When looking at an image, the direction of phase encoding can always be determined by the direction of the phase mismapping or ghosting artefact.

MRI in Practice, Fourth Edition. Catherine Westbrook, Carolyn Kaut Roth, John Talbot.
© 2011 Blackwell Publishing Ltd. Published 2011 by Blackwell Publishing Ltd.

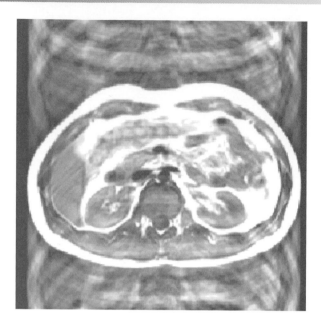

Figure 7.1   Axial image through a breathing abdomen showing phase mismapping.

Cause

Phase mismapping is produced by anatomy moving along the phase encoding gradient during the pulse sequence. It only occurs along this gradient for the following reasons.

- The phase encoding gradient has a different amplitude every TR, while frequency and slice select gradients have the same amplitude every TR (*see* Chapter 3). Therefore as anatomy moves during the scan it is misplaced in phase encoding direction as the phase gradient changes. Imagine the chest wall moving during the scan, as shown in Figure 7.2. The chest wall is located at a position along the phase encoding gradient during expiration, but may have moved to another position during the next phase encoding at inspiration. The chest wall is given different phase values depending on its position along the gradient, e.g. 3 o'clock and 2 o'clock. Therefore moving anatomy is mismapped into the FOV along the phase encoding gradient.
- There is a time delay between phase encoding and readout (Figure 7.2). Therefore anatomy may have moved between phase encoding and when the signal is read during frequency encoding and put into K space. No mismapping occurs along the frequency axis as frequency encoding is performed as the signal is read and digitized.

Remedy

There are several ways of reducing phase mismapping. Total elimination, is, however, impossible unless of course you are imaging a cadaver. The remedies of mismapping are associated with their individual causes.

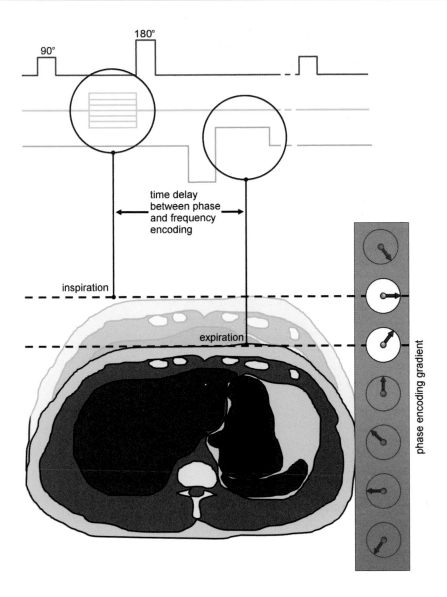

Figure 7.2 The causes of phase mismapping.

Swapping phase and frequency

As ghosting only occurs along the phase axis, the direction of phase encoding can be changed, so that the artefact does not interfere with the area of interest. For example, in a sagittal cervical spine, frequency encoding is usually performed by the Z gradient (head to foot) as this is the longest axis of the patient in the sagittal plane (Figure 7.3). Phase is therefore anterior–posterior and performed by the Y gradient. Swallowing and pulsatile motion of the carotids along the phase axis produces ghosting over the spinal cord. Swapping phase and frequency so that the Y gradient (anterior–posterior) performs frequency encoding and the Z gradient performs phase encoding,

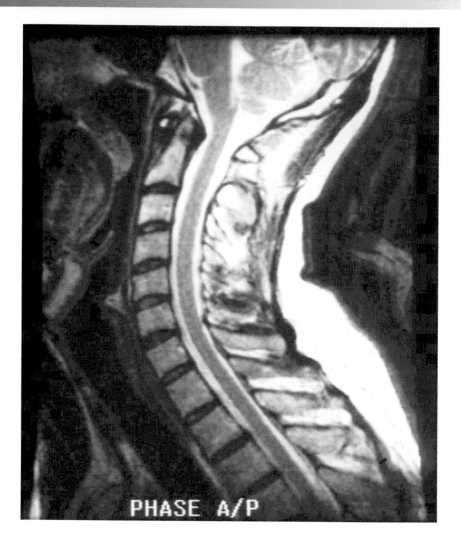

PHASE A/P

Figure 7.3 Sagittal T2 weighted image of the cervical spine with phase and therefore phase ghosting mapped anterior to posterior.

places the artefact head to foot so that it does not obscure the spinal cord (Figure 7.4). This remedy is also useful in sagittal imaging of the knee to remove artefact originating from the popliteal artery, and in axial imaging of the chest where anterior mediastinal structures are obscured by the aorta. Which way do you think phase and frequency should be located in these examples?

Using pre-saturation pulses

Pre-saturation (discussed in Chapter 6) nulls signal from specified areas. Placing pre-saturation volumes over the area producing artefact nullifies signal and reduces the artefact. For example, in sagittal imaging of the cervical spine, swallowing produces ghosting along the phase axis

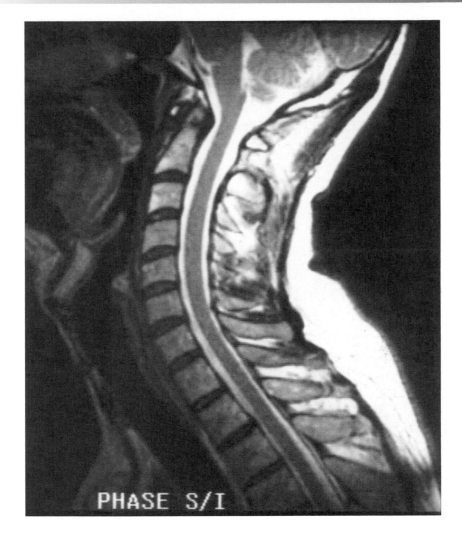

PHASE S/I

Figure 7.4   Sagittal T2 weighted image of the cervical spine with phase and therefore phase ghosting mapped superior to inferior. Note how visibility of the cervical cord has been slightly improved compared with Figure 7.3.

(anterior–posterior) and obscures the spinal cord. Bringing a pre-saturation pulse into the FOV and placing it over the throat reduces the artefact. In addition, pre-saturation reduces artefact from flowing nuclei in blood vessels. Pre-saturation produces low signal from these nuclei and is most effective when placed between the origin of the flow and the FOV.

Using respiratory compensation techniques

When imaging the chest and abdomen, respiratory motion along the phase axis produces phase mismapping. In fast sequences it is possible for the patient to hold their breath, eliminating

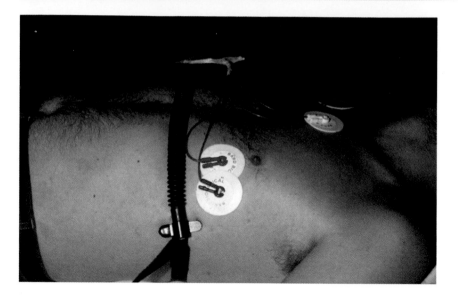

Figure 7.5   Placement of respiratory compensation bellows and cardiac gating leads.

artefact. In longer sequences a method known as **respiratory compensation** or respiratory ordered phase encoding (ROPE) can greatly reduce ghosting from respiration. This entails placing a set of bellows around the patient's chest when imaging the chest or abdomen. These bellows are cor-rugated in their middle portion and expand and contract as the patient breathes (Figure 7.5). This expansion and contraction causes air to move back and forth through the bellows. The bellows are connected by hollow rubber tubing to a transducer located on the system. A transducer is a device that converts the mechanical motion of air flowing back and forth along the bellows to an electrical signal. The system therefore analyzes this signal, the amplitude of which corresponds to the maximum and minimum motion of the chest wall during respiration. Respiratory compensa-tion does not affect the scan time or the image contrast. The only penalty of this method is that the number of slices available for a given TR may be slightly reduced.

Learning point: respiratory compensation and K space filling

As described in Chapter 3, the central lines of K space are filled after shallow phase encoding gradient slopes (which result in good signal and contrast), while the outer lines are filled after steep phase encoding gradient slopes that result in high spatial resolution. Anatomy that moves along a shallow phase encoding slope produces maximum ghosting because there is a higher signal to mismap in the image. Anatomy that moves along a steep phase encoding gradient slope, however, produces less ghosting as there is a smaller signal to mismap.

The system is able to read the electrical signal from the transducer and perform the shallow phase encoding gradient slopes, which fill the central lines of K space when the chest or abdominal wall movement is at a minimum. In this way most of the data that provide image signal and contrast are acquired when chest wall motion is low. The steep phase encoding slopes that fill the outer lines are reserved for when the chest wall movement is at a maximum (Figure 7.6). Essentially the data laid out in K space in this manner look non-periodic and therefore ghosting artefact from respiratory motion is reduced. Look at Figures 7.7 and 7.8. Phase mismapping seen in Figure 7.7 is reduced by using respiratory compensation in Figure 7.8.

Systems also use a method known as **respiratory gating** or **triggering** that times the excitation RF with a certain phase of respiration. Each slice of the acquisition is therefore obtained at the same phase of respiration. However, this method has several drawbacks. First, the TR and therefore the contrast is determined by the rapidity of respiration and second, since respiratory rates are generally longer than the TR, the scan time is lengthened and image contrast may change. **Respiratory navigator echoes** can also be used to reduce phase mismapping caused by respiratory

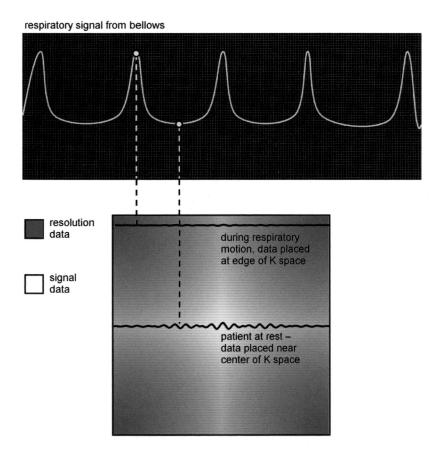

Figure 7.6   Respiratory compensation and K space.

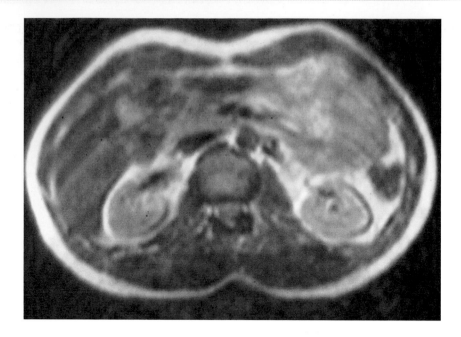

Figure 7.7   Axial T1 weighted image of the chest showing phase ghosting from respiration.

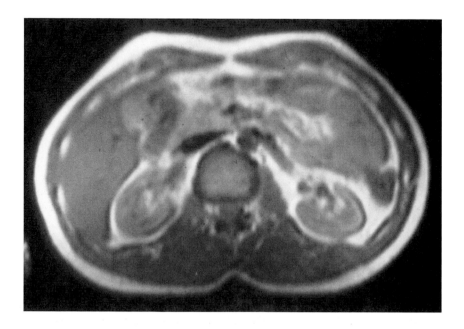

Figure 7.8   Axial T1 weighted image of the chest with respiratory compensation. Phase ghosting is reduced.

motion. In this technique, a region of interest (ROI) is placed across the diaphragm in either coronal or sagittal localizers. The system monitors the signal intensity within this ROI and throws out data acquired outside prescribed boundaries. While this is an effective method, as data are removed, the scan time may increase and/or the SNR decreases.

Cardiac gating

Gating is a very general term used to describe a technique of reducing phase mismapping from the periodic motion caused by respiration, cardiac and pulsatile flow motion. Just as respiratory gating monitors respiration, cardiac gating monitors cardiac motion by co-ordinating the excitation pulse with the R wave of systole. This is achieved by using an electrical signal generated by the cardiac motion to trigger each excitation pulse. There are two forms of gating.

- *Electrocardiogram (ECG, EKG) gating* uses electrodes and lead wires that are attached to the patient's chest to produce an ECG (Figure 7.5). This is used to determine the timing of the application of each excitation pulse. Each slice is acquired at the same phase of the cardiac cycle and therefore phase mismapping from cardiac motion is reduced. ECG gating should be used when imaging the chest, heart and great vessels.
- *Peripheral gating* uses a light sensor attached to the patient's finger to detect the pulsation of blood through the capillaries. The pulsation is used to trigger the excitation pulses so that each slice is acquired at the same phase of the cardiac cycle. Peripheral gating is not as accurate as ECG gating, so is not very useful when imaging the heart itself. However, it is effective at reducing phase mismapping when imaging small vessels or the spinal cord, where CSF flow may degrade the image. ECG and peripheral gating are discussed in more detail in Chapter 8.

Gradient moment nulling

This reduces ghosting caused by flowing nuclei moving along gradients (discussed in Chapter 6). It produces a bright signal from these flowing nuclei and also reduces ghosting significantly. It is most effective in slow, regular flow within the imaging plane.

Other motion reducing techniques

Some types of voluntary motion, such as eye movement, can be reduced by asking the patient to focus their eyes on a particular part of the magnet/room. Other involuntary motion, such as bowel motion, is reduced by administering antispasmodic agents (Figures 7.9 and 7.10). Increasing the NEX may also help, as this increases the number of times the signal is averaged. Motion artefact is averaged out of the image as it is more random in nature than the signal itself. In addition Propeller (*see* Chapter 3) effectively uses multiple NEX on the central K space regions and fills multiple areas of K space per TR thereby reducing the scan. Both of these mechanisms reduce motion artefact. Voluntary motion can be reduced by making the patient as comfortable as possible, and immobilizing them with pads and straps. A nervous patient always benefits from thoughtful explanation of the procedure and a constant reminder over the system intercom to keep still. A relative or friend in the room can also help in some circumstances. In extreme cases, sedation of the patient may be required.

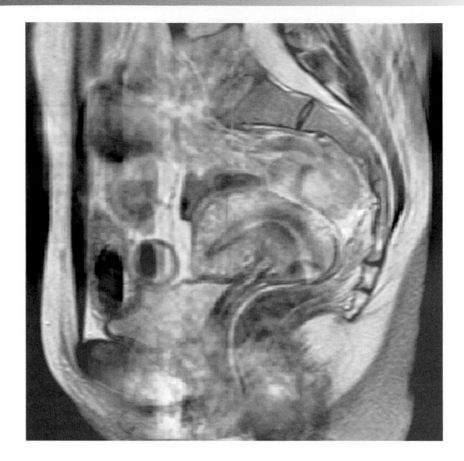

Figure 7.9   Sagittal T2 weighted images of the pelvis. Bowel motion has caused blurring of structures.

Aliasing or wrap around

Appearance

Wrap or aliasing produces an image where anatomy that exists outside the FOV is folded onto the top of anatomy inside the FOV. In Figure 7.11 the FOV in the phase direction is smaller than the anterior–posterior dimensions of the head. Therefore signal outside the FOV in the phase direction is wrapped into the image.

Cause

Aliasing is produced when anatomy that exists outside the FOV is mapped inside the FOV. Anatomy outside the selected FOV still produces a signal if it is in close proximity to the receiver coil. Data from this signal must be encoded, i.e. allocated a pixel position. If the data are under-sampled,

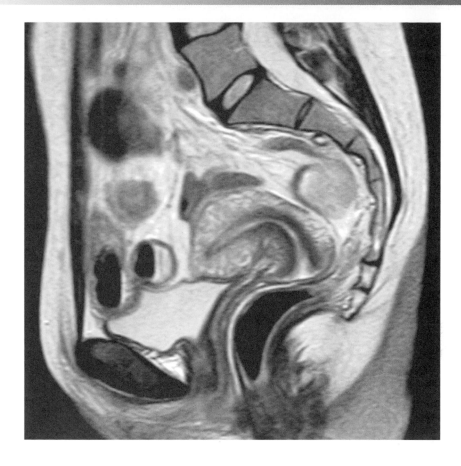

Figure 7.10 Sagittal T2 weighted image of the pelvis after administration of anti-spasmodic agents. Bowel motion has been reduced.

the signal is mismapped into pixels within the FOV rather than outside. Aliasing can occur along both the frequency and phase axis.

Frequency wrap

Aliasing along the frequency encoding axis is known as **frequency wrap**. This is caused by under-sampling the frequencies that are present in the echo. These frequencies originate from any signal, regardless of whether the anatomy producing it is inside or outside the selected FOV. Ideally, only the frequencies originating from inside the FOV are allocated a pixel position. This only occurs if the frequencies are sampled often enough. According to the Nyquist theorem (*see* Chapter 3), frequencies must be sampled at least twice per cycle to map them correctly. If the Nyquist theorem is not obeyed and frequencies are not sampled enough, signal from anatomy outside the FOV in the frequency encoding direction is mapped into the FOV (Figure 7.12, bottom image). Wrap around results along the frequency encoding axis.

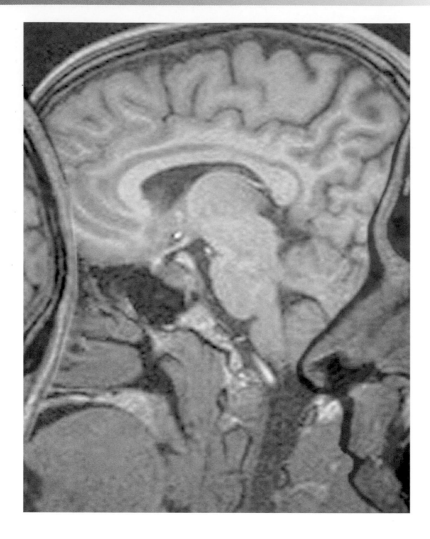

Figure 7.11   Sagittal image of the brain showing aliasing or wrap around.

Phase wrap

Aliasing along the phase axis of the image is known as **phase wrap**. This is caused by under-sampling along the phase axis. After FFT every phase value from 0° to 360° (or 12 o'clock through to the following 12 o'clock) must be mapped into the FOV in the phase encoding direction (Figure 7.13). This phase curve is repeated on both sides of the FOV along the phase axis. Any signal is allocated a phase value according to its position along this curve. As the curve is repeated, signal originating outside the FOV in the phase direction is allocated a phase value that has already been given to signal originating from inside the FOV. There is, therefore, a duplication of phase values. This duplication causes phase wrap along the phase axis.

Look at Figure 7.14 where the FOV in the right-to-left phase axis of the image is smaller than the dimensions of the axial abdomen. The phase encoding gradient has been applied in this

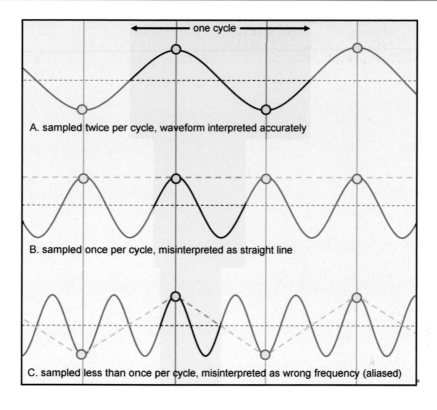

A. sampled twice per cycle, waveform interpreted accurately

B. sampled once per cycle, misinterpreted as straight line

C. sampled less than once per cycle, misinterpreted as wrong frequency (aliased)

Figure 7.12   Aliasing and under-sampling.

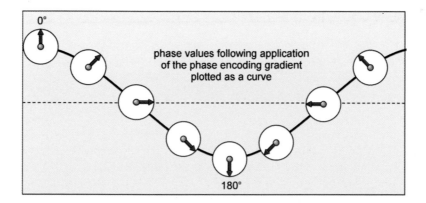

Figure 7.13   The phase curve.

237

238

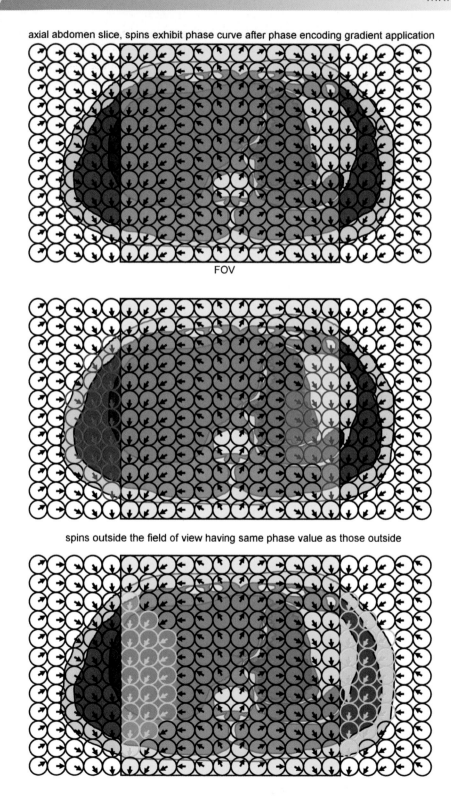

axial abdomen slice, spins exhibit phase curve after phase encoding gradient application

FOV

spins outside the field of view having same phase value as those outside

Figure 7.14 Phase wrap.

direction and produces a change of phase across the X-axis of the bore of the magnet. At this particular gradient slope, spins outside the FOV have the same phase position as spins inside the FOV (red and blue areas in the diagram). As they have the same phase value these red and blue areas are wrapped inside the image because they have a phase value exactly the same as spins within the FOV.

Remedy

Aliasing along both the frequency and phase axis can totally degrade an image and should be compensated for. Enlarging the FOV so that all anatomy producing signal is incorporated within the FOV achieves this, but also results in a loss of spatial resolution. Bringing pre-saturation bands onto areas outside the FOV that may wrap into the image can sometimes sufficiently null signal from these areas and reduce aliasing. There are, however, two anti-aliasing software methods available that compensate for wrap.

Anti-aliasing along the frequency axis

Increasing the sampling rate so that all frequencies are digitized sufficiently would eliminate aliasing in the frequency direction. However, doing so would also increase noise in the image. Therefore a frequency filter is used to filter out frequencies that occur outside the selected FOV. Signal originating from outside the FOV along the frequency axis is no longer mismapped as it is filtered out (Figure 7.15). Most systems automatically apply this option so that aliasing never occurs along the frequency encoding axis, which is similar to filtering out the bass and treble on a music system with a graphic equalizer.

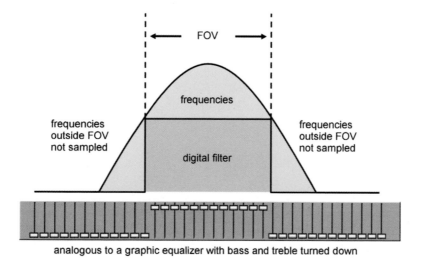

Figure 7.15   Anti-aliasing along the frequency axis.

Anti-aliasing along the phase axis

This is termed **no phase wrap**, **phase over-sampling** or **anti-foldover**. No phase wrap over-samples along the phase encoding axis by increasing the number of phase encodings performed. This is achieved by enlarging the FOV in the phase direction so that the phase curve extends over a wider area of anatomy. There is now no duplication of phase values as signal outside the FOV has a different phase value to that inside. Anatomy is no longer mismapped and aliasing does not occur (Figure 7.16). However, as enlarging the FOV results in a loss of spatial resolution, the number of phase encodings is increased to compensate for this. Increasing the number of phase encodings in turn increases the scan time and so some systems automatically reduce the NEX or signal averages to compensate for this. Others, however, do not, so using this option increases the scan time.

In the systems where the NEX is automatically reduced to maintain the scan time, the extended portion of the FOV is discarded during reconstruction so that only the selected FOV is displayed. In systems that do not automatically reduce the NEX, the extended portions are not discarded and the phase FOV therefore increases in size. Although the SNR is not noticeably altered in either option, image quality may suffer slightly with no phase wrap. As a decrease in NEX reduces the number of signal averages, motion artefacts may be more apparent. Look at Figures 4.25 and 4.26 in Chapter 4 that were acquired with 1 and 4 NEX. In Figure 4.25 you may notice some ghosting along the superior sagittal sinus. This is reduced in Figure 4.26 because a higher NEX was used.

Learning point: no phase wrap, K space and the chest of drawers

The chest of drawers analogy describes this option well. The height of the chest of drawers determines the number of pixels in the phase direction of the image (i.e. if a 256 matrix has been selected then drawers +/–128 are filled with data, the top and bottom drawers). To reduce this artefact, more phase encodes must be performed, therefore more drawers must be filled. To fill more drawers and still keep the height of the chest of drawers the same, each drawer must be thinner (as discussed in Chapter 4). The depth of the drawer is inversely proportional to the FOV in the phase direction as a percentage of the frequency FOV, so halving the depth of each drawer doubles the FOV in the phase direction compared with the frequency direction, allowing anatomy to be included in a larger FOV and prevent aliasing. Doubling the number of phase encoding steps or drawers doubles the scan time, and some systems halve the NEX (the number of times each drawer is filled) to compensate (Figure 7.16). Hence on these systems this option eliminates aliasing (as long as anatomy is outside the larger FOV) and maintains the original resolution, FOV and scan time (Figures 7.17 and 7.18).

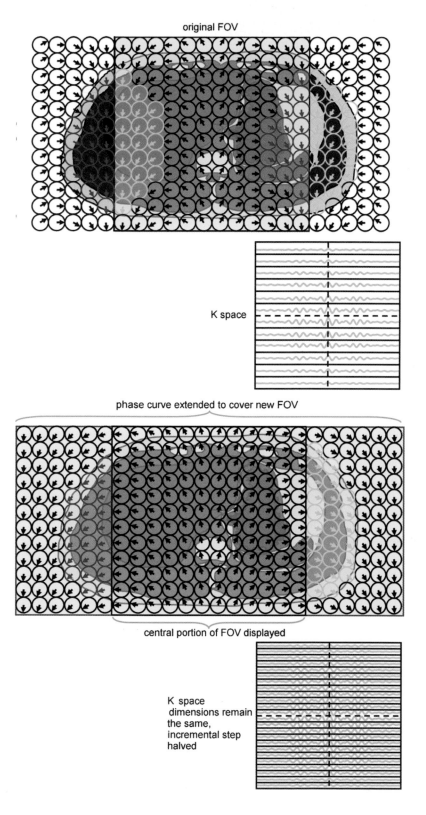

original FOV

K space

phase curve extended to cover new FOV

central portion of FOV displayed

K space dimensions remain the same, incremental step halved

Figure 7.16 Anti-aliasing along the phase axis.

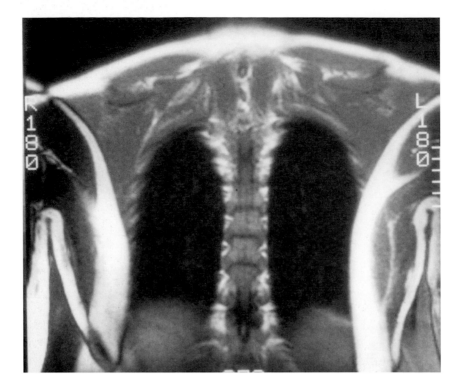

Figure 7.17   Coronal image of the chest showing phase wrap.

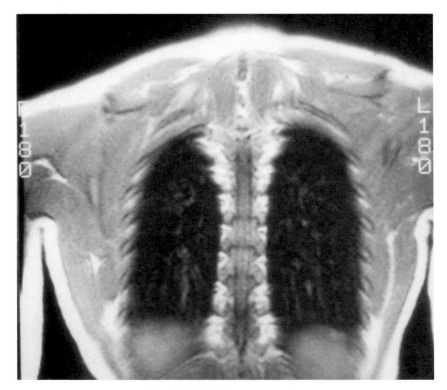

Figure 7.18   Coronal image of the chest with anti-aliasing. Wrap has been eliminated.

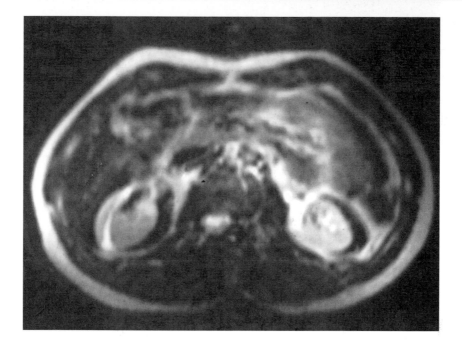

Figure 7.19   Chemical shift artefact seen as a black band to the right-hand side of each kidney.

Chemical shift artefact

Appearance

Chemical shift artefact produces a dark edge at the interface between fat and water. It occurs along the frequency encoding axis only. Figure 7.19 shows a black band to the right of both kidneys. This is chemical shift artefact.

Cause

Chemical shift artefact is caused by the different chemical environments of fat and water. Although fat and water are both made up of hydrogen protons, fat consists of hydrogen arranged with carbon, while in water, hydrogen is arranged with oxygen (*see* Chapter 2). As a result, fat precesses at a lower frequency than water. This difference in precessional frequency is proportional to the main magnetic field strength, B_0. For example, at 1.5 T the difference in precessional frequency is 220 Hz. That is, fat precesses 220 Hz less than water. At 1.0 T this difference is 147 Hz and at lower field strengths (0.5 T or less) it is usually insignificant. However, at higher field strengths, it can lead to an artefact known as **chemical shift**. The amount of chemical shift is often expressed in arbitrary units known as parts per million (ppm) of the main magnetic field strength. Its value is always independent of the main field strength and equals 3.5 ppm. From this, the chemical shift between fat and water can be calculated at different field strengths.

The receive bandwidth determines the range of frequencies that must be mapped across the FOV. The FOV is divided into pixels, the number of which is determined by the matrix size. If 256 frequency samples are selected, the receive bandwidth must be mapped across 256 pixels in the FOV. The receive bandwidth and the number of frequency samples determine the bandwidth of each pixel or frequency column.

For example, if the receive bandwidth is +/−16 KHz, 32000 Hz are mapped across the FOV. If 256 frequency samples are collected, the FOV is divided into 256 frequency columns or pixels. Each column therefore has an individual frequency range of 125 Hz per pixel (32000/256 Hz) (Figure 7.20). At a field strength of 1.5 T, the precessional frequency difference between fat and water is 220 Hz and therefore using the above example, fat and water protons existing adjacent to one other in the patient are mapped 1.76 pixels apart (220/125) (Figure 7.20, middle diagram). This pixel shift of fat relative to water is called chemical shift artefact. The actual dimensions of this artefact depend on the size of the FOV, as this determines the size of each pixel. For example, a FOV of 24 cm and 256 frequency columns results in pixels 0.93 mm in size. A pixel shift of 1.76 results in an actual chemical shift between fat and water of 1.63 mm (0.93 × 1.76 mm). As the FOV is enlarged this dimension increases.

Remedy

Chemical shift can be limited by scanning at lower field strengths and by keeping the FOV to a minimum. At high field strengths, the size of the receive bandwidth is one way of limiting chemical shift. As the receive bandwidth is reduced, a smaller frequency range must now be mapped across the same number of frequency columns, for example 256. The individual frequency range of each pixel therefore decreases, and so the 220 Hz difference in precessional frequency between fat and water is translated into a larger pixel shift (Figure 7.20, lower diagram). For example, if the receive bandwidth is reduced to +/− 8 KHz, only 16000 Hz is now mapped across 256 frequency columns. Each pixel has a range of only 62.5 Hz (16000/256 Hz). The 220 Hz precessional frequency difference between the two adjacent fat and water protons is now translated into a pixel shift of 3.52 pixels (220/62.5) (Figure 7.20, lower diagram).

To reduce chemical shift artefact always use the widest receive bandwidth in keeping with good SNR (see Chapters 3 and 4) and the smallest FOV possible (Figure 7.21). If the bandwidth is reduced to increase the SNR, use chemical saturation to saturate out the signal from either fat or water (see Chapter 6). By doing so, as either fat or water is nulled, there is nothing for one tissue to shift against and therefore chemical shift artefact is eliminated. These measures are really only necessary at higher field strengths. At 0.5 T or less, chemical shift artefact is insignificant and usually does not need to be compensated for.

Out of phase artefact (chemical misregistration)

Appearance

When fat and water are in phase their signals add constructively, and when they are out of phase their signals cancel each other out. This cancellation effect is known as **out of phase artefact** or **chemical misregistration**, which produces a ring of dark signal around certain organs where fat and water interfaces occur within the same voxel, for example the kidneys (Figure 7.22). It is most degrading to the image in gradient echo pulse sequences, where gradient reversal is very ineffective.

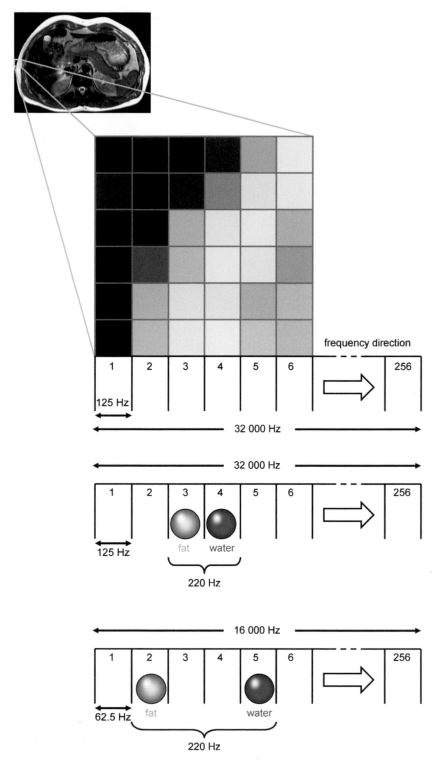

Figure 7.20   Chemical shift and pixel shift.

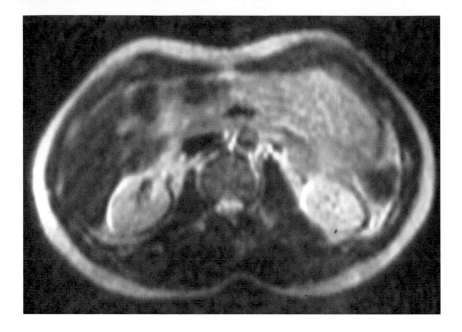

Figure 7.21 Axial image through the abdomen acquired with a wide receive bandwidth. Chemical shift artefact seen on Figure 7.19 has been reduced.

Cause

Out of phase artefact is an artefact produced as a result of the precessional frequency difference between fat and water. The artefact is caused because fat and water are in phase at certain times and out of phase at others, due to the difference in their precessional frequency. As they travel at different speeds around their precessional paths, they are at various positions on the path but periodically they are at the same position and therefore in phase.

Learning point: chemical misregistration and the watch analogy

This is analogous to the hour and minute hand of a clock. Both hands travel at different speeds around the clock: the hour hand moves through 360° in 12 hours, while the minute hand moves the same distance in one hour. However, at certain times of the day, the hands are superimposed or in phase, i.e. approximately at 12 noon, 1.05 am, 2.10 am, 3.15 am, etc. (Figure 7.23).

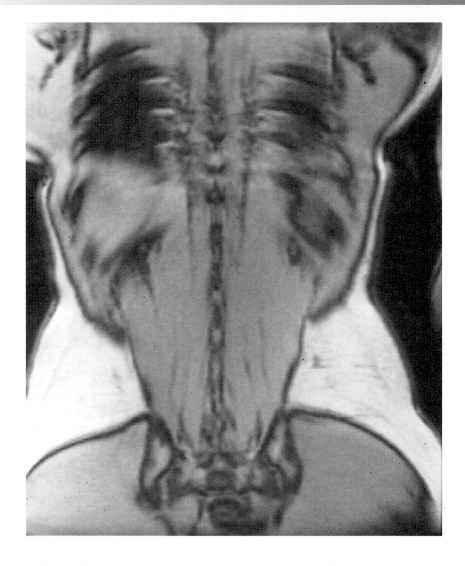

Figure 7.22   Chemical misregistration seen as a black line around the abdominal organs.

Remedy

Select a TE that matches the periodicity of fat and water at your field strength. The periodicity of fat and water depends on the field strength (Figure 7.24). At 1.5 T, for example, selecting a TE that is a multiple of 4.2 ms reduces chemical misregistration artefact, while at 0.5 T the periodicity of fat and water is 7 ms. In addition, use spin echo sequences rather than gradient echo as 180° RF pulses are very effective at compensating for differences in phase between fat and water, while gradient echo sequences are generally very poor at this.

Refer to animation 7.1 on the supporting companion website for this book: www.wiley.com/go/mriinpractice

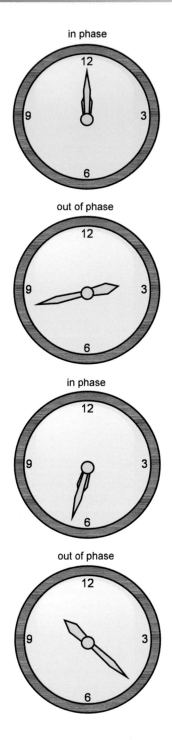

Figure 7.23   Out of phase artefact and the watch analogy.

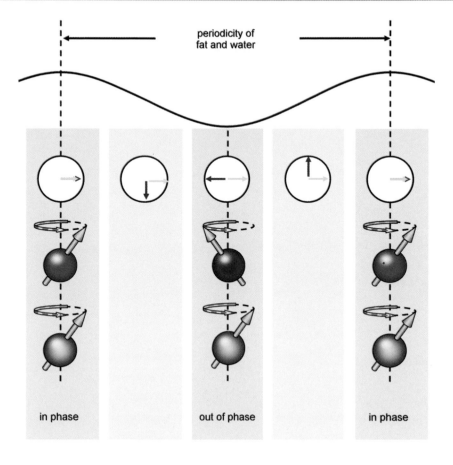

Figure 7.24   The periodicity of fat and water.

Truncation artefact

Appearance

This artefact produces a banding artefact at the interfaces of high and low signal. Figure 7.25 shows this at the edges of the brain where high signal from fat in the scalp lies adjacent to low signal from the skull.

Cause

This artefact results from under-sampling of data (too few K space lines filled) so that inter-faces of high and low signal are incorrectly represented on the image. Truncation artefact occurs in the phase direction only and produces a low intensity band running through a high intensity area.

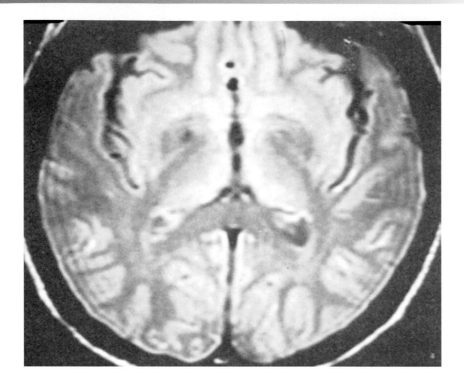

Figure 7.25 Axial image of the brain showing truncation artefact seen as faint lines adjacent to the skull–brain interface.

Remedy

Under-sampling of data must be avoided. To do so, increase the number of phase encoding steps. For example, use a 256 × 256 matrix instead of 256 × 128.

Magnetic susceptibility artefact

Appearance

This artefact produces distortion of the image together with large signal voids. Figure 7.26 shows magnetic susceptibility artefact from a hairgrip present within the image volume.

Cause

Magnetic susceptibility is the ability of a substance to become magnetized. Different tissues magnetize to different degrees, which results in a difference in precessional frequency and phase. This causes dephasing at the interface of these tissues and a signal loss. In practice, the main causes of this artefact are metal within the imaging volume, although it can also be seen from naturally

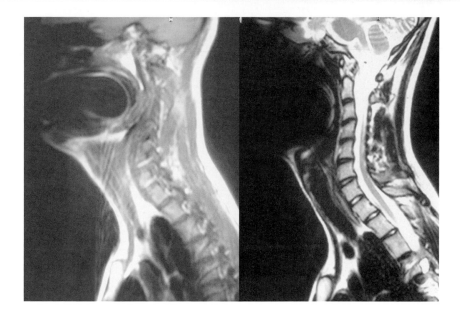

Figure 7.26   Magnetic susceptibility from a hairgrip causing massive distortion of the image.

occurring iron content of hemorrhage, as these magnetize to a much greater degree than the surrounding tissue. Ferromagnetic objects have a very high magnetic susceptibility and cause distortion of the image. Magnetic susceptibility artefact is more prominent in gradient echo sequences as the gradient reversal cannot compensate for the phase difference at the interface.

Remedy

This artefact can, under some circumstances, aid diagnosis. In particular, small hemorrhages are sometimes only seen because they produce a magnetic susceptibility effect. However, in general this artefact is undesirable and can ruin an image. There are several remedies available.

- *Remove all metal objects.* Always ensure that the patient has removed all metal objects where possible before the scan. Always check whether the patient has aneurysm clips or metal implants. Most implants can be scanned but may cause local heating effects (*see* Chapter 10).
- *Use spin echo sequences instead of gradient echo.* The 180° rephasing pulse used in spin echo sequences is very affective at compensating for phase differences between fat and water, while gradient echo sequences are very poor at this. In Figures 7.27 and 7.28 gradient echo and spin echo sequences have been used respectively. Metal artefact in the tibia produces magnetic susceptibility artefact on both images but this is significantly reduced in the spin echo sequence. The same effect is also produced when using SS–FSE as opposed to standard FSE. The long echo train used in single shot imaging produces increased rephasing from added 180° rephasing pulses. The artefact is therefore significantly reduced.
- *Decrease the TE.* Longer echo times allow for more dephasing between tissues with susceptibility differences, therefore using a short TE reduces this artefact. Broad receive bandwidths

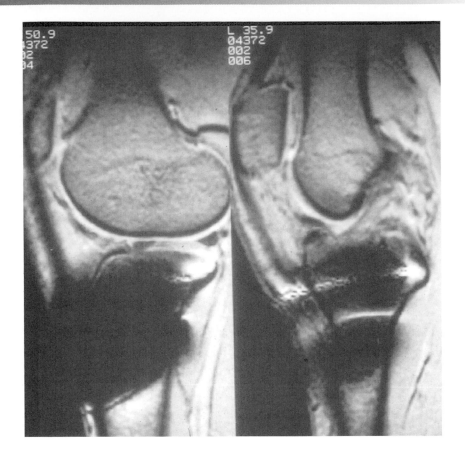

Figure 7.27   Sagittal gradient echo images of the knee with pins in the tibia. Magnetic susceptibility has produced a large distortion of the image.

also reduce the TE (*see* Chapter 3), so this is also a useful remedy when faced with this artefact.

Cross-excitation and cross-talk

Appearance

Adjacent slices in an acquisition have different image contrasts (Figure 7.29).

Cause

An RF excitation pulse is not exactly square. The width of the pulse should be half its amplitude, but this normally varies by up to 10%. As a result, nuclei in slices adjacent to the RF excitation

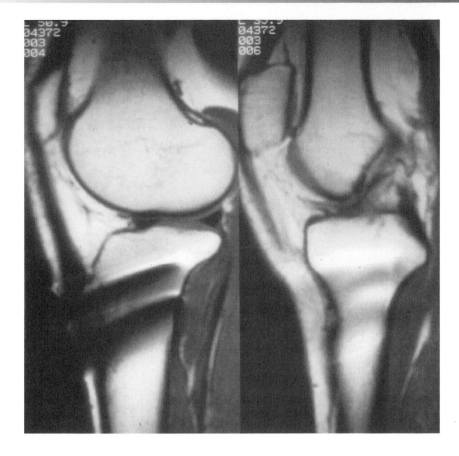

Figure 7.28   Sagittal spin echo images of the same patient as shown in Figure 7.27. The artefact is reduced.

pulse may become excited by it. Adjacent slices receive energy from the RF excitation pulse of their neighbors (Figure 7.30).

This energy pushes the NMV of the nuclei towards the transverse plane, so that they may become saturated when they themselves are excited. This effect is called **cross-excitation** and affects image contrast. The same effect is produced by energy dissipation to adjacent slices, as nuclei within the selected slice relax to B_0. These nuclei lose their energy due to spin lattice relaxation and may dissipate this energy to nuclei in neighboring slices. This is specifically called **cross-talk** and should not be confused with cross-excitation.

Remedy

Cross-talk can never be eliminated as it is caused by the natural dissipation of energy by the nuclei. Cross-excitation can be reduced by ensuring that there is at least a 30% gap between the slices. This is 30% of the slice thickness itself, and reduces the likelihood of RF exciting adjacent slices.

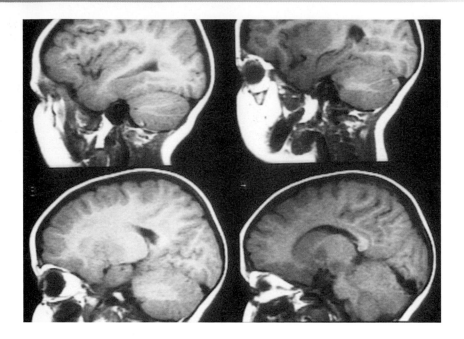

Figure 7.29   Contrast changes between slices as a result of cross-excitation.

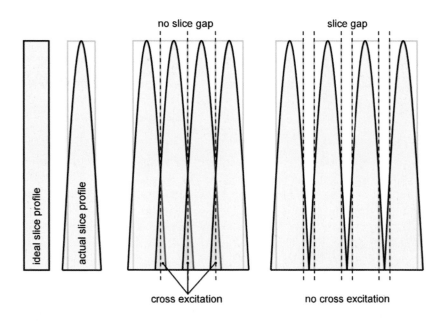

Figure 7.30   Cross-excitation.

For example, if the slice thickness selected is 5 mm, use a skip or gap of 2 mm (40% of 5 mm) rather than a 1 mm gap (20% of 5 mm). In addition, most systems excite alternate slices during the acquisition so that there is some time for cross-excitation in adjacent slices to decay before it is their turn to be excited. For example, excitation order of slices is 1, 3, 5, 7, 2, 4, 6, 8. Slices 1 to 7 have time to decay their cross-excitation, while slices 2 to 8 are being excited (approximately half the TR).

A process known as **interleaving** or **concatenation** extends this time even further. When interleaving slices, alternate slices are excited and divided into two acquisitions. In this way, cross-excitation created in adjacent slices has the time of a whole acquisition to decay before it is its turn to be excited. For example, excitation order of slices is 1, 3, 5, 7 in the first acquisition and 2, 4, 6, 8 in the second. Slices 1 to 7 have the time of a whole acquisition (several minutes) to decay while slices 2 to 8 are being excited. When using interleaving, no gap is required between the slices.

Some systems use software to 'square off' the RF pulses so that the adjacent nuclei are less likely to become excited. This reduces cross-excitation but often results in some loss of signal, as a proportion of the RF pulse is lost in the squaring off process. It is still wise to use a small gap of 10%, when employing this software.

Zipper artefact

Appearance

Zipper artefact appears as a dense line on the image at a specific point (Figure 7.31).

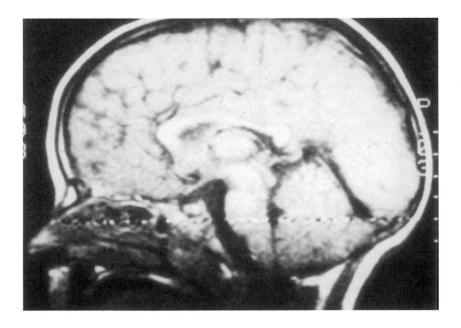

Figure 7.31   Zipper artefact seen as a horizontal line across the image.

Cause

This is caused by extraneous RF entering the room at a certain frequency and interfering with the inherently weak signal coming from the patient. It is caused by a leak in the RF shielding of the room.

Remedy

Call the engineer to locate the leak and repair it.

Shading artefact

Appearance

This produces a difference in signal intensity across the imaging volume.

Cause

Shading is an artefact that produces a loss of signal intensity in one part of the image. Its main cause is the uneven excitation of nuclei within the patient due to RF pulses applied at flip angles other than 90° and 180°. Shading is also caused by abnormal loading on the coil or by coupling of the coil at one point. This may occur with a large patient who touches one side of the body coil and couples it at that point. Shading can also be caused by inhomogeneities in the main magnetic field, which can be improved by shimming (*see* Chapter 9).

Remedy

Always ensure that the coil is loaded correctly, i.e. that the correct size of coil is used for the anatomy under examination, and that the patient is not touching the coil at any point. The use of foam pads or water bags between the coil and the patient will usually suffice. In addition, also ensure that appropriate pre-scan parameters have been obtained before the scan (*see* Chapter 3), as these determine the correct excitation frequency and amplitude of the applied RF pulses.

Moiré artefact

Appearance

This is shown as a black and white banding artefact on the edge of the FOV in Figure 7.32. It is always seen in gradient echo imaging.

Cause

This is a combination of wrap and field inhomogeneity in gradient echo sequences. In coronal imaging of the body, especially if the patient's arms are touching the bore of the magnet, pixels are wrapped on top of each other because anatomy exists outside the FOV but is producing signal. Inhomogeneities cause this wrap to be in and out of phase causing the banding appearance.

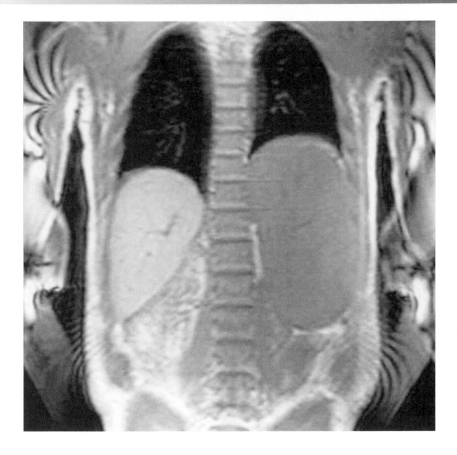

Figure 7.32   Moiré artefact seen as zebra lines on the edge of the FOV.

Remedy

Use spin echo sequences or ensure the patient keeps their arms within the FOV.

Magic angle

Appearance

This is seen in tissues that contain collagen (such as tendons) as high signal intensity. In Figure 7.33 this is seen in the patellar tendon and may mimic pathology.

Cause

This is caused when structures that contain collagen lie at an angle of 55° to the main field. The anisotropic shape of the molecules in collagen causes the reduction of spin–spin interactions to

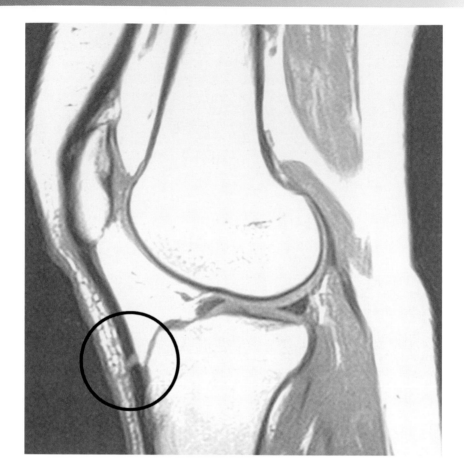

Figure 7.33 Magic angle artefact seen has high signal intensity at the lower border of the patellar tendon.

zero so that the T2 decay time increases when collagen containing structures lie at this angle to B_0. This causes an increase in the signal intensity in the structure when short TEs are used.

Remedy

Alter the angle of the structure or change the TE.

There are some other artefacts caused by major equipment malfunction. The loss of a gradient, for example, causes distortion of the image, and eddy currents induced in the gradient coils can cause phase artefacts as they create additional unwanted phase shifts. In addition, data acquisition errors cause a variety of different artefacts, most of which mimic cloth or tweed. These usually disappear if the scan is repeated.

On the whole, however, artefacts produced in MR can be compensated for to some extent, and this is summarized in Table 7.1.

Table 7.1 Artefacts and their remedies.

Artefacts	Axis	Remedy	Penalty
Flow motion	phase	swap phase and frequency	may need anti-aliasing
		gating	variable TR
			variable image contrast
			increased scan time
		pre-saturation	may lose a slice
		gradient moment rephasing	increases minimum TE
Chemical shift	frequency	increase bandwidth	decrease minimum TE available
			decrease SNR
		reduce FOV	reduces SNR
			increases resolution
		use chemical saturation	reduces SNR
			may lose slices
Out of phase artefact	frequency and phase	select a TE at periodicity of fat and water	may lose a slice if TE is significantly increased
Aliasing	frequency and phase	no frequency wrap	none
		no phase wrap	may reduce SNR
			may increase scan time (Siemens)
			increases motion artefact (GE/Philips)
		enlarge FOV (Siemens)	reduces resolution
Zipper	frequency	call engineer	irate engineer!
Magnetic susceptibility	frequency and phase	use spin echo	not flow sensitive
			blood product may be missed
		remove metal	none

MRA techniques include:

- digital subtraction MRA (acquired with and without gadolinium)
- time of flight (TOF-MRA, 2D and 3D)
- phase contrast (PC-MRA, 2D and 3D)
- contrast enhanced MRA, multiphase and ciné acquisitions.

MRI and MRA techniques rely on the motion of blood within the vessel (rather than the anatomy of the vessel itself) to demonstrate vasculature on MR images. In addition, imaging of blood flow relies primarily on the first order of motion for optimal image quality (*see* Chapter 6).

Blood does not usually flow at a constant velocity but is pulsatile. Pulsatile motion is nearer third or second order of motion rather than first order motion (*see* Chapter 6 for more information on flow phenomenology). For this reason, there are a number of practical considerations associated with vascular imaging in MRI. This chapter discusses techniques used for vascular imaging in MR, including MRI and MRA.

Conventional MRI vascular imaging techniques

Since flowing blood appears differently on various types of pulse sequence, conventional MRI can be used to evaluate vascular structures. MR imaging techniques for vascular imaging include a number of imaging sequences including:

- spin echo
- fast spin echo
- inversion recovery
- gradient echo techniques (Figure 8.1).

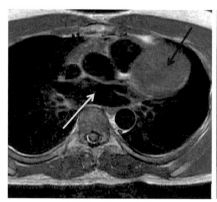 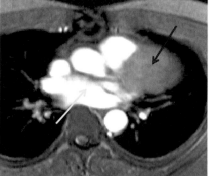

axial T1 SE acquisition   axial T1 GE acquisition

Figure 8.1   This image demonstrates spin echo (SE) black blood images (left) and gradient echo (GE) bright blood images (right) of the chest at the level of the pulmonary arteries (indicated with the yellow arrow). Note that the vasculature appears bright on the GE acquisition and dark on the spin echo sequence. This patient has developed a mass in the right atrium of the heart (indicated with the red arrow) that has the same contrast characteristics (gray) on both SE and GE images.

Spin echo, fast or turbo spin echo and inversion recovery sequences (acquired with combinations of 90° and 180° RF pulses) typically render images in which the signal from blood has been largely eradicated, known as **black blood imaging**. Gradient echo sequences render images with bright blood, known as bright blood imaging (*see* Chapter 5).

These pulse sequences can be supplemented with options such as gradient moment nulling (GMN – to reduce phase mis-mapping from the high-signal inflowing blood) and spatial pre-saturation (SAT – to reduce signal from the inflowing blood). As discussed in Chapter 6, there are options that can be used to reduce motion artefact from flowing nuclei and/or to create hypo-intense or hyper-intense signal from the lumen of blood vessels. These imaging options increase contrast between the vessel lumen and the surrounding tissue by exploiting flow-related enhancement or high velocity signal loss. These techniques can therefore be very useful to demonstrate vascular disease as a supplement to MRA and/or when MRA sequences are unavailable. Imaging sequences (SE, FSE, IR and GE) and imaging options (GMN and SAT) are now described in the context of vascular imaging.

263

Black blood imaging

In flow-dependent MRA, the key aim is to increase vascular conspicuity, the lumen being made to appear brighter or darker than the surrounding tissue. Several techniques can be used to produce images where vessels appear dark. These include spin echo acquisitions (with the application of pre-saturation pulses outside of the imaging volume) and/or inversion recovery sequences (with multiple IR pulses, known as double IR or triple IR sequences).

In spin echo sequences, flowing blood often appears dark, enabling visualization of the vessel relative to surrounding tissues (Figure 8.2). To detect signal on MR images acquired with spin echo, nuclei must receive a combination of (at least) two RF pulses. The most efficient combination of RF pulses includes a 90° excitation pulse followed by a 180° refocusing pulse. In spin echo sequences, the 90° and 180° RF pulses are slice selective pulses, so that only the tissues within the selected slice receives and is affected by both pulses. Flowing nuclei, however, may only receive one of these pulses but this depends on the slice thickness, velocity of flow and the TE (*see* Chapter 6).

Imagine blood flowing within a vessel such as the abdominal aorta. If an axial slice is acquired through the liver, stationary tissues in the liver receive the 90° and 180° pulses. The spins in flowing blood (in the aorta) are moving perpendicularly through the axial slice. Depending on the slice thickness, TE and velocity of flow, flowing spins may not receive both pulses. This is known as Time of Flight signal loss, referring to the time taken for spins to move across a certain distance (the slice thickness) in a certain time (TE). The result is hypo-intense flow within the aorta (Figure 8.3).

In addition to conventional spin echo imaging, FSE sequences can also provide images with intraluminal signal void as, like spin echo sequences, the 90° excitation pulse, and the train of 180° refocusing pulses, are slice selective.

Since inversion recovery sequences are acquired with combinations of 90°/180° RF pulses, they can also provide images with black blood. However, IR sequences can be associated with scan times that can reach upwards of 20 minutes, depending on the scan parameters selected. To reduce scan times, fast inversion recovery can be used (*see* Chapter 5). In IR sequences the inversion pulse can be applied prior to the FSE sequence. In this case, an inverting 180° pulse is applied, followed by a typical fast spin echo 90°/180°/180°/180°/180° combination. This is known as a fast IR sequence or a FSE-IR sequence. Remember, the number of 180° pulses applied after the 90° excitation pulse is known as the echo train length (ETL) or turbo factor and influences scan time.

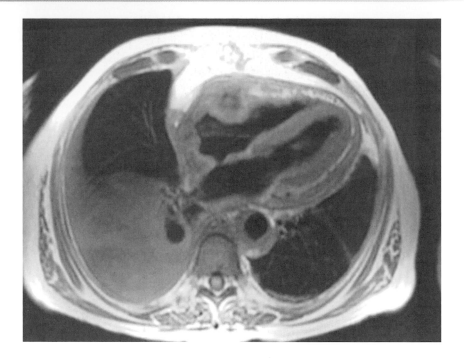

Figure 8.2 Axial black blood image of the heart. Blood in the chambers of the heart and the thoracic aorta demonstrate low signal intensity.

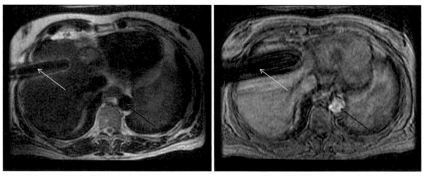

axial T1 SE acquisition   axial T1 GE acquisition

Figure 8.3 Fast spin echo black blood images (left) and gradient echo bright blood images (right) of the abdomen at the level of the liver. Note that the vasculature (aorta – red arrow) appears bright on the gradient echo acquisition and dark on the spin echo sequence. This patient is having a liver biopsy by MR guidance. Note that the biopsy needle (within the liver) presents a larger susceptibility artefact on the gradient echo sequence.

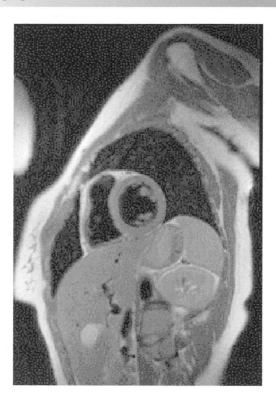

Figure 8.4   This image was acquired with a double IR prep sequence. This imaging plane demonstrates a short axis view of the heart. Since the heart is oriented 'obliquely' within the chest cavity, a double oblique acquisition is required to enable the visualization of an axial view of the heart itself.

In fast IR sequences, flowing blood can appear even darker by the application of multiple inversion pulses. A technique known as double IR prep applies a non slice-selective 180° pulse followed by a slice selective 180° pulse that immediately restores longitudinal magnetization within the slice. A TI equivalent to the null point of flowing spins in blood entering the slice enables saturation of this flow by the 90° excitation pulse (Figure 8.4). An additional slice selective inverting pulse may also be applied during the TI to null the signal specifically from fat within the slice. This third 180° RF pulse must be timed so that the null points of fat and flowing spins coincide. In this way both blood and fat are saturated (triple IR prep).

All types of spin echo sequences can be further improved by the application of pre-saturation (SAT) pulses (*see* Chapter 6). Spin echo imaging with the use of pre-saturation pulses outside of the imaging volume, is highly effective at reducing the signal from in-flowing blood, especially when T1 weighting is used. As a fluid, blood is inherently hypo-intense on T1 weighted images and the saturation pulses ensure that in-flowing spins have minimal transverse magnetization before entering the imaging volume. This technique is particularly suited to demonstrating dissection of the intima, easily distinguishing between hypointense flow and any relatively hyperintense haemorrhage in the subintimal area.

Spatial pre-saturation (also known as SAT pulses or SAT bands) can be used to evaluate vascular patency throughout the cardiovascular system. Since pre-saturation uses additional RF pulses, the specific absorption rate (SAR, discussed in Chapter 10) is increased, and the number of slices (typically available for a given TR) may be reduced. Pre-saturation pulses applied outside the slice (or outside the FOV or outside the imaging volume) flip the magnetization of flowing spins 90° into the transverse plane (Figure 8.5). Flowing spins then flow into the slice and receive an additional 90° RF pulse. The magnetization of flowing spins is therefore flipped an additional 90°. Therefore spins flowing into the slice or imaging volume are saturated because they have received both the 90° saturation pulse and the 90° excitation pulse (total 180°). Signal saturation from flowing spins occurs because no time is allowed for the recovery of magnetization. Given that

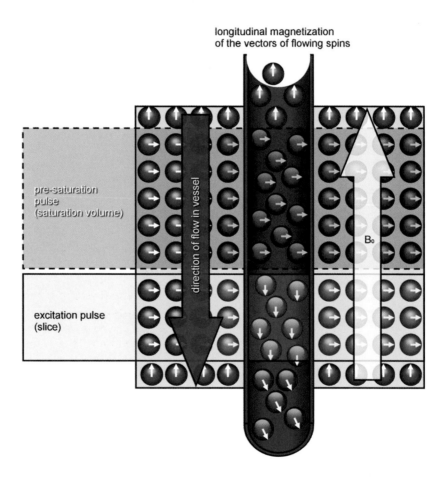

Figure 8.5 Spatial pre-saturation to produce black blood. Note that the magnetic moments of nuclei in the vessel (at the top of the illustration) are aligned with the magnetic field (B_o) along the Z axis. As the blood within the vessel flows down into the saturation volume or SAT band they receive a 90° RF pulse and their NMVs enter the transverse (XY plane). As the blood continues to flow down (into the slice) the nuclei receive yet another 90° RF pulse. Note that the the magnetic moments of the nuclei are now aligned 180° from their original position (at the top of the image). At this point (and with no time to recover) the nuclei within the blood within the slice, are saturated (and appear black on the image).

flowing blood in vessels should appear black, persistent signal within vessel lumen after the application of SAT pulses indicates slow flow, a blood clot or vascular occlusion.

Bright blood imaging

Vascular structures can also be visualized by making vessels appear hyper-intense rather than hypo-intense. Several techniques can be used to enhance the signal from flowing blood in MRI, including gradient echo pulse sequences, imaging options such as gradient moment rephasing (also known as gradient moment nulling, GMN) and contrast enhancement.

In gradient echo sequences, flowing blood appears bright, enabling visualization of the vessel relative to surrounding tissues. To detect signal acquired with gradient echo acquisitions, nuclei must receive at least one RF excitation pulse, followed by gradient rephasing. The excitation pulse can be a 90° RF pulse or a different flip angle (depending on the desired image contrast). The RF excitation pulse is slice selective but gradient is applied to the entire imaging volume. Therefore flowing spins are refocused irrespective of their position within the imaging volume and return a high signal.

Imagine blood flowing within a vessel, such as the abdominal aorta. If an axial slice is acquired through the liver, all spins within the slice receive the 90° excitation pulse. The spins within flowing blood in the aorta are moving perpendicularly through the axial slice and will also receive this excitation pulse. The gradient rephasing pulse is then applied to the entire imaging volume. This will cause all of the flowing spins to produce signal, providing they have been excited at some point in time. As an example, a spin may have been located in slice 1 when the excitation pulse was applied, but will still emit signal if rephased by the gradient as it passes through slice 10. As a result, this technique can be referred to as **bright blood imaging** (Figure 8.6)

In addition to conventional gradient imaging, there is a technique that uses a steady state free precession sequence in combination with balanced gradient system (*see* Balanced gradient echo in Chapter 5). The utilization of this balanced gradient technique yields a net phase shift of zero within the spins. Balanced gradient echo images are acquired with a very short TR and TE. In fact, the TE is generally half the TR value. For example, if the TR is 8 ms then the TE is 4 ms (depending on the gradient capabilities of the imaging system). A steady state acquisition yields image contrast that is weighted to T2/T1. Tissues with a high T2/T1 ratio (in stationary and/or moving fluids such as CSF and blood) appear bright. Balanced sequences are used for cardiac imaging (Figure 8.7), for MR cholangiopancreatography (MRCP), MR myelography and for the evaluation of the internal auditory canals (IACs) (*see* Figures 5.40 and 5.41).

Gradient echo imaging can be further improved by the application of an imaging option known as gradient moment nulling (GMN) or gradient moment rephasing (GMR) (*see* Chapter 6). GMN is generally considered to be a first order velocity compensation technique used to refocus moving spins, and hence visualize slow-moving protons. Even though moving protons (associated with flowing venous blood or flowing CSF) are not 'perfectly' first order motion, they tend to respond to this imaging option. The response is that the moving spins are rephased along with stationary spins, reducing intra-voxel dephasing. GMN complements flow by making vessels (containing slow-flowing spins) appear bright and therefore enhancing the signal from flowing blood and CSF.

GMN is widely used in the brain, body (chest and abdomen) and extremities, and for the myelographic effect of CSF in T2 weighted images of the spine. There are, however, several trade-offs for using gradient moment rephasing. One such trade-off is that it requires a longer minimum TE due to the use of additional gradients, and results in a reduction in the number of slices available. Another trade-off is that gradient moment rephasing is not particularly effective on rapid flow (such as arterial flow within the chest or abdomen). However, GMN is helpful for the visualization of slow flow found in these areas.

can assist in the reduction of swallowing, and hence motion artefacts. Pulsation artefacts can be reduced by timing the acquisition to the cardiac cycle. This technique is known as gating and will be discussed later in the chapter.

To overcome the limited coverage provided by 3D TOF-MRA, one can either acquire images in another plane or combine a number of 3D acquisitions in a technique known as MOTSA. This combines a number of high-resolution 3D acquisitions to produce an image that has good resolution and a large area of coverage. Venetian blind artefacts associated with MOTSA can be reduced by selecting an appropriate slab overlap, ensuring that each slab is not too thick, and by the use of mathematical image processing algorithms.

MRA image reformation

The manner in which the data from MRA images are reformatted plays a large part in determining the way in which vascular anatomy is perceived in the images. Several techniques are used, including **maximum intensity projection (MIP)** and shaded surface display (SSD). Each technique has its benefits and caveats. MIP results in a reformatted image that appears to be projected onto a 2D surface. There is no depth cueing, and the observer may find it difficult to appreciate which vessels are to the foreground and which vessels lie behind. Shaded surface display improves 3D perception of the data by using a formula from the world of 3D computer graphics known as Phong's formula. This technique segments the data using edge detection; in simple terms a boundary between a high and low signal area is treated as a surface. This surface is then presented on the reformatted data as though illuminated by a directional light source. The benefit of this is that structures appear to be solid and those vessels closer to the observer's point of view appear to lie in front of the structures behind.

As the name suggests, maximum intensity projection simply assigns a numerical value to each pixel in terms of its grey-scale and then projects the maximum intensity from each row or column within every slice onto a two-dimensional plane. This allows the data to be viewed as though from different angles, and in the case of inflow angiography this tends to be at right angles to the acquisition plane. This relates to the fact that inflow studies require the slices to be perpendicular to the vessel for reasons mentioned earlier in the chapter. In this instance the slice thickness affects the spatial resolution of the reformatted image, and this is the principal reason for the use of 3D, rather than 2D inflow techniques.

The resulting projection is orthographic due to the fact that the data used to reconstruct the image are in parallel rows and columns. The resulting lack of perspective tends to obscure any sense of depth, but this can be partially offset by reconstructing the data from different angles. By reformatting each image with an incremental change in angle, the resulting images can be run as a cine loop. This allows for a more three-dimensional visualization of the data (Figures 8.11, 8.12 and 8.13).

Phase contrast MRA

The vascular signal produced in phase contrast MRA (PC-MRA) relies on velocity induced phase shifts. This means that the vascular enhancement seen in PC-MRA is related to the change in phase of flowing blood. Phase shift is related to the blood flow velocity, flow direction and the

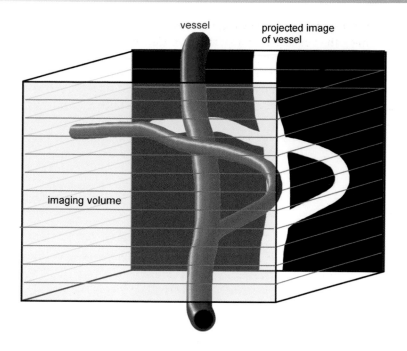

Figure 8.11   MIP reformatting, with a 'projection' of the vessel displayed. After the mathematical MIP process is complete (Figure 8.12), an image of the vessel is produced.

type of scan acquired. Therefore, PC-MRA provides information about vascular anatomy, flow velocity, multidirectional blood flow and flow direction. Blood flow velocity is related to the type of vessel, the size of the vessel, pathology within the vessel and physiologic conditions (such as the phase of the cardiac cycle). The changes in the velocity of blood flow cause phase shift to occur.

Phase shifts can also be generated in the pulse sequence by the application of additional gradient pulses. PC-MRA uses a gradient echo pulse sequence with small flip angles and additional gradient pulses to create changes in the phases of the nuclei within flowing blood. The gradient pulses used in PC-MRA are bipolar gradient pulses. Bipolar gradients include pulses with two lobes that are equal in strength: one negative gradient pulse and one positive gradient pulse. Although bipolar gradient pulses are applied to *all* of the tissues within the volume, application of bipolar gradient pulses allows for the distinction between stationary tissues and spins within flowing blood.

Bipolar gradients are applied in multiple 'steps'. The first step is to apply a positive lobe followed by a negative lobe (Figure 8.16). The next step is to apply a negative lobe followed by a positive lobe. During initial application of the first bipolar gradient there is a shift of phases of stationary and flowing spins (both are affected equally). The bipolar gradient is then applied with opposite polarity (or direction) but at the same strength (or amplitude). So that the same variants occur in phase contrast MRA, contrast is obtained between moving and stationary tissue by manipulating the phase position of the spins. A gradient echo sequence is used, having a small flip angle to prevent saturation, and an additional bipolar gradient known as a velocity encoding gradient or VENC.

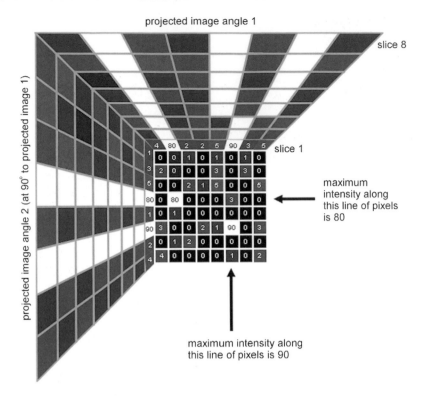

Figure 8.12 MIP reformatting. The maximum intensity projection ascertains the maximum intensity in each row or column of pixels and assigns this value to a pixel in a projected plane. In the diagram there are two such planes representing an anterior and lateral projection of the data. Note that due to the orthogonal nature of the projected image, there is no diagnostic value in having more than 180° of rotation as any further images would be perfectly symmetrical copies of their 180° counterparts.

The purpose of the VENC is to cause a greater phase shift in moving spins than in stationary spins. This relies on the fact that stationary spins will momentarily become phase-advanced (or phase-retarded) as their precessional frequency is affected by the first lobe of the VENC but importantly will be restored to their original phase position by the equal and opposite second lobe.

Moving spins on the other hand will have changed their position between the applications of the first and second lobes, and will not experience an equal and opposite second lobe. The result will be an data set where the stationary spins may be at the 12 o'clock phase position while the moving spins are at 6 o'clock.

The entire procedure requires several data acquisitions in order to sensitize flow in all three orthogonal directions, and create a flow-compensated data set for digital subtraction.

Gradient moment nulling is used during acquisition of the subtraction mask, resulting in a data set in which the moving spins have the same phase position as the stationary background spins. When this mask is digitally subtracted from the flow sensitized data, an image is created in which only the moving spins are visualized.

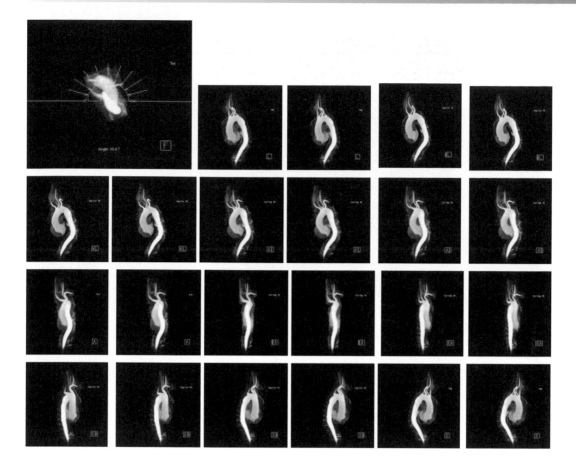

Figure 8.13   These images were post processed with 'radial' MIP. In this case there are 24 images reformatted in 15° increments between images. This provides a 180° degree rotation of the vasculature.

Velocity encoding (VENC)

The strength and duration of the velocity encoding gradient pulse is selected based on the blood flow velocity that is to be imaged. The unit used in VENC settings is centimeters per second (cm/s) and should be selected to produce signal from blood flowing at that velocity. For example, to evaluate slow flow in venous structures where blood flows at 10 cm/s low VENC settings of 10 cm/s are selected. To evaluate high velocity flow in arterial structures where blood flows 80 cm/s high VENC settings of 80 cm/s are selected. Generally, medium VENC settings of 50 cm/s are commonly used to evaluate both arterial and venous flow (Figure 8.15).

VENC settings determine the amplitude and/or duration of the bipolar gradient pulses. When arterial blood flow is to be imaged (flow has high velocity) a high VENC is required. Although this does not seem obvious, high VENC uses low amplitude gradient pulses, and vice-versa. To understand this concept, imagine the phases of flowing spins in both fast and slow flow when a phase shift of 45° is desired. In fast-flowing blood, spins travel rapidly along the gradient, so the gradient need only be shallow (low amplitude) to achieve this degree of shift. Conversely, in slow flow, a

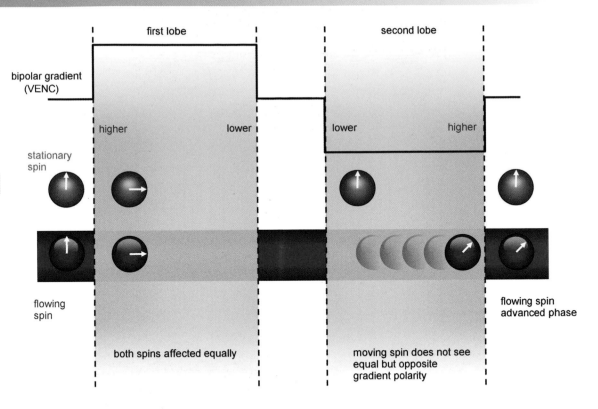

280

Figure 8.14   Bipolar gradients in PC-MRA demonstrating blood flowing through a vessel before the bipolar gradient pulse, during the positive lobe and during the negative lobe. Note the phase changes during the application of these gradient pulses.

high gradient amplitude is required to achieve the same degree of phase shift. Consider now a spin in a slow flowing vessel (Figure 8.15).

If the VENC selected is lower than the velocity of blood flow within the vessel, aliasing can occur. This results in low signal intensity in the center of the vessel, but better delineation of the vessel wall itself. Aliasing occurs because in laminar flow the viscosity of blood results in drag, or friction, against the vessel wall. This means that the highest velocity of flow is found in the center of the vessel, and the signal is aliased or mis-mapped out of the vessel lumen. However, even though there is signal void within the vessel lumen, there is better delineation of the vessel wall above background noise levels. Conversely, with high VENC settings, intraluminal signal is improved but vessel wall delineation is compromised (Figure 8.16).

Flow encoding axes

Sensitization to flow is obtained along the direction of the applied bipolar gradient. If the bipolar gradient pulses are applied along the Z-axis, phase shifts are induced in blood flowing from superior to inferior or vice versa, so sensitizing the PC-MRA to flow that runs from head to foot. Since flow can occur in other directions (known as multidirectional flow), bipolar gradients are applied

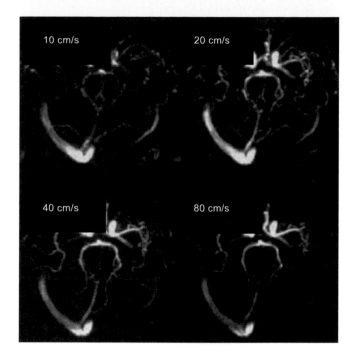

Low VENC

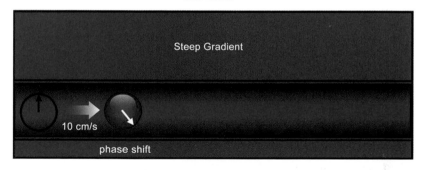

High VENC

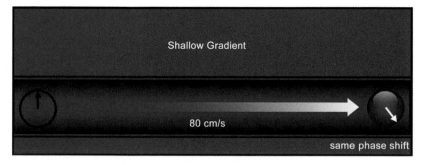

Figure 8.15   These images were acquired with PC-MRA with various velocity encoding (VENC) settings (10, 20, 40 and 80 cm/s). Note that the images acquired with low VENC settings (10 cm/s) demonstrate vessels with slower flow velocities (venous structures). Images acquired with higher VENC settings (80 cm/s) demonstrate vessels with higher flow velocities (arterial) vasculature in the Circle of Willis). Although it seems backwards, high VENC uses bipolar gradient pulses with low amplitudes and vice versa.

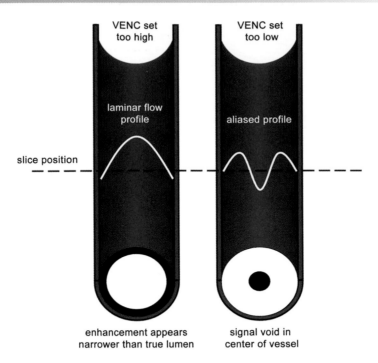

Figure 8.16 The results of inaccurate VENC settings. On the left, the VENC was set higher than the velocity of the blood flowing within the vessel. Due to the laminar flow profile of the high velocity blood flow, the signal from flowing blood results in an image whereby the vessel 'appears' smaller than its actual diameter. When the VENC setting is too low, aliasing can occur rendering images with intraluminal signal void in the center of the vessel (right-hand image).

in all three dimensions, and in doing so sensitize flow in all directions X, Y and Z (Figures 8.17 and 8.18). These are known as **flow encoding axes**. However, an increase in the number of flow encoding axes also increases the imaging time (as images are acquired without bipolar gradients (first acquisition), with the application of gradients in the 'Z' direction (second acquisition), with the application of gradients in the 'Y' direction (third acquisition) and with the application of gradients in the 'X' direction (fourth acquisition)).

One of the benefits of PC-MRA is its ability to evaluate multidirectional blood flow (unlike TOF-MRA, which can only visualize flow that is perpendicular to the slice plane). If the evaluation of blood flowing from head to feet (or feet to head) is required, gradients are applied along the Z-axis. If the evaluation of blood flowing from right to left (or left to right) is required, gradients are applied along the X-axis. If the evaluation of blood flowing from anterior to posterior (or posterior to anterior) is required, gradients are applied along the Y-axis. If the evaluation of multidirectional blood flow is required, bipolar gradients are applied in all three directions (Z, Y and X).

An advantage of phase contrast MRA is that the the technique allows the creation of two types of image – known as *magnitude* and *phase* images.

Magnitude images look much like other MRA images with high signal vessels and a suppressed background, phase images on the other hand have a somewhat pixelated noisy-looking back-

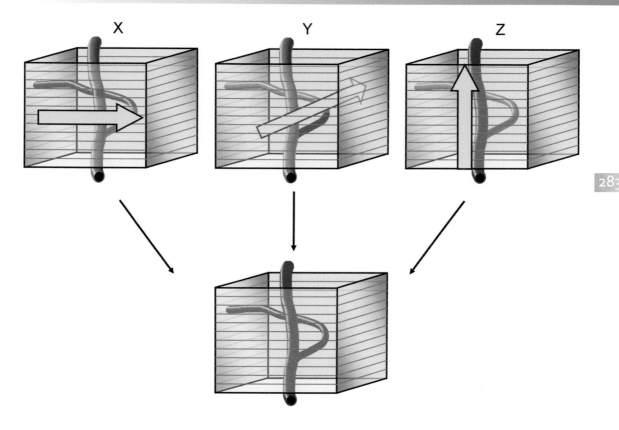

Figure 8.17 Flow encoding axes, where gradients are applied along the X, Y and Z axes. If all three encoding axes are selected, multidirectional flow is demonstrated.

ground but are able to show direction of flow. Flow that is in the same direction as the VENC looks white whereas flow in the opposite direction looks black.

2D and 3D PC-MRA

PC-MRA sequences have the ability to evaluate vasculature with blood flow in multiple directions and with varying flow velocities. In addition, PC-MRA can be acquired with the use of either 2D or 3D acquisition strategies. 3D offers SNR and spatial resolution superior to 2D imaging strategies, and the ability to reformat in a number of imaging planes retrospectively.

Three-dimensional, phase contrast MR angiography (3D PC-MRA) acquisitions are generally acquired for smaller vessels, and multidirectional vascular information such as flow velocity and flow direction is required. Examples include the evaluation of arteriovenous malformation (AVM) and intracranial aneurysms. The trade-off, however, is that in 3D PC-MRA, imaging time increases with the TR, NEX, the number of phase encoding steps, the number of slices and the number of flow encoding axes selected. For this reason, scan times can approach 15 min or more.

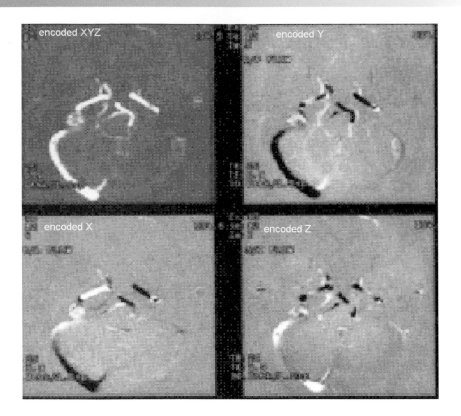

Figure 8.18 Images acquired with PC-MRA encoded with various flow encoding axes. The top left image is known as a magnitude image and was encoded in all three orthogonal axes. The upper right and the bottom images are phase images, and were encoded along one axis. The upper right image was encoded along the Y-axis (anterior to posterior). On this upper right image, blood that is flowing from anterior to posterior (along the encoding direction) appears bright and blood flowing posterior to anterior (against the encoding direction) appears black, on 'phase images'. The lower left image was encoded along the X-axis (right to left). On this lower left image, blood that is flowing from right to left (along the encoding direction) appears bright and blood flowing left to right (against the encoding direction) appears black, on 'phase images'. The lower right image was encoded along the Z-axis (superior to inferior). On this lower right image, blood that is flowing from superior to inferior (along the encoding direction) appears bright and blood flowing inferior to superior (against the encoding direction) appears black, on 'phase images'.

Two-dimensional, phase contrast MR angiography (2D PC-MRA) techniques provide flow direction information, flow velocity and multidirectional flow in acceptable imaging times (1–3 min). If a 2D PC-MRA acquisition has been flow encoded from superior to inferior, blood flowing from the head to the feet appears white, while flow from the feet appears black. For example, for the evaluation of possible sagittal sinus thrombosis, the superior sagittal sinus could be imaged with 2D PC and encoded along one single direction. For imaging of the superior sagittal sinus with 2D

PC-MRA sequences, images can be encoded anterior to posterior. 2D acquisitions, however, are generally acquired with lower resolution than 3D acquisitions and cannot be reformatted and viewed in other imaging planes.

Parameters and clinical suggestions for PC-MRA

When flow velocity, multidirectional flow and flow direction must be evaluated, PC-MRA should be considered. For this reason, PC-MRA can be used effectively in the evaluation of arteriovenous malformations (AVMs), aneurysms, venous occlusions, congenital abnormalities and traumatic intracranial vascular injuries. 3D volume acquisitions can be used to evaluate intracranial vasculature (Figure 8.19). Suggested parameters are:

- 28 slices volume, with 1 mm slice thickness
- flip angle   20° (if a 60-slice volume is selected, flip angle is reduced to 15°)
- TR   less than or equal to 25 ms
- VENC   40 to 60 cm/s
- flow encoding in all directions.

2D techniques offer more acceptable imaging times of approximately 1–3 min. For intracranial applications of 2D PC-MRA suggested parameters are:

- TR   18–20 ms
- flip angle   20°
- slices thickness   20–60 mm
- VENCs   20–30 cm/s for venous flow
                              40–60 cm/s for higher velocity with some aliasing
                              60–80 cm/s to determine velocity and flow direction.

For carotids 2D PC-MRA parameters include:

- flip angles   20–30°
- TR   20 ms
- VENCs   40–60 cm/s for better morphology with aliasing
                              60–80 cm/s for quantitative velocity and directional information.

Velocity encoding techniques

Velocity encoding techniques are designed to evaluate flow velocity and direction providing information similar to Doppler ultrasound. The projection plane is located at right angles to the excitation plane. Essentially, this technique does not produce images, but rather 'blips' like on an ECG tracing. The location of vascular 'blips' on the projection plane shows flow direction (blip up represents arterial flow and blip down represents venous flow) and the length of the projection (or height of the 'blip') defines the velocity of flow. High 'blips' represent arterial flow (high flow

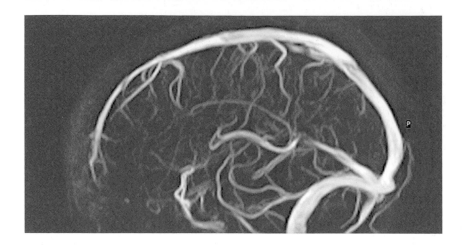

286

Figure 8.19   Sagittal PC-MRA image of the superior sagittal sinus. This image was acquired with 3D PC with encoding along all three axes (X, Y and Z).

Advantages of PC-MRA

- Sensitivity to a variety of vascular velocities (can evaluate blood flow velocity)
- Sensitivity to flow within the FOV (can evaluate multidirectional blood flow)
- Reduced intra-voxel dephasing
- Increased background suppression
- Magnitude and phase images (can evaluate flow direction)

Disadvantages of PC-MRA

- Long imaging times in 3D
- More sensitive to turbulence

velocity) and lower 'blips' represent venous flow (low flow velocity). These velocity encoding techniques are not commonly utilized, but deserve brief mention.

Contrast enhanced MRA

TOF and PC-MRA have become the standard for the evaluation of vascular structures of the head. However, there are a number of disadvantages associated with TOF-MRA and PC-MRA, particularly for vascular structures of the body. Caveats for body MRA (with TOF-MRA and/or PC-MRA) include motion artefact and the potential signal loss in vascular structures due to in-plane flow. For this reason, the standard for the evaluation of vessels within the neck, body (chest, abdomen and pelvis) and peripheral vascular system is contrast enhanced MRA (CE-MRA). Contrast enhanced MRA uses T1 3D gradient echo, followed by a bolus injection of gadolinium and dynamic imaging.

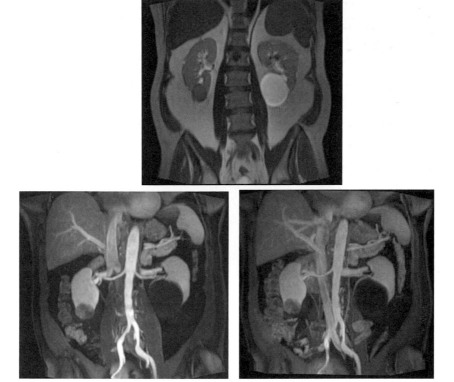

Figure 8.20 Coronal CE-MRA images of the abdomen acquired before (top) and after (bottom) contrast administration. The image on the bottom left is the arterial phase and the image on the bottom right is acquired after that (intermediate or cortico-venous phase).

Images are acquired before, during and after injection and/or timed to the arterial, intermediate and venous phases of the vascular cycle (Figure 8.20). Technical considerations for enhanced MRA include:

- protocol parameters.
- injection method
- contrast type and dosage
- scan timing.

Parameters and options for CE-MRA

For CE-MRA acquisitions, parameters are selected to reduce signal from stationary tissues in acceptable imaging times, then gadolinium is administered to enhance signal from blood flow. Optimal CE-MRA acquisitions require both high spatial resolution (small voxels) and high temporal resolution (rapid imaging times). Unfortunately, high spatial resolution and high temporal resolution are mutually exclusive. For example, images acquired with high spatial resolution generally require longer scan times (for optimal SNR, CNR and image quality) (*see* Chapter 4). Fast imaging techniques are generally acquired at the 'expense' of resolution. In an attempt to acquire images with high spatial resolution in acceptable imaging times, CE-MRAs are acquired with fast, 3D T1 gradient echo sequences during breath-hold, dynamically during contrast administration. TRs are selected for fast scan times and combined with appropriate flip angles to saturate the signals from stationary tissues (much like TOF-MRA sequences) thereby maximizing T1 contrast. TEs are selected as short as possible to reduce intra-voxel dephasing and minimize T2 contrast. Intra-voxel dephasing renders images with suboptimal signal within vascular structures. Another method for reducing intra-voxel dephasing is the use of small voxels (small FOV, thin slice thickness, high matrix). CE-MRA images acquired with small voxels also yield high spatial resolution. Although high-resolution images are required for the visualization of smaller vessels, they generally have lower SNR. For this reason, appropriate RF coil selection is essential. Generally multi-coil arrays are used for contrast enhanced MRA of the body.

The scan plane for CE-MRA is selected relative to the vascular anatomy to be imaged. It is advantageous to acquire images in the plane that best covers the anatomy. For example, to adequately cover the aortic arch the sagittal (or sagittal oblique) plane is optimal. The coronal plane is better for the evaluation of the pulmonary arteries, renal arteries, the abdominal aorta and the peripheral vascular system.

Injection method for CE-MRA

Although hand injection is possible, bolus injections of gadolinium (Gd) during CE-MRA acquisitions are generally administered using a power injector. Power injectors provide an accurate 'bolus' injection, consistency among injection rates (for patients who require follow-up examinations) and the ability to complete CE-MRA procedures with one technologist.

Contrast type and dosage

The recommended dosage of Gd is 0.1 millimoles per kilogram (mmol/kg) of body weight (0.2 ml/kg or approximately 0.1 ml/lb). Several specific agents have been approved for up to 0.3 mmol/kg or three times the dose compared with the majority of Gd agents. Many facilities use a double dose of Gd or a higher relaxivity agent for CE-MRA imaging. For example, a 100 lb (45.5 kg) patient would receive 9.1 ml of gadolinium as a standard dose. In this case, a double dose of 18.2 ml (or an estimated dose of 20 ml) could be considered appropriate for vascular imaging. It is also recommended to follow the contrast injection with a rapid bolus of saline.

Scan timing

Timing is essential for optimal CE-MRA imaging. In fact, to optimize the visualization of vascular structures, scan timing should be such that the center of K space is filling while the contrast fills the vessels of interest. CE-MRA images acquired too soon after injection could yield images without the visualization of Gd contrast and images acquired too late will provide images of the venous structures (not arteries). Therefore, scan time and K space filling (normal, linear, centric, spiral) should be considered for determining accurate delay times (*see* Chapter 3 for more on K space). For example, if scan time is 30 s and centric K space filling is used, the scan delay is 30 s and imaging can begin immediately after injection.

There are several options for the optimization of scan timing, including test bolus, bolus tracking and 'fluoro' triggering. Automated methods of determining scan delays include scan options such as bolus tracking (where a tracker pulse is positioned to measure signal from within the lumen of the aorta, and which initializes the scan when the increased signal from contrast is detected) and/ or fluoro triggering which uses a navigator-type acquisition having a high temporal resolution. Images are displayed in real time allowing the operator to witness the arrival of the contrast agent bolus in the vessel of interest and manually initiate the main MRA acquisition. These options can provide accurate scan delays for CE-MRAs. Another method for determining scan timing is with the use of a test bolus. With the test bolus method, a small injection of 1 or 2 ml of Gd is injected and scans are repeated in intervals to detect the exact time to begin scanning. In this case the technologist notes the time when the contrast reaches the vessels of interest and scans accordingly.

CE-MRA images can be post-processed (like TOF-MRAs) with either MIP or SSD techniques. Even with post-processed MIP images, the background suppression on CE-MRA acquisitions can be suboptimal. To visualize contrast enhanced MRA images without obstruction of background tissues, subtraction techniques can be used. This technique takes the image acquired without contrast, and 'subtracts' the image from that acquired during contrast enhancement. The resultant image demonstrates vascular signal free from background signal (Figure 8.21).

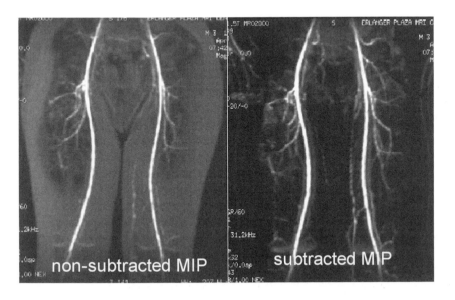

Figure 8.21   Images acquired with 3D T1 gradient echo CE-MRA that have been post-processed with MIP technique. The image on the left is the un-subtracted MIP image and the image on the right is the subtracted MIP image. Note that the visualization of the vasculature and the background suppression is optimized by the subtraction technique.

Magnetic resonance angiography summary

The information provided by PC-MRA and TOF-MRA differs from that of conventional contrast angiography as MRA produces a flow-sensitive image rather than a morphological image. Consequently, clinical situations that require hemodynamic information are more suited to MRA than those requiring fine anatomic detail. Using MRA, laminar flow can be clearly imaged. However, as turbulent flow contains dispersion velocities that result in dephasing within a voxel, a loss of signal intensity results. In many respects, information provided by MRA is a combination of the flow information obtained in a Doppler ultrasound examination and the morphological information contained in conventional contrast angiography. This is especially true when PC-MRA and TOF-MRA are used in combination with velocity encoding techniques.

Cardiac MRI

Cardiac anatomy

Cardiac imaging poses a number of imaging challenges including motion and the position of the heart within the chest cavity. Motion consists of periodic, physiologic motion (such as pulsatile heart motion, vascular motion and respiratory motion) and aperiodic motion (such as patient motion and gastric motion). The relative position of the heart is in a 'double-oblique' position within the chest. For these reasons, cardiac imaging can be challenging, even for the seasoned technologist, radiographer, radiologist or even the cardiologist.

The heart is a triangular-shaped organ that is positioned such that the triangle is 'upside down' within the chest. The 'base' of the heart is located superiorly and the 'apex' inferiorly. Generally, we define the word 'base' as it refers to the bottom of a structure, and the apex as the top. In this case, however, the terms (apex and base) are used to describe a 'triangle'. In geometry, the flat portion of the triangle is the base and the 'point' the apex.

The heart contains four chambers, including two atria and two ventricles, separated by septae. The atria are located superiorly, posterior and toward the right, and the ventricles are located inferiorly and toward the left. The base of the triangle contains the right and left atria (separated by the atrial septum) and the apex contains the right and left ventricles (separated by the ventricular septum). In addition to its unusual shape, the heart is located in a 'double oblique' orientation within the chest cavity. The oblique position of the cardiac muscle renders it oblique 'P–A' (posterior to anterior), oblique 'L–R' (left to right) and oblique 'S–I' (superior to inferior). The most inferior chamber of the heart is the left ventricle (LV) and the most superior chamber is the right ventricle (RV). The RV is located superior, towards the posterior of the chest and slanted to the right.

Imaging planes for cardiac MRI

To properly evaluate the heart, images should be acquired in planes that are relative to the heart itself, and not to the chest. For example, an axial view of the thorax or chest will not produce an image that is axial to the plane of the heart muscle and chambers. Therefore, to evaluate the heart multi-oblique images are required. These views (or planes) demonstrate the chambers of the heart in profile and include short axis view (axial to the plane of the heart), long axis or two-chamber view (sagittal to the plane of the heart) and four-chamber view (coronal to the plane of the heart). To scan at right angles to the heart itself, multiple obliques are selected. If the system does not allow for multiple oblique imaging (acquired automatically) these sequences can be prescribed manually. Once the short axis image is acquired, two-chamber and four-chamber views can be prescribed. Two-chamber views are acquired where the slices are selected parallel to the inter-ventricular septum. Four-chamber views are acquired where the slices are selected perpendicular to the inter-ventricular septum.

Imaging options for cardiac MRI

Cardiac imaging poses a number of imaging challenges including motion and heart position. Although scan planes can be orientated so that they are axial, sagittal and coronal to the plane of the heart, periodic, physiologic motion and aperiodic motion still play a significant role in the degradation of image quality on cardiac MR images. To image the heart and great vessels specifically, motion during cardiac activity must be compensated for if good quality images are to be obtained. A compensation technique known as cardiac gating can be used to reduce the unwanted artefacts caused by physiologic motion. To visualize the cardiac anatomy and vasculature accurately, it is essential that cardiac images are acquired with cardiac gating. Improper gating produces poor image quality.

Cardiac gating

Cardiac gating is a method that reduces motion artefact in cardiac MR images caused by the phase mis-mapping produced as a result of heart motion and pulsatile blood flow. It uses the electrical signal of the heart, or the mechanical flow of the vascular bed, to trigger each pulse sequence (Figure 8.23). Two methods are used.

- *Electrocardiogram* (ECG, EKG) gating uses electrodes and lead wires placed on to the patient's chest to detect the electrical activity of the heart.
- *Peripheral gating* uses a photo-sensor placed on the patient's finger to detect a pulse in the capillary bed.

The ECG

The ECG is acquired by measuring the voltage difference between two (three or four) electrodes attached to the patient's chest (known as ECG leads). Most systems color code the electrodes so that they can be placed correctly on the patient. The red and the white electrodes are usually placed at the level of the heart to measure the voltage difference between two points. The green electrode is the ground, and should be placed near to (but not touching) either the red or the white electrode. Electrodes and suggested positioning can vary by vendor. Be sure to review the system requirement and recommendations to avoid potential patient burns. The ECG consists of:

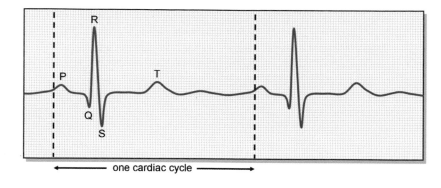

Figure 8.22   The ECG.

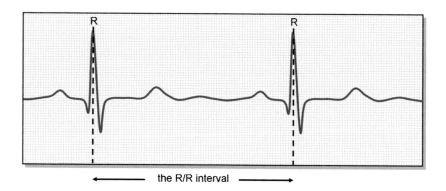

Figure 8.23   The R to R interval and hence the *effective* TR on cardiac gated images.

- a P wave that represents atrial systole (contraction)
- a QRS complex that represents ventricular systole
- a T wave that represents ventricular diastole (relaxation) (Figure 8.22).

When cardiac gating is utilized, the RF pulse (and hence the pulse sequence) is initiated by the R wave. The peak of the R wave is used to initiate (trigger) each pulse sequence, because electrically it has the greatest amplitude (Figure 8.23). This technique is known as prospective gating. Prospective means that the scan is timed to, and triggered from, the beats of the heart during the acquisition. Prospective gating is the technique that occurs during image acquisition, as opposed to retrospective gating. Retrospective gating (performed during many cardiac ciné acquisitions) acquires image data and times to the cardiac cycle during reconstruction (after the scan acquisition – retrospectively).

The effective TR

As cardiac gating uses each R wave to trigger the pulse sequence, the TR depends entirely on the time interval between each R wave. This is called the **R to R interval** and is controlled by the patient's heart rate (Figure 8.23). If a patient has a fast rate, the RR interval is shorter than if the patient has a slow heart rate. Since the scan is initiated by the R wave the time between the R waves is the TR. Therefore, the TR, and hence the image weighting and number of slices, depends *totally* on the heart rate. The TR is now termed 'effective' as the heart rate is not perfectly constant and varies from one heartbeat to another.

For example, if the heart rate is 60 beats per minute then:

$$R \text{ to } R \text{ interval} = 60\,000\,ms \div 60 = 1000\,ms.$$

(There are 60 seconds per minute and 1000 milliseconds per second or 1 heartbeat every second.)

$$R \text{ to } R \text{ interval} = 1\,s \text{ or } 1000\,ms, \text{ and } TR = 1000 \text{ ms.}$$

If the patient's heart rate is 120 beats per minute then:

$$R \text{ to } R \text{ interval} = 0.5\,s \text{ or } 500\,ms, \text{ and } TR = 500\,ms.$$

With prospective cardiac gating, gating can be restrictive in terms of weighting (TR) and slice number. To a certain extent this is true, in that there is no control of the R to R interval itself. In some patients the effective TR is 500 ms and in others the TR is more than 1000 ms, which reduces the T1 weighting considerably. This has to be tolerated when using prospective cardiac gating techniques as a penalty for producing images with reduced cardiac motion artefact.

Obtaining T2 weighted images can be more troublesome, but most systems use a method where every second or third R wave can be used as a trigger. In this way, the effective TR is lengthened (long effective TR) so that saturation (and therefore T1 weighting) does not prevail, and proton density (short TE) and T2 (long TE) images can be obtained.

For example, if the heart rate is 60 beats per minute, the R to R interval is 1000 ms:

½ R to R selected effective TR = 500 ms
1 R to R selected effective TR = 1000 ms
2 R to R selected effective TR = 2000 ms
3 R to R selected effective TR = 3000 ms.

To achieve T1 weighting images that are acquired with cardiac gating, trigger occurs with each R wave ($1 \times RR$). In the example above ($1 \times RR$), selection yields images with ($1 \times 1000\,ms$) = 1000 ms R to R interval, hence 1000 ms TR.

For a shorter TR value, some vendors allow for the option of ($\frac{1}{2} \times RR$). In the example above, where the patient's heart rate is 60 beats per minute, the result would be:

heart rate = 60 beats per minute
60 s to the minute
1 s = 1000 ms
1 s between R waves
R to R interval = 1 s
R to R interval = 1000 ms
($\frac{1}{2} \times RR$) or ($\frac{1}{2} \times 1000\,ms$)
effective TR = 500 ms

For proton density and T2 weighting, every second ($2 \times RR$) or third ($3 \times RR$) R wave is used to trigger, resulting in an effective TR of 2000–3000 ms.

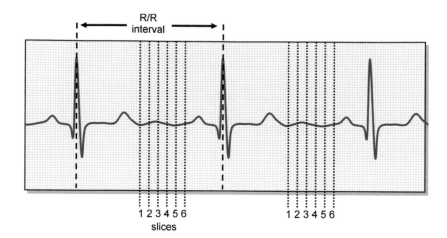

Figure 8.24 An ECG gated sequence where six slices are acquired, with each slice location acquired at the same 'phase' of the cardiac cycle. For example, each phase encoding step for slice 1 is acquired just after the T wave. For this reason, every phase encoding step will be acquired at the same time during the cardiac cycle (after the T wave). The resultant image will appear as if the heart was stationary, frozen in that particular phase.

Slice acquisition

The slices are acquired during the effective TR in the same way as in conventional imaging. As TR increases the number of available slices increases. Phase encoding data from each slice are acquired during the R to R interval. During the next interval data from another phase encoding step are acquired (Figure 8.24). This is repeated until the acquisition of data (or all the phase encoding steps) for each slice is complete. Data from each slice are always acquired when the heart is at the same phase of cardiac activity. In other words, slice 1 is always acquired when the heart is at a certain position in its cycle, and so are slices 2, 3, etc. In this way, the motion artefact of each slice is reduced.

This of course, only applies if the patient's heart rate remains perfectly constant throughout the scan. If the heart rate changes at all, data are obtained at different times during the cardiac cycle and image quality suffers. Even in healthy patients, there are mild variations in the heart rate that occur periodically. Most patients' heart rates do not remain 'perfectly' constant, but fluctuate due to anxiety and/or the gradient noise during the sequence.

To compensate for this, certain safeguards are built in to the effective TR so that gating is more efficient. These safeguards are waiting periods around each R wave. Many imaging systems automatically build these waiting periods into the pulse sequences. Others provide these as user-selectable parameters. These two waiting periods are known as the trigger window and the delay after trigger (or trigger delay).

The trigger window

The waiting period before each R wave is often called the trigger window. This is a time delay, usually expressed as a percentage of the total R to R interval, where the system stops scanning and waits for the next R wave (Figure 8.25).

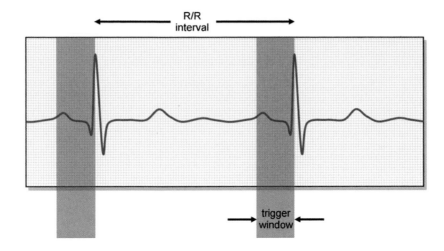

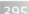

Figure 8.25 A trigger window within an ECG tracing. If the trigger window is set at 10%, the actual delay is 1000 ms (effective TR) minus 10% and the resultant time for slice acquisition is 900 ms. This is known as the available imaging time (AIT).

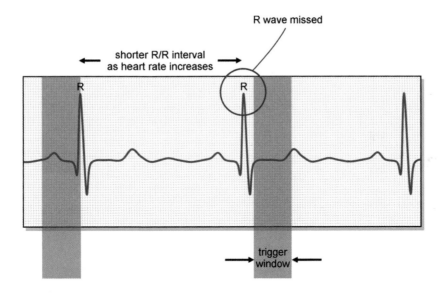

Figure 8.26 An ECG gated sequence in which the R wave was missed during image acquisition. A missed R wave occurs, in this case, as the heart rate increases.

This delay allows for the fact that the patient's heart rate may increase during the scan, moving the R wave nearer to the beginning of the window. If the system has stopped scanning and is waiting for the next R wave, it triggers the pulse sequence, regardless of whether the R wave is occurring sooner than expected. If the heart rate speeds up even more, so that the R wave occurs while the system is still acquiring data, the R wave is missed and the effective TR suddenly lengthens (Figure 8.26).

Sometimes the patient falls asleep during image acquisition. When the patient sleeps the heart rate often slows down so that the R wave moves further away from the beginning of the window. However the system is still waiting to trigger the scan and does so when it detects the next R wave. The effective TR is lengthened but the R wave is not missed (Figure 8.27).

The trigger window is usually expressed as a percentage of the R to R interval. Clearly, the correct window must be selected so that any increase in the heart rate is compensated for. Selecting a very large window, however, reduces the amount of time available to acquire slices, and so a balance is required. In practice, most patients' heart rates vary by about 10% during the scan, so selecting a window of about 10–20% compensates adequately for any variations in the heart rate and still allows a reasonable number of slices to be acquired (Figure 8.28). In patients

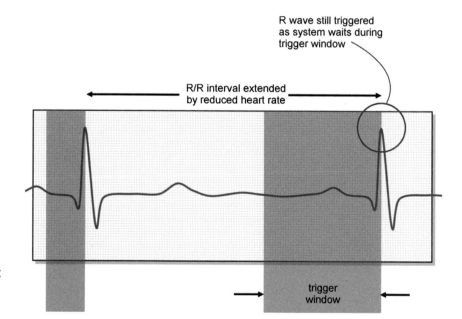

Figure 8.27 The R wave is not missed at the heart rate decreases.

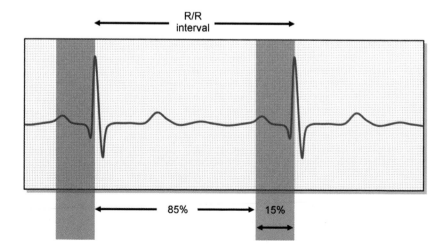

Figure 8.28 What would the trigger window be if the R to R interval was 1000 ms?

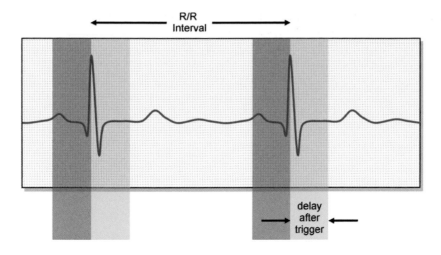

Figure 8.29   The waiting period known as delay after trigger.

with known arrhythmias, an increase in trigger window (up to 25%) will allow for the optimization of gated images in arrhythmic patients.

The trigger delay

The waiting period after each R wave is often termed the delay after trigger or trigger delay. There is always a slight hardware delay between the system detecting the R wave and transmitting RF to excite the first slice. This is usually in the order of a few milliseconds. This period can often be extended, however, to delay the acquisition of the slices until the heart is in diastole and is therefore relatively still (Figure 8.29).

The available imaging time

The available imaging time is the time available to acquire slices. It is defined as the effective TR minus the trigger window and the delay after trigger.

$$\text{available imaging time} = \text{R to R interval} - (\text{trigger window} + \text{trigger delay})$$

If the R to R interval is 1000 ms, the trigger window 10% and the trigger delay 100 ms, the time available to acquire the data is:

$$1000\,\text{ms} - 100\,\text{ms} - 100\,\text{ms} = 800\,\text{ms}.$$

The available imaging time is *not* the effective TR. The effective TR is the time between the excitation of slice 1 in the first R to R interval, to its excitation in the second R to R interval. The available imaging time is purely the time allowed to collect data, and governs the number of slices that can be obtained (Figure 8.30).

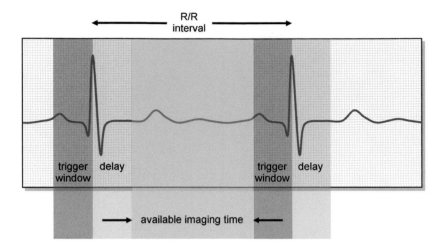

Figure 8.30   The available imaging time.

Peripheral gating

Peripheral gating works in exactly the same way as ECG gating. A photo-sensor attached to the patient's finger detects the increase in blood volume in the capillary bed during systole. This in turn, affects the amount of light reflected back to the sensor and a wave form is obtained. The peaks of the waves are now termed the R waves, but these represent the peripheral pulse that occurs approximately 250 ms after the R wave of the ECG. The trigger window, trigger delay and available imaging time still apply.

Parameters used in gating

T1 weighting:

- short TE
- 1 R to R interval.

PD/T2 weighting:

- short TE (PD)/long TE (T2)
- 2 or 3 R to R intervals.

Safety aspects of gating

The electrodes used in gating are attached to cables that are conductors and are therefore capable of carrying relatively high currents. The cables lie within the high intensity region of the gradient field and RF fields applied during image acquisition. As a result, currents may be induced in the cables, which can potentially store and transfer heat to the patient. It is therefore possible to burn or blister the patient if strict safety rules are not adhered to.

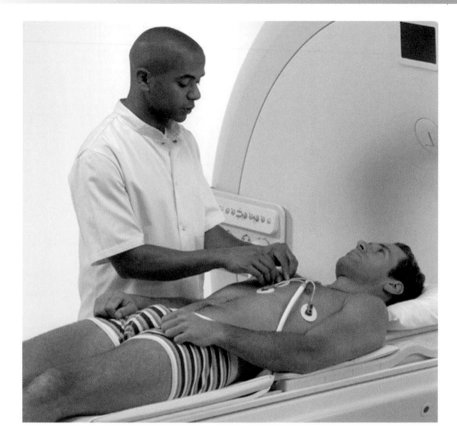

Figure 8.31   Suggested placement of gating leads for a particular gating system.

Always check the cables and electrodes for damage. If they are frayed or splitting, do not use them under any circumstances. When positioning the cables avoid looping or crossing them over. The point of cross-over creates extra heat that could burn through the insulating material of the cable. When positioning the patient within the bore of the magnet, make sure that the cables do not touch either the patient or the bore of the magnet. Running the cables down the center of the patient avoids contact with the bore, and placing pads between the cables and the patient prevents possible injury (Figure 8.31). For safety information regarding coils and cables *see* Chapter 10.

The uses of gating

Gating is useful when imaging any area that contains pulsatile flow or the heart itself. This includes the chest and great vessels, the abdomen, the spinal cord (CSF pulsations) and the brain. Virtually any area where pulsatile motion degrades the image lends itself to gating of some sort. The decision to use ECG or peripheral gating is often difficult. ECG gating is more time-consuming because of the electrode placement, and because arrhythmias can alter the ECG to such an extent that the system cannot detect an adequate R wave. These difficulties are usually not present with peripheral gating, but this is not adequate when imaging the heart itself. Generally, peripheral gating is adequate for the brain, spine and vessels away from the heart. ECG gating should be used for the heart itself.

Gating is a rather lengthy process as the scan time is determined by the patient's heart rate (among other things). Usually there is no control over the TR, weighting or slice number when using gating. Gating is relatively time-consuming, especially if the heart rate is slow. For this reason, a patient with bradycardia poses a challenge in MRI because scan times are very long. Gating in patients with bradycardia will result in longer R to R intervals and hence longer effective TRs and longer scan times. For this reason, many sites reserve gating for cardiac and/or chest imaging only.

Pseudo-gating

ECG gating requires electrode and lead placement on the patient to reduce the effects of motion so that anatomy can be well demonstrated and images are artefact free. Pseudo-gating is a very simple method of gating that involves selecting a TR that matches the R to R interval. ECG and peripheral gating is not required for pseudo-gating. Instead, the patient's heart rate is measured by taking the pulse prior to the examination. The R to R interval is then calculated and the corresponding TR is selected. As long as the heart rate does not significantly change during image acquisition (as it would if the patient anxiety level increases and/or the patient falls asleep), data from each slice is acquired at exactly the same time during the cardiac cycle as in conventional gating. This technique may be useful when conventional gating fails due to a poor ECG signal or low peripheral pulse. However, to be most effective, the heart rate must remain unaltered during the examination.

Gating is essential when studying the anatomy and pathology of the heart and great vessels. This technique allows for the acquisition of cardiac images for the evaluation of anatomic and pathologic information. However, it is possible to acquire images of the heart for functional information as well. A study of heart function requires multiple images (at the same slice location) acquired at multiple phases of the cardiac cycle. This can be achieved using multiphase imaging or ciné acquisitions.

Multiphase cardiac imaging

Figure 8.22 demonstrates a typical ECG tracing. When scans are timed to the cardiac cycle, the motion artefact from physiologic cardiac motion is reduced. This is known as single phase, prospective gating. Gated (single phase) images are acquired to reduce motion artefacts for the evaluation of anatomy and pathology of the heart. Multiphase cardiac images can be acquired for the evaluation of physiology or function. In multiphase imaging, images are acquired at a given location during each phase of the cardiac cycle. For example, in Figure 8.22, there could be images acquired at the same slice location and up to seven phases of the cardiac cycle. Multiphase images can be 'played' as a ciné acquisition for the evaluation of heart beating. Examples of multiphase functional images are demonstrated.

The multiphase images can be performed with either single-slice or multi-slice acquisition techniques. In multi-slice acquisition, the first slice location is acquired in each of four phases of the cardiac cycle. This is then repeated at the other slice locations. All of the images acquired at each slice location can be played in a 'loop' so that they may be viewed rapidly one after the other, like a ciné acquisition (a movie). In this way, cardiac wall motion can be visualized and cardiac function evaluated. One drawback is that the imaging time increases with the number of slice locations and/or phases imaged. For example, a 2-minute spin echo acquisition, acquired

Table 8.1   Multiphase imaging with spin echo compared with ciné acquisitions acquired with gradient echoes.

Multiphase imaging – gradient echo	Multiphase imaging – spin echo
Ciné with retrospective gating	SE with prospective gating
Requires ECG leads	Requires ECG leads
Uses a method of collecting data continuously throughout all phases of the cardiac cycle	Uses a method where scan acquisitions are timed to and triggered by the R wave – prospectively
Phases are post processed, after the scan – retrospectively	Data from each slice location can be acquired at different phases of the cardiac cycle
GE – blood flow yields bright signal	SE – blood flow yields dark signal

with four slice locations, with four phases results in a 32-minute scan. By today's standard, this is an unacceptable scan time.

Ciné

Multiphase images can be acquired for the evaluation of cardiac wall motion and heart function (functional imaging). Multiphase spin echo acquisitions have already been discussed. Another method, for the evaluation of heart function is with gradient echo ciné acquisitions. Most cardiac ciné acquisitions are acquired with a gradient echo sequence with retrospective gating techniques. ECG or peripheral gating must be used, but data collection is continuous (and separated later, retrospectively, into images displaying various cardiac phases) not triggered. The ECG is purely used to determine the phase of the cardiac cycle for reconstruction into multiple phases. After the gradient echo acquisition the system can sort the data and reconstruct the images across the whole of the cardiac cycle. Ciné acquisitions are usually performed with gradient echo sequences, where flowing blood appears bright. Both prospective and retrospective gating produce images that can be 'played' in a ciné loop (or a movie). This enables the visualization of moving myocardium, and hence heart function. The two functional techniques are compared in Table 8.1.

Table 8.1 compares typical combinations of multiphase techniques. Bear in mind, however, that it is possible to acquire gradient echo ciné acquisitions with prospective gating. It is also possible to acquire spin echo multiphase acquisitions with retrospective gating.

Parameters used in ciné

Good contrast between the vessel to be imaged and the surrounding tissue is needed for optimal ciné. T2* weighted coherent gradient echo sequences are used so that blood or CSF appears bright. Gradient echo sequences are flow sensitive, because gradient reversal is not slice selective (as in spin echo). Therefore, a flowing nucleus produces signal after gradient rephasing regardless of its slice location during excitation (see Chapter 6). Using a pulse sequence that employs coherent transverse magnetization in conjunction with the steady state maximizes T2* weighting. A short TR (in the order of 40 ms) in conjunction with flip angles of 30–45° should be selected to maintain the steady state.

Using a short TR ensures that the stationary spins within the slice become saturated or beaten down by rapid successive RF pulses, while the flowing spins enter the slices relatively fresh. This saturates the background stationary tissue and enhances the brightness of the flowing nuclei. The TE should be relatively long to enhance T2* weighting (about 20 ms), and the use of gradient moment rephasing maximizes contrast even further. Some systems also permit ciné acquisitions with incoherent gradient echo sequences. These can be used to give T1 weighted ciné images. To optimize vascular contrast, however, use:

- coherent gradient echo sequences
- TR   less than 50 ms
- flip angles   30–45° (to maintain the steady state and saturate stationary nuclei)
- TE   15–25 ms (to maximize T2)
- gradient moment rephasing (to enhance bright blood).

Data collection

During retrospective gating, image data are collected from each slice at a certain interval across the cardiac cycle. The R to R interval and the effective TR for each slice determines how many times (phases of the cardiac cycle) these data can be collected during each cardiac cycle. Each individual ciné image could be acquired (evenly spaced) between the R to R interval. In addition, the number of phases of the cardiac cycle required to make up the ciné loop can be selected.

In Figure 8.32 there is an example of the following scenario. If 16 phases are selected each slice must demonstrate 16 different positions of the heart in one cardiac cycle (compared with four phases in multiphase imaging). In this case, four slice locations are acquired, each at four phases, for a total of 16 images. If these images are acquired evenly spaced across the R to R interval, then images should be acquired at specific time points. In this example, the TR is 50 ms. To evenly space the phase acquisitions, the 16 phases/images are acquired evenly spaced in the R to R interval of 1000 ms.

$$\text{heart rate} = 60 \text{ beats per minute}$$

$$\text{R to R interval} = 1000 \text{ ms}$$

$$TR = 50 \text{ ms}$$

$$\text{slice interval} = 1000 \text{ ms} \div 16 \text{ phases} = 62.5 \text{ ms})$$

The first image/phase would be acquired at 62.5 ms, then 125 ms, 187.5 ms, 250 ms and so on, in 62.5 ms intervals. To do this accurately, the collection of data must correlate as much as possible to each cardiac phase (Figure 8.32). Each data point must coincide with each cardiac phase. If a desired phase of the cardiac cycle is to be reconstructed, optimal image reconstruction can be achieved if data are collected at that time. If the system cannot match the data points and the phases, it takes some data from one point and some from another to form the image at a certain phase position. In the above example, if a 100 ms image is desired, data from the 62.5 ms image would be combined with data from the 125 ms image to interpolate an image at 100 ms. Under these circumstances, ciné is not as efficient as is could be (Figure 8.33).

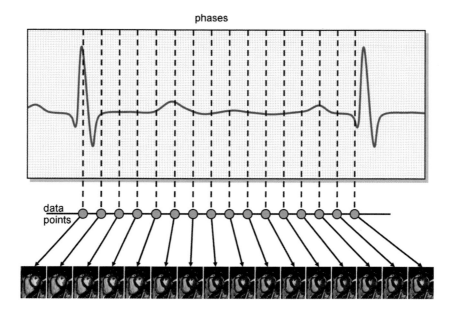

Figure 8.32 Data acquisition in cine imaging. Ciné acquisitions acquired with four slice locations at four phases, so a total of 16 images are acquired.

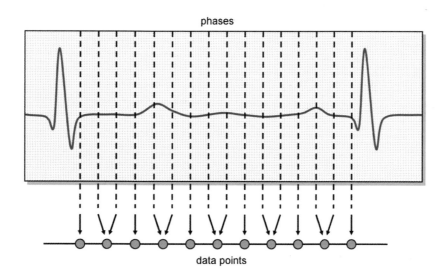

Figure 8.33 When a particular image is desired and image data for that time point has not been acquired, interpolation of nearby data points are used. This results in mismatching of the data points.

In this example, if a given ciné sequence is acquired with a TR of 25 ms and the patient's heart rate is 60 beats per minute, there is the potential for 40 phases to be acquired. In this example 1000 ms R to R interval is divided by the 25 ms TR, allowing for 40 evenly spaced phases to be acquired, at the exact time points during the cardiac cycle.

This is analogous to frames per second, but in ciné it refers to the number of phases per cardiac cycle. Currently, ciné acquisitions are capable of producing sequences with 64 phases of the cardiac cycle. As the number of phases increases, the temporal resolution increases. Improved temporal resolution is increased with the number of phases

In practice, therefore, it is important to calculate how many data points the system can collect for a given R to R interval, and ensure that the number of phases selected does not exceed this. The number of data points can be calculated by dividing the R to R interval by the effective TR. In ciné, the effective TR for each slice is the TR selected multiplied by the number of slices prescribed.

For example, if a TR of 40 ms is selected and two slices are prescribed, the effective TR is 80 ms. The effective TR in ciné is therefore very different from that used in gating, and the two should not be confused. In gating, the TR is not selectable as it is determined by the R to R interval. Although gating is used in ciné, the data are collected across the whole of the cardiac cycle and a TR is selectable. The ECG trace is purely used by the system to measure the cardiac cycle, not to trigger the pulse sequence.

The effective TR of each slice in ciné imaging is the time between the collections of data for each slice. The number of data points collected is therefore determined by this and by the R to R interval of each cardiac cycle. If the effective TR is 80 ms and the R to R interval is 800 ms, 10 data points can be collected during each cardiac cycle. To ciné efficiently, the number of cardiac phases reconstructed should not exceed 10 in this example.

The uses of ciné

Ciné is useful for dynamic imaging of vessels and CSF. For example, ciné can evaluate aortic dissection and cardiac function. In the brain, it may be useful to demonstrate dynamically the flow of CSF in patients with hydrocephalus.

SPAMM

In addition to the classic cardiac imaging techniques there are new advances currently used in research. One of these techniques is known as spatial modulation of magnetization (SPAMM). SPAMM modulates the magnetization thus creating a saturation effect on the image. This effect can be seen on the image, appearing as cross-hatching of stripes. SPAMM is used in association with a multi-slice multiphase acquisition and acquires data along the short axis of the left ventricle. In normal hearts, the stripes move along with the cardiac muscle. However, in cases of infarction, the infarcted area does not contract along with the normal muscle and can therefore be easily identified in relation to the stripes (Figure 8.34).

Cardiac and vascular imaging can be a useful tool in the evaluation of a whole host of clinical situations. However, there are many logistical drawbacks. Motion artefact is a constant problem and patient co-operation is essential. In addition, radiographer education is a fundamental necessity if consistently diagnostic cardiac and vascular images are to be obtained. The quality and applications of cardiac MRI have increased with the use of EPI sequences and software options

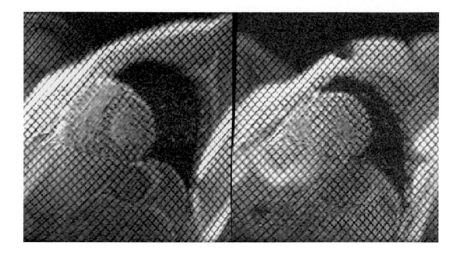

Figure 8.34   These images were acquired with SPAMM tagging, normal (left) and hypertrophic cardiomyopathy (right).

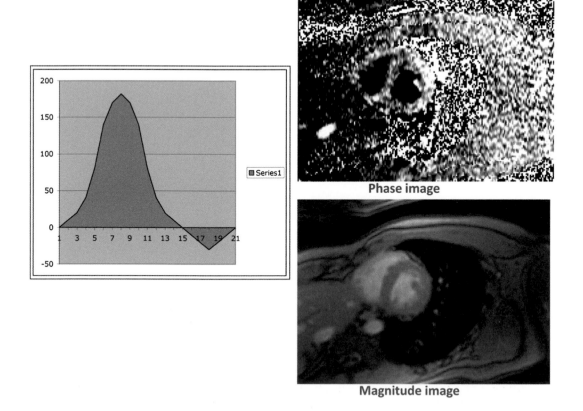

Phase image

Magnitude image

Figure 8.35   This dataset is acquired with phase (upper image) and magnitude (lower) imaging. The graph demonstrates phase changes.

that allow rapid filling of K space (*see* Chapters 3 and 5). In addition to magnitude imaging, phase imaging has become a useful tool for the evaluation of the cardiovascular system (Figure 8.35).

 For questions and answers on this topic please visit the supporting companion website for this book: www.wiley.com/go/ mriinpractice

9

Instrumentation and equipment

Introduction

Several processes must be completed to produce magnetic resonance images, including image acquisition and image formation. To complete these processes a number of system components are required, including hardware (instrumentation or equipment) and software programs (pulse sequences and image formation programs). The processes include nuclear alignment, radio frequency excitation, spatial encoding and image formation, and the hardware required to complete such processes includes:

- a magnet – for nuclear alignment
- a radio frequency source – for RF excitation
- a magnetic field gradient system – for spatial encoding
- a computer system – for the image formation process and the user interface
- an image processor – to convert 'signals' into images.

The magnet aligns the nuclei into low-energy (parallel) and high-energy (anti-parallel) states (*see* Chapter 1). The stronger the magnet, the more spins in the low-energy state. The more low-energy spins the greater the spin excess, the higher the signal and hence the better the image quality (*see* Chapter 4). To maintain magnetic evenness or homogeneity, a shim system is necessary. The more homogeneous the magnetic field, the better the image quality. A radio frequency (RF) source

MRI in Practice, Fourth Edition. Catherine Westbrook, Carolyn Kaut Roth, John Talbot.
© 2011 Blackwell Publishing Ltd. Published 2011 by Blackwell Publishing Ltd.

perturbs or excites nuclei. The RF system requires a transmitter and a receiver. To achieve resonance the frequency of the RF excitation pulse must be similar to the precessional frequency of
the magnetic moments of the nuclei in the slice (*see* Chapter 1). Magnetic field gradients determine spatial location of RF signals (*see* Chapter 3). The MR signal is changed to an understandable
format from a FID into a spectrum by a series of mathematical equations known as Fourier trans-
formations. This process occurs via the array processor. The signals from the array processor are
then converted into shades of gray, represented as pixels in the MR image. This process occurs in
the image processor. The host computer oversees the process and allows a means for operator
interface with the system (Figure 9.1). This chapter discusses magnetic resonance instrumentation
in more detail. First, however, magnetism and magnetic properties in general are described, as
this helps to understand different magnet types.

308

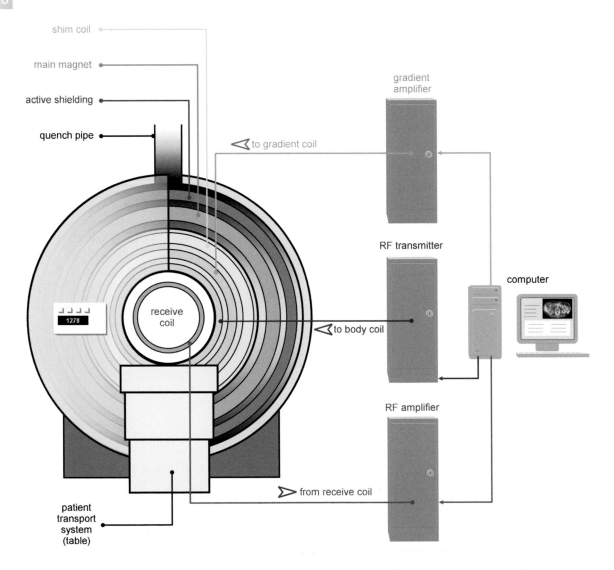

Figure 9.1   The closed bore MRI scanner in axial cross section reveals the principal components
to be arranged in concentric circles, most of these being solenoid electromagnets.

Magnetism

Like the mass and electrical charge of a particular substance, **magnetism** is a fundamental property of matter. All substances will interact with an applied magnetic field, even those that one might consider non-magnetic. The way that materials behave in the presence of an external magnetic field is determined by a property known as *magnetic susceptibility*.

Magnetic susceptibility

The word susceptibility refers to how easily something can be influenced by an external factor. For example, someone who is susceptible to hypnotism can be easily hypnotized. In the context of MRI this translates into a concept whereby materials that are susceptible to magnetism can be readily magnetized. As you might imagine, there is a spectrum here, including materials that cannot be magnetized, and even those that actively repel an external magnetic field.

The degree of magnetism exhibited by a substance is related to a property known as the atomic magnetic dipole (or moment). These dipoles are generated in an atom by the movement of electrons. In the classical model of the atom, electrons exhibit two principal kinds of movement – an orbital motion around the nucleus and a spinning motion around their own axes. The law of electromagnetic induction indicates that whenever a charged particle such as an electron exhibits motion, a corresponding magnetic field is induced (*see* Chapter 1). The net magnetic moment of an atom is a combination of the magnetic moments of all the electrons present.

Electrons present in the energy shells of atoms can be described as 'spin-up' or 'spin-down', depending on the direction in which they spin. Typically there are equal numbers of each type in a fully filled electron shell. The opposing polarities of these electrons will cancel out leaving no net magnetic moment. In certain atoms with partially filled shells there will be unpaired electrons, the presence of which will create a net magnetic effect in the atom.

The magnetic behavior of an atom is therefore dictated by the configuration of the orbiting electrons. Elements can be classified as belonging to one of four main categories, depending on their electron configuration. In increasing order of magnetic strength these categories are:

- diamagnetism
- paramagnetism
- superparamagnetism
- ferromagnetism.

Diamagnetism

Diamagnetic materials have paired electrons. With no external magnetic field present, diamagnetic substances such as lead and copper show no net magnetic moment. This is due to the fact that the electron currents caused by their motions add to zero. However, when an external magnetic field is applied, diamagnetic substances show a small magnetic moment that opposes the applied field. Substances of this type are therefore not attracted to, but are slightly repelled by, the magnetic field. For this reason, diamagnetic substances have low negative magnetic susceptibilities and show a slight decrease in magnetic field strength within the sample (Figure 9.2). Examples of diamagnetic substances include bismuth, carbon (diamond), carbon (graphite), copper, mercury, lead and water.

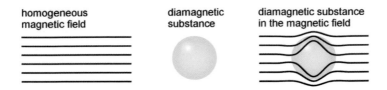

Figure 9.2   Diamagnetic materials in a homogeneous magnetic field.

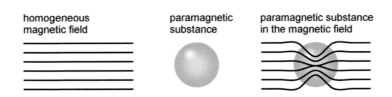

Figure 9.3   Paramagnetic materials in a homogeneous magnetic field.

Paramagnetism

Paramagnetic materials have unpaired electrons. As the result of unpaired electrons within the atom, paramagnetic substances have a small magnetic moment. With no external magnetic field, these magnetic moments occur in a random pattern and thus cancel each other out. However, in the presence of an external magnetic field, paramagnetic substances align with the direction of the field and so the magnetic moments add together (Figure 9.3). Therefore paramagnetic substances affect external magnetic fields in a positive way, by attraction to the field resulting in a local increase in the magnetic field. Paramagnetic substances have a low, positive susceptibility. Examples of paramagnetic materials include tungsten, cesium, aluminum, lithium, magnesium and sodium. Another more commonly known paramagnetic material is gadolinium chelates used as MR contrast agents.

Diamagnetic effects appear in all substances. However, in materials that possess both diamagnetic (low negative) and paramagnetic (low positive) properties, the positive paramagnetic effect is greater than the negative diamagnetic effect and therefore the substance appears paramagnetic. The apparent magnetization of an atom can be shown by the following equation:

$$B_0 = H_0(1+x)$$

where

B_0 is the magnetic field
H_0 is magnetic intensity.

A substance is diamagnetic when $x < 0$ (low negative). A substance is paramagnetic when $x > 0$ (low positive).

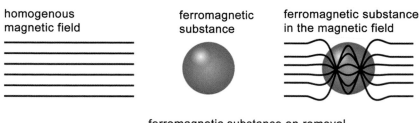

homogenous
magnetic field

ferromagnetic
substance

ferromagnetic substance
in the magnetic field

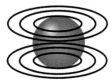

ferromagnetic substance on removal
from external magnetic field

Figure 9.4   Ferromagnetism.

Ferromagnetism

Ferromagnetic materials have half-filled electron shells. For this reason, ferromagnetic substances differ a great deal from diamagnetic and paramagnetic substances. When a ferromagnetic substance such as iron comes in contact with a magnetic field the results are strong attraction and alignment. Objects made of substances of this type can become dangerous projectiles when inadvertently brought near a strong magnetic field. Also, ferromagnetic materials retain their magnetization even when the external magnetic field has been removed. Therefore, ferromagnetic substances remain magnetic, are permanently magnetized and subsequently become **permanent magnets**. The magnetic field in permanent magnets can be hundreds or even thousands of times greater than the applied external magnetic field (Figure 9.4). So in comparison to diamagnetic (low negative susceptibility) and paramagnetic (low positive susceptibility) materials, ferromagnetic materials have a very high positive susceptibility. Examples of ferromagnetic materials include iron, steel and gadolinium when in its native state and below its curie temperature.

Superparamagnetism

Superparamagnetic materials have an intermediate positive magnetic susceptibility that is greater than that exhibited by paramagnetic materials (low positive) and less than that of ferromagnetic materials (high positive). Such substances include iron oxide particles, which can be used as T2 or T2* agents for MRI. Superparamagnetic materials have 'medium' positive susceptibility. Examples of superparamagnetic materials include iron oxide contrast agents.

Magnets

Once a ferromagnetic material is exposed to an external magnetic field it retains magnetization and therefore becomes magnetized. As this magnetic field remains in place when the external field is no longer present, it is known as a permanent magnet. Permanent magnets commonly have two poles, designated north and south. The magnetic field exerted by a permanent magnet produces magnetic field lines or lines of force running from the magnetic south to the north poles of the magnet. The magnetic field of the earth also illustrates this phenomenon, which can be demonstrated with the use of a compass. The magnetic needle of the compass aligns with the lines of force of the earth and points toward the magnetic North Pole.

The magnetic field strength is measured in one of two units: gauss (G), or tesla (T). The unit gauss is used to measure low field strengths. For example, the strength of the Earth's magnetic field is approximately 0.6 G (depending on one's location relative to the equator). In MRI, the gauss is the unit used to measure the fringe magnetic field that extends beyond the bore of the main magnet. The FDA limits the strength of the stray field, located in areas accessible by the general public, to 5 G. The tesla (T), on the other hand, is the unit used to measure higher magnetic field strengths. In MRI, the strength of the magnetic field within the bore is expressed in units of tesla. The units of measurement are related as follows:

$$1\,T = 10\,kG = 10\,000\,G.$$

Most clinical MR systems operate from as low as 0.2 T to as high as 4 T. There are also imaging systems used clinically known as ultra-low magnetic fields (0.01 T) and ultra high (10 T), but they are uncommon. About 85% of the clinical scanners used worldwide are 1.5 T. Until July 2004, the FDA limited clinical imaging in the USA to 2 T. As of July 2004, the Food and Drug Administration Criteria for Significant Risk Investigations of Magnetic Resonance Diagnostic Devices (FDA CDRH) increased to a limit of 4 T for infants up to one month of age and up to 8 T for any age above this. This has allowed for an increase in the development and clinical usage of high field systems (mainly 3 T at present).

The magnetic field generated inside an MRI scanner is not perfectly homogenous. Inhomogeneity within a particular magnetic field is expressed in an arbitrary unit known as parts per million (ppm). An inhomogeneity of 1 ppm in a 1 T magnet (where 1 T = 10 000 G) yields a range in field strength from 10000.00 G to 10000.01 G. Another way to express the amount of inhomogeneity is in Hz. In a 1.0 T scanner, a frequency of 42.57 MHz is used to achieve resonance (this was discussed in Chapter 1). As 42.57 MHz = 42.57 million Hertz, a 1 ppm inhomogeneity will result in a difference in frequency of 42.57 Hz (or one, one-millionth of the original frequency).

Now that various magnetic properties of matter have been described, different types of magnet (that can be used as MR imagers) will be discussed. These include:

- permanent magnets
- electromagnets (solenoid)
- resistive magnets
- superconducting magnets
- hybrid magnets.

Permanent magnets

Since ferromagnetic substances retain magnetism after being exposed to a magnetic field, these substances are used in the production of a **permanent magnet**. Examples of substances used are iron, cobalt and nickel. The most common material used to produce a permanent magnet is an alloy of aluminum, nickel and cobalt known as **alnico**. There are also some ceramic bricks possessing ferromagnetic properties that can be magnetized and used to produce permanent magnets.

The main advantage of permanent magnets is that they require no power supply or cryogenic cooling and are therefore relatively low in operating costs. In addition, the magnetic field created by a permanent magnet has lines of flux running vertically from the south to the north pole (bottom to the top) of the magnet, keeping the magnetic field virtually confined within the boundaries of the system (between the upper and lower magnetic plates) and hence well within the scan room (Figure 9.5). As a result, permanent magnet systems have almost no discernable fringe field. This means that they have fewer safety considerations with respect to fringe fields (that could cause projectiles in the MR scan room) compared to high field systems (*see* Chapter 10).

313

Siting for permanent magnet systems

As permanent systems have small fringe fields, they can usually be sited near public areas. However there can be problems associated with the weight of these systems. The weight of a

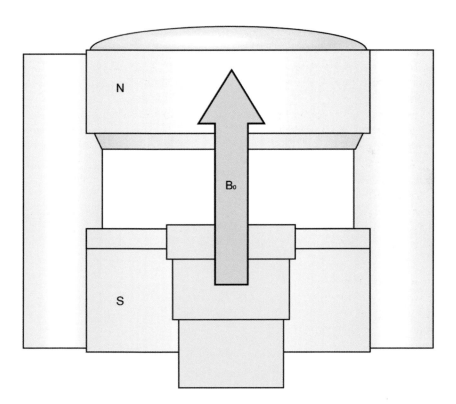

Figure 9.5   A permanent magnet. Note that the B$_o$, or static magnetic field, is vertical in this type of scanner.

permanent magnet can be on the order of 15 000 kg, as compared with some superconducting electromagnets that weigh 5000 kg. Magnet weights do vary by vendor and system configuration, and lighter configurations are being designed for both permanent and electromagnets.

Permanent magnet scanners are temperature sensitive, and to maintain homogeneity and image quality a constant temperature must be maintained. In fact, such is their sensitivity, the temperature fluctuation should not fluctuate by more than 1 kelvin for optimal operation of the permanent magnet MR system.

Permanent magnet systems are typically designed so that the magnetic plates are located above and below the patient, providing good all-round access. These are known as open MRI systems. Despite comparatively low field strengths and associated lower SNR, open systems have become popular for lower initial cost and lower operational costs when compared with high field electromagnets. In addition, there is a large patient population, including pediatric, claustrophobic and obese patients, that has difficulty with conventional 'tube-shaped', electromagnets. Finally, there are a variety of imaging procedures that require larger openings within the scanner to complete these procedures. These include, but are not limited to, kinematic musculoskeletal studies and interventional procedures, which are difficult in a closed configuration.

Although these permanent magnet systems appear to have an open configuration (side to side across the patient), the vertical opening (anterior to posterior in relation to the patient) can be as narrow as 48 cm in some systems. This is small compared with some closed configurations that have diameters of up to 70 cm. Also, not all systems with an open configuration are necessarily low field permanent magnets. In fact, there are a number of high field (1.0 T) superconducting systems with an open configuration.

Electromagnets

Michael Faraday's law of electromagnetic induction states: 'The induced electromotive force in a closed loop equals the negative of the time rate of change of magnetic flux through the loop.' Put simply, if one considers the variables of charge, motion, and magnetism, the interaction of any two of these variables will automatically result in the creation of the third. Therefore, if a current (or a moving charge) is passed through a long straight wire, a magnetic field is created around that wire (Figure 9.6). The strength of the resultant magnetic field is proportional to the amount of current moving through the wire. So, more current means a higher magnetic field strength. The magnetic field strength created by introducing current through a wire is calculated using the following equation:

$$B_0 = kI$$

where

I   is the current flowing through the wire
k   is the proportionality constant (quantity of charge on each body)
B_0 is the strength of the magnetic field.

Therefore the current passing along the wire is proportional to the magnetic field induced around it. The direction of the magnetic field induced can be expressed by the right-hand thumb rule.

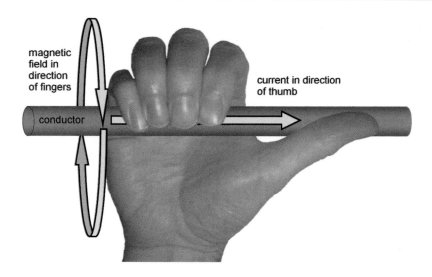

magnetic
field in
direction
of fingers

current in direction
of thumb

conductor

Figure 9.6   The right-hand thumb rule.

This rule states that if the fingers of the right hand are curled around a wire and the thumb points in the direction of the current, the fingers point in the direction of the magnetic field. In the case of a coil, the fingers represent the windings *and* the direction of the current, and the thumb represents the net magnetic field direction (Figure 9.6).

If current is passed through two parallel straight wires in opposing directions, the two magnetic fields tend to cancel each other out in the region between the two wires. Conversely, if the current passing along the parallel wires is flowing in the same direction, contributions to the resultant magnetic field are additive (the magnetic fields add). This property is exploited for the generation of large magnetic fields by using many current-carrying wires to create larger magnetic fields.

Solenoid electromagnets

To create a strong magnet, a number of current-carrying wires can be placed side by side. Instead of using several parallel wires, one wire can be wrapped around to form many loops (like a spring). The loops of wire form a coil and act as though they are parallel straight wires. This 'spring-like' electromagnet is called a **solenoid electromagnet**. In this case the strength of the magnetic field is determined by the amount of current passed through the wire, the number of loops in the spring and the distance between the loops (in addition to the temperature and other characteristics of the wire).

A factor that governs the efficiency of the passage of current is the inherent resistance of the coil. The degree of resistance along a wire is determined by **Ohm's law**. Ohm's law states:

$$V = IR$$

where

V is equal to the applied voltage (which for our purposes is constant)
I is the current
R is the resistance within the wire.

An electromagnet at room temperature is subject to Ohm's law and is said to be a **resistive magnet.**

Resistive magnets

The magnetic field strength in a resistive magnet depends on the current that passes through its coils of wire. The direction of the main magnetic field in a resistive magnet follows the right-hand thumb rule, and can be either horizontal or vertical depending on the configuration of the magnet. For example, if the loop of wire is configured such that the system produces magnetic field lines running from the head to the foot of the magnet (Figure 9.7), the direction of the field (B_0) is

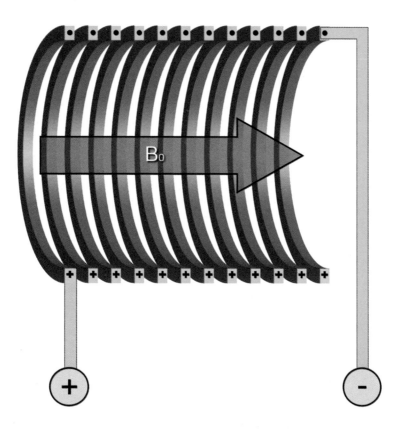

Figure 9.7   A simple electromagnet. Note that the direction of the static magnetic field B_0 is *horizontal* in this configuration. A closed-bore MRI system would typically feature two solenoids such as this, one at each end of the bore.

horizontal. The direction of B_0 in resistive systems can be either horizontal or vertical, depending on the orientation of the magnet coils.

The maximum field strength in a system of this type is less than 0.2 T or 0.3 T, due to the fact that any increase in magnetic field would require an increase in current. This would create more resistance in the windings which, in turn, would raise the temperature to a level that would ultimately destroy the electromagnet. The resistive system is unique in that the magnetic field associated with it can be turned off instantly at the flick of a switch (unlike permanent magnets and/or superconducting magnets). Depending on the orientation of the wires (and hence the direction of the magnetic field) there can be considerable stray magnetic field in horizontal B_0 systems but these are of lesser concern in vertical B_0 systems.

As a resistive system primarily consists of current-carrying loops of wire, it is lighter in weight than the large ferromagnetic pole-shoes used in a permanent magnet. Also, although its capital costs are comparatively low, the operational costs of the resistive magnet are quite high due to the large quantities of power required to maintain the magnetic field. To keep the magnetic field on, the power to the system must be on.

Superconducting electromagnets

As previously mentioned, many electromagnets are configured using wire in the shape of a coil. The current required to maintain a magnetic field in an electromagnet is significant and it can therefore be expensive to run. The reason for the high power requirement is that, in order to achieve a high field strength, a high current must be applied to the solenoid. Unfortunately conductors such as copper exhibit resistance to a flowing current due to vibrations in the molecular lattice and imperfections in the metal. As the resistance increases, the temperature of the conductor also increases, and this in turn causes more resistance. Picture an electric bar fire as an example of this process in action. Eventually a conductor such as this would be destroyed by the heat – the windings would oxidize or simply melt.

To get around this problem, and to allow the high current necessary to obtain a very high magnetic field, the coils are constructed from an alloy of niobium and titanium. This material exhibits a property known as **superconductivity** when cooled to below a certain critical temperature.

A superconductor has virtually zero resistance and will continue to carry a powerful electrical current indefinitely and without heating up.

When used to produce MR systems, the superconducting magnet produces relatively high magnetic field strengths with virtually no power requirements (after the magnetic field has been ramped up). With resistance virtually eliminated, no additional power input is required to maintain the high magnetic field strength.

Although the superconducting magnet has a relatively low operating cost, a system of this type is expensive to buy. However, the whole body superconducting system offers field strengths of 0.5 T (considered mid-field) to 3 T (considered high field) for clinical imaging. There are also systems operating as high as 14 T (considered ultra-high field) for research, spectroscopic and high-resolution studies. Higher-field imaging systems are available for research of specimens at even higher field strengths, but with bore sizes to accommodate test tubes and/or tiny specimens.

In the majority of high-field superconducting whole body scanners the direction of the main magnetic field runs horizontally. Horizontal field systems have B_0 that is along the bore of the scanner, from the head to the feet of the patient. Figure 9.8 shows a typical solenoid magnet, but note that in a MRI scanner, there are typically two solenoids to generate the main static field, one at each end of the magnet bore. There are further windings located along the length of the bore – known as bucking coils – to improve homogeneity. The entire structure is known as the *bobbin*.

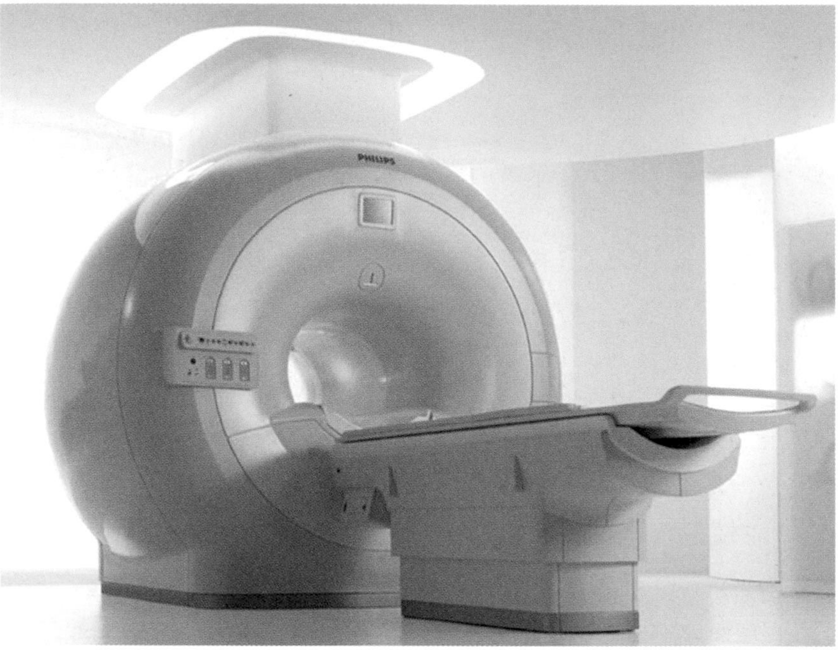

Figure 9.8   A superconducting system. With permission from Philips Medical.

Refer to animation 9.1 on the supporting companion website for this book: www.wiley.com/go/mriinpractice

The process of creating an electromagnetic field initially involves passing current through the main superconducting coil of the scanner. This process is called ramping up. When the scanner is delivered and fixed in place, the magnetic field is ramped up by the service engineer. The temperature at which the niobium-titanium wire becomes superconducting is 4 K (Kelvin) (approximately −269°C or −450°F). To maintain superconductivity the current-carrying loops of wire are super-cooled with substances known as **cryogens** to eliminate resistance. Cryogens used in MRI include liquid helium (He) and in some cases liquid nitrogen (N). Helium is used to create superconductivity and, if two cryogens are used, nitrogen is used to keep the helium cold. The superconductive loops of wire are submerged in the cryogen. Helium is an increasingly rare resource that is extracted from natural gas. There are only a handful of helium-rich sites on the planet. When this is coupled with the fact that liquid helium boils away to gas fairly quickly at room temperature it becomes apparent that MRI scanners must be able to contain the helium in such a way as to prevent it being lost to the atmosphere.

This is achieved by the use of a cryostat, a stainless-steel tank configured in the shape of a hollow cylinder. The inside of the cylinder contains layers known as heat shields, and the helium reservoir is isolated from the outer walls of the cryostat by an evacuated chamber.

Finally the entire structure is cooled by a refrigeration unit. These features reduce heat transfer by radiation, convection and conduction respectively. Modern cryostats also have a helium re-

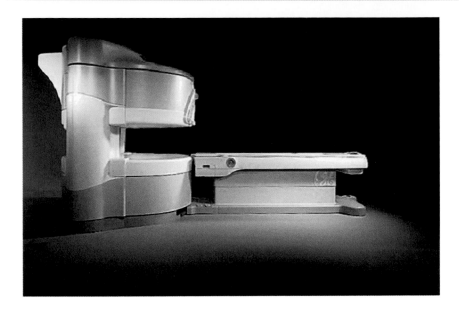

Figure 9.9   A high-field open system. Image courtesy of GE Medical Systems.

condenser that recycles any boil-off. This conserves the helium and negates the need for cryogen refills.

The prime safety concern related to helium gas is the fact that it displaces oxygen. There has been at least one recorded fatality attributed to breathing helium in the recent past, the cause of death being anoxia.

One liter of liquid helium produces 748 liters of helium gas when allowed to boil off. The capacity of an MRI cryostat varies with machine design, but a volume of 1500 liters would probably be a good average. In the event of a spontaneous helium boil-off over 1 000 000 liters of gas are liberated. This event is known as a quench (due to the fact that the magnetic field is rapidly stifled) and can be fairly explosive in nature. **Quenching** will be discussed in Chapter 10.

High-field open systems

Advances in technology have led to the production of high-field open MRI systems. These 1T systems give the advantage of a patient-friendly, spacious scan environment, coupled with the benefits of high-field scanning – high SNR and ideal T1 contrast. The scanner construction uses superconducting solenoid magnets above and below the patient, creating a vertical magnetic field (Figure 9.9).

Niche magnets

Since shortly after the inception of MR imaging, system manufacturers have tried to invent variations in system designs for specialty imaging concerns. These types of imager have become

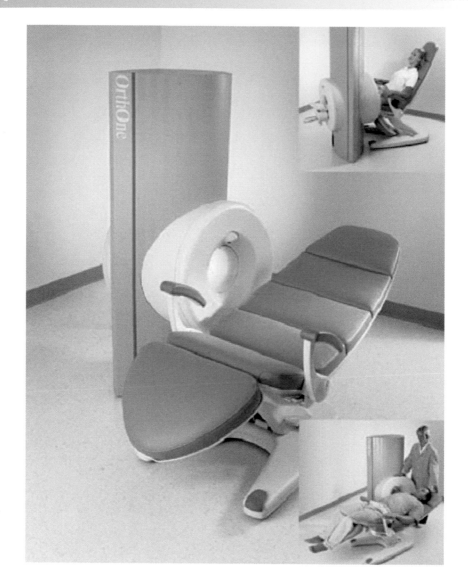

Figure 9.10   An example of a niche magnet for imaging extremities. This scanner is a high-field (1.0 T) superconducting imaging system. Image courtesy of ONI Medical Systems Inc, MA, USA.

known as niche magnets. For example, several imaging companies have developed ultra-low imaging systems and/or high-field magnets for orthopedic applications. Some of these operate at field strengths as low as 0.01 T and others as high as 1.0 T. (An example of a 1.0 T extremity system is shown in Figure 9.10.) In the ultra-low field (0.01 T) scanners, the field strength is very low and there are SNR restrictions. To improve SNR in low B_0 systems, trade-offs should be made in imaging parameters. Modification in imaging parameters (to increase SNR) often result in an increase in scan time. This is not the case in the high-field extremity systems. High-field (1.0 T) extremity scanners generally yield images with high SNR.

Summary

Permanent magnets

- remain magnetized permanently
- are usually open design where flux lines run vertically/static field B_o is vertical
- require no power supply
- low operational costs
- small fringe fields
- heavy
- low field strengths (SNR lower, usually longer scan times)

Resistive magnets

- field can be switched on or off as required
- flux lines horizontal or vertical/static field B_o can be horizontal or vertical
- on-going costs for the power supply
- larger fringe field

Superconducting magnets

- flux lines horizontal/static field B_o is horizontal
- lower power requirements
- expensive to buy
- high field strength (higher SNR/usually shorter scan times)

Fringe fields

The static magnetic field has no respect for the confines of conventional walls, floors or ceilings. The stray magnetic field outside the bore of the magnet is known as the stray field or **fringe field.** An illustration of this concept is shown in the next chapter, in Figure 10.2. To some extent all magnets have a fringe field. The field associated with a permanent magnet is relatively low, but in un-shielded high-field electromagnets the fringe field can extend over an area of many metres. These fringe fields must therefore be taken into account when siting a magnet, so that they do not extend into areas where potential projectiles (ferromagnetic metal objects), potentially contraindicated patients, monitoring devices and other mechanical and magnetically activated devices are present.

Magnetic shielding

Magnetic shielding can significantly reduce the area affected by the fringe field. There are two methods of magnetic shielding – passive and active. Generally speaking active shielding implies current/activity, whereas passive shielding implies no current/passivity. Current standards state that shielding must restrict the fringe field to a limit of 5 G within the scan room (walls, floor and ceiling).

Passive shielding is accomplished by surrounding the magnet (or lining the magnet room) with steel plates. This method is both expensive and inconvenient. Passive shielding can weigh up to 40 tonnes, necessitating a ground floor magnet room with specially prepared foundations. Passive shielding is therefore only used when absolutely necessary – to maintain the fringe field of ultra-high-field MRI systems such as 7T research scanners. This is facilitated by the construction of a thick-slabbed steel arch over the scanner.

Actively shielded ultra-high-field systems will undoubtedly be introduced in the near future.

For convenience, most superconducting systems are now actively shielded. **Active shielding** uses additional solenoid electromagnets located around the outside of the main magnet coils at each end of the magnet bore. These are located inside the cryostat and are superconducting coils. They exhibit an equal but opposite effect to the main magnet, which results in a significant reduction in the size of the fringe field footprint. The 5G threshold is only a few feet from the isocentre.

When comparing superconducting electromagnets with no shielding, passive shielding and active shielding, one can use the following illustration. If an MR system is non-shielded, it would take a space typically as large as a 'doubles' tennis court to contain the confines of the field to 5 G within the scan room walls. If it is passively shielded, a typical tennis court would do. However, if the system was actively shielded, one quarter of a doubles tennis court would contain the 5G area within the scan room. This is noteworthy if siting is an issue and because space is costly (i.e. smaller scan rooms cost less).

Refer to animation 9.2 on the supporting companion website for this book: www.wiley.com/go/mriinpractice

Shim coils

Due to the tolerances of manufacture, an MRI superconducting magnet has field homogeneity of approximately 1000 ppm on delivery from the factory. Imaging requires homogeneity of approximately 4 ppm across the imaging volume to provide good geometric sharpness and to allow even spectral fat saturation. Spectroscopic procedures require better than 1 ppm.

To achieve this, a process known as **shimming** is used. The term shimming comes from the discipline of carpentry where it refers to the use of wooden wedges (or shims) to level a surface. Like shielding, shimming can be achieved either actively or passively or by a combination of both. In the context of MRI, shimming makes the field even and is achieved by the use of metal discs/ plates (**passive shimming**) and an additional solenoid magnet (**active shimming**).

Passive shimming is achieved by placing small ferromagnetic plates in specially constructed non-ferrous metal trays located around the circumference of the warm bore of the magnet. This refers to the circumference of the *inner* wall of the cryostat, inside which are housed the shims, gradient coils and RF transmitter. These trays are typically 16 in number and each can hold about 15 shims.

Passive shimming is performed by scanning a phantom and adjusting the position of the shim plates until optimum field homogeneity is achieved. Passive shimming is performed at the time of installation and also counteracts any inhomogeneity due to the physical location of the magnet (due to nearby metal structures in the building or room construction).

Active shimming is performed by an electromagnetic coil and can be used to shim the system for each patient or even each sequence within a protocol. This ensures that the magnetic field is as homogeneous as possible irrespective of patient size.

322

Most imaging systems use a combination of passive and active shimming. Generally passive shimming is used to get the magnetic field to a particular level of homogeneity and then active shimming is used to optimize for each patient examination.

Gradient coils

The next component to be found in the warm bore of the magnet is the gradient set. This is a cylindrical structure containing three individual electromagnets. On modern scanners this component also includes (for example) 18 individual solenoids that make up the active shim system mentioned in the previous section.

The gradient coils are each supplied by at least one, if not two, powerful amplifiers. As the gradient set is at room temperature (i.e. not superconducting) high-power gradients may require water-cooling. Each of the three components of the gradient set can be activated to create a slope in the static field in the x, y or z axes respectively.

Gradient coils are used for **spatial encoding** and in certain imaging options such as GMN. In gradient echo sequences they are also used to rephase spins and produce echoes (*see* Chapters 2 and 5).

By definition, a gradient is simply a slope, in this case a very linear slope in magnetic field strength across the imaging volume in a particular direction. To understand how the strength of a magnetic field can be altered, we need to consider the factors that change the strength of an electromagnet. They are:

- the current passing through the windings
- the number of windings in the coil
- the diameter of the wire used in the windings
- the distance or spacing between the windings.

Altering any of the first three factors would change the amplitude or strength of a magnetic field induced around the coil uniformly. To slope the magnetic field (i.e. change the amplitude of the magnetic field from one end of the coil to the other), one could theoretically alter the spacing between the loops. For example, if loops were spaced far apart at one end of the gradient coil and gradually closer got together towards the other end, then the magnetic field strength would change gradually from a low to a higher field.

In practice, however, coils tend to be more symmetrical in design and rely on a three-terminal arrangement to achieve the gradient field. There are a number of gradient coil configurations. To understand this concept, it is first necessary to visualize a simple electromagnet coil as shown in Figure 9.7. This coil has 12 windings uniformly spaced and is attached to an electrical terminal at each end. Current therefore flows in one direction through the coil and the resulting direction of the magnetic field can be demonstrated with the right-hand rule, in this case left to right. Note that the direction of flow is represented by a dot and a cross indicating flow towards and away from the observer respectively (think of an arrow with a dot as its point and a cross as its tail feathers).

If this design is altered slightly to include a third terminal in the center of the coil (Figure 9.11), the polarity of the terminals can be arranged so that current flows in opposite directions at each end of the coil. This generates two magnetic fields of equal but opposite direction.

Consider a combination of these two coils as shown in Figure 9.12. The first coil represents the main magnet, and the second represents the Z gradient coil. To the left, the secondary coil is

To accomplish the goals of spatial encoding, refocusing and other 'tasks' during image acquisition in acceptable imaging times, gradient systems need to be fast and strong. To evaluate speed and strength of gradients, gradient characteristics need to be understood. These gradient characteristics include: gradient strength, gradient speed, the combination of strength and speed, and the duty cycle.

- **Gradient strength** or **gradient amplitude** defines how steep or strong a particular gradient is. It is measured in milliTesla per meter (mT/m) or gauss per centimeter G/cm
- **Gradient speed** or **gradient rise time** defines the time it takes for a given gradient to reach maximum amplitude. Rise time is measured in microseconds (μs).
- **Slew rate** defines the time it takes for a given gradient to reach maximum amplitude and what that amplitude is. Slew rate is the speed and strength of the gradient and is measured in units of milliTesla per meter per second (mT/m/s)
- **Duty cycle** defines the percentage of time that the gradient is permitted to work. Duty cycle is expressed in units of percentage (%).

Gradient amplitudes vary but typical gradient strengths are between 10 and 40 mT/m, depending on the power of the gradients within the system. In a 10 mT/m gradient system, the strength of the magnetic field changes 10 mT over each meter along the gradient field. In a 40 mT/m gradient system, the strength of the magnetic field changes 40 mT for every meter along the magnet. The maximum amplitude or strength of a gradient is important when good spatial resolution is required. To achieve small voxels that are necessary for good spatial resolution, all three gradients must be able to achieve a high amplitude. Gradient strength can be expressed in units of G/cm or mT/m, where 1 G/cm = 10 mT/m.

How quickly a gradient can attain a particular gradient slope is called the rise time. This affects how fast a gradient can be switched on and off and this in turn affects the scan time. Gradient rise times are in the order of 120 μs. If the rise time is reduced, time is saved within the pulse sequence, which is then translated into shorter overall imaging times (Figure 9.14). The stronger

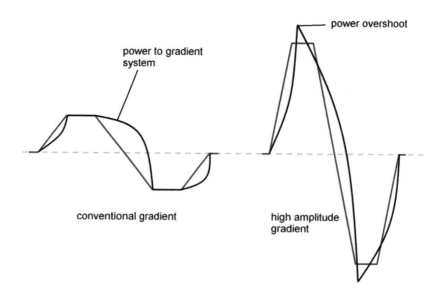

power overshoot

power to gradient system

conventional gradient

high amplitude gradient

Figure 9.14   Gradient amplitude versus rise time.

the gradient the longer it takes to get the gradient to achieve that strength (longer rise time). Stronger gradients therefore generally equal longer rise times. However, there are methods that allow for shorter rise times. These will be discussed in the section on high-speed gradient systems.

An understanding of the gradient amplitude and rise time is helpful in understanding MR system characteristics. For example, if a given imaging system has a high amplitude gradient it is not efficient if the rise time is long. Conversely, having a rapid rise time is helpful for reducing scan time, but not optimal if gradient amplitude is low. Therefore, to evaluate the gradient characteristics properly, the amplitude and rise time must be measured together. This measurement is known as slew rate.

Typical gradient slew rates are in the order of 70 mT/m/s. High-speed gradients can be as high as 200 mT/m/s. Some investigational slew rates approach 240 mT/m/s but at present this can exceed the FDA guidelines for gradient strength. As slew rates increase, the potential for time varied magnetic field effects (TVMF) effects increases (TVMF effects are described in Chapter 10).

The duty cycle increases with slew rate, but as the duty cycle increases, gradient heating can increase and the number of attainable slices can be reduced. In spin echo imaging the typical duty cycle is 10%, while in echo planar imaging (EPI) it is closer to 50% of the TR period.

The acoustic noise generated by the scanner is caused by vibration of the gradient set. Higher amplitude gradient values and rapid gradient activation will therefore increase acoustic noise. Therefore in addition to stronger gradients, manufacturers have modified gradient systems in an attempt to reduce gradient noise. These are known as quiet systems. Regardless of the gradient system it is always recommended to provide hearing protection, in the form of headphones or ear plugs, for patients and visitors in the scan room during image acquisition.

Balanced gradient systems

In a balanced gradient system, each gradient pulse is balanced by an equal but opposite gradient pulse. This is known as a **bipolar** or **balanced gradient system**. For example, a positive gradient pulse is followed by a negative pulse to undo the changes caused by the positive lobe. Therefore, in a balanced gradient system, the area under the positive lobe of the gradient equals the area under the negative lobe (Figure 9.15).

During readout, the amplitude of the lobes are limited by the desired resolution chosen by the FOV (bandwidth and sampling time). The time that the gradient is on (determined by the sampling time) is determined by the readout/receive bandwidth. If this time is doubled by the application of positive and negative lobes of the same amplitude and sampling, time is wasted within the pulse

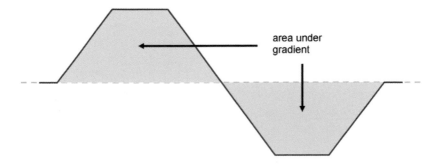

Figure 9.15   Balanced or bipolar gradient pulses.

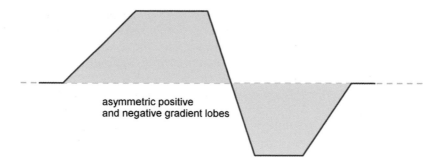

Figure 9.16   Asymmetric gradients.

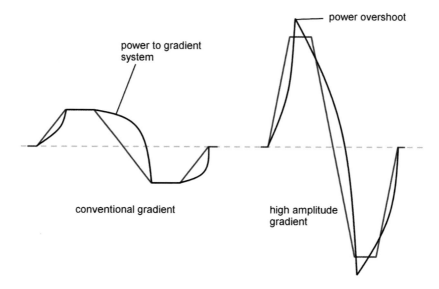

Figure 9.17   Comparison of the power supply to conventional and high-speed gradient systems.

sequence. This wasted time results in fewer slices or, in the case of fast spin echo or EPI, shorter turbo factors and/or fewer slices. However, since it is the area under the lobes that must be equal, the negative (refocusing) lobe can have higher amplitude and shorter sampling time and still complete the same area. This asymmetric gradient paradigm permits time savings in the sequence and hence more slices and/or longer turbo factors can be used (Figure 9.16). This is one step in the production of high-speed gradients.

High-speed gradient systems

To acquire high gradient amplitudes with shorter rise times, modifications to the power can be considered. As shown in Figure 9.17, the application of enough power to create high gradient amplitudes shortens rise times but yields a power *overshoot*. In addition, high gradient amplitudes permit high amplitude balancing lobes, allowing for time savings within pulse sequences. Therefore for ultra-fast and/or ultra-high-resolution images, higher gradient amplitudes of 25 mT/m or greater are required. High power gradients with asymmetric refocusing lobes will reduce the time lost within the sequence and result in higher resolution rapid images. A technique known as ramp sampling can also be used to reduce 'valuable' time within a pulse sequence that can be traded for faster scans. This is described later in this chapter.

High-speed gradient switching necessitates high-quality gradient amplifiers. Resonant gradient systems that oscillate at a particular frequency provide a suitable alternative. Such systems produce a sinusoidal readout gradient, which reduces gradient demands, but are often incompatible with other imaging techniques that benefit from gradient switching.

Sampling

MR signals are sampled during readout when the frequency encoding gradient is applied. Signals are sampled only after the gradient has reached maximum amplitude. This type of sampling is known as conventional sampling and occurs at the TE time. Unfortunately, time is wasted within the pulse sequence waiting for the frequency encoding gradient to change. In addition, since sampling occurs at the TE time, minimum allowable TEs are longer, and longer TEs result in changes in image contrast and fewer allowable slices.

Time within the sequence is reduced if sampling is performed while the frequency encoding gradient is changing. This is accomplished with a technique known as **ramp sampling**, in which data points are collected when the rise time is almost complete. Sampling occurs while the gradient is still reaching maximum amplitude, while the gradient is at maximum amplitude and as it begins to decline (Figure 9.18). However, this technique requires reconstruction programs to reduce artefacts, and resolution may be lost. Resonant gradient systems that oscillate at a particular frequency produce a sinusoidal readout gradient that permits sinusoidal sampling. This technique provides an efficient sampling mechanism but is not compatible with all imaging sequences (Figure 9.19).

High-speed gradients (with characteristics including combinations of high power gradients, asymmetric refocusing lobes and ramp sampling) allow for rapid imaging sequences. All the previously described time savings within pulse sequences can be translated into practical applications for MR system users. Such savings result in shorter imaging times, more slices and higher resolution than in conventional imaging.

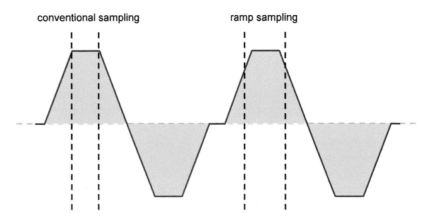

Figure 9.18
Conventional vs ramped sampling.

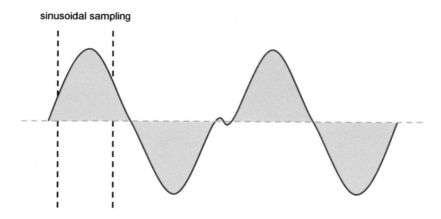

sinusoidal sampling

Figure 9.19   Sinusoidal sampling.

Radio frequency (RF)

To produce MR images, energy must be added to the system. The energy required to produce resonance of nuclear spins is expressed as a frequency and can be calculated by the Larmor equation ($\omega_0 = B_0\gamma$). At field strengths used in MRI, energy within the radio frequency (RF) band of the electromagnetic spectrum is necessary to perturb or excite the spins. As shown by the Larmor equation, the magnetic field strength (B_0) is proportional to the radio frequency (ω_0), the energy of which is significantly lower than that of X-rays. To produce an image, RF must first be transmitted at the resonant frequency of hydrogen, so that resonance can occur. The transverse component of magnetization created by resonance must then be detected by a receiver coil (this concept was described in Chapter 1).

RF coils

The instrumentation (hardware) required to achieve resonance is the RF coil assembly, which includes RF transmitter coils and RF receiver coils. Coils that transmit signals are known as RF transmit (or transmitter) coils, and those that detect signal are the RF receive (or receiver) coils. There are coils that both transmit and receive signal known as transceivers.

RF transmitters

Energy is transmitted at the resonant frequency of hydrogen in the form of a short intense burst of electromagnetic radiation known as a **radio frequency** (or RF) pulse. This is achieved by an RF transmitter that sends radio waves with enough energy to create phase coherence and flip some of the spins from a low- energy state to a high-energy state. This RF pulse transfers the NMV from a position along the Z axis into the transverse X, Y plane. Such a pulse is therefore called a 90° RF pulse. The 90° RF pulse is created by an oscillating secondary magnetic field (B_1) formed as a result of alternating current flowing through a loop of wire called an **RF transmitter coil**.

The primary RF transmitter in a closed-bore MRI system is the closest component to the magnet bore. Colloquially known as the body coil, this cylindrical array of conducting coils is capable of transmitting and receiving RF. This transceiver is connected to an RF synthesizer, a computer-controlled device that digitally constructs a high-frequency sine wave which is then passed through a digital-to-analogue converter. The result is an oscillating current in the transceiver, which in turn creates an RF pulse at 90° to the main magnetic field. This is an electromagnetic wave, the magnetic component of which is termed B1.

RF transmission is not confined to the body coil; in many systems there are volume coils provided that are also capable of transmitting RF. To summarize:

- A **body coil**, a cylindrical array of electrically conductive elements positioned around the inner circumference of the magnet bore. The body coil is the main RF transmitter and transmits RF for most examinations that are acquired without a transmit/receive coil.
- A **head coil**, which can be of a saddle-shaped, or birdcage type configuration, or a multichannel coil (multichannel head coils are generally receive only).
- **Extremity coils**, which are generally of a saddle configuration and are configured to accommodate the size of the adult knee. Extremity coils are generally used to image the lower extremities (knee, ankle, foot), but can also be used to image the upper extremities (elbow and wrist).

Receiver coils

As previously discussed, passing current through a wire produces a magnetic field. Conversely, if a loop of wire is exposed to an oscillating field, a current is induced in the loop. This is proven by Faraday's law of induction:

$$dB/dt = dv \text{ or } \Delta B/\Delta \tau = \Delta v$$

where

dB is the changing magnetic field (oscillating magnetic field caused by RF signals)
dt is the changing time
dv is the changing voltage (MR signal).

This induced current and the resulting voltage constitute the MR signal. Receiver coils must be placed properly to detect the MR signal adequately. To accomplish signal reception, the secondary B_1 field must be situated at right angles to the main magnetic field B_0 (*see* Figure 4.28).

 Refer to animation 9.3 on the supporting companion website for this book: www.wiley.com/go/mriinpractice

The configuration of the RF transmitter and receiver coils directly affects the quality of the MR signal and hency the image quality. Generally speaking, the smaller the coil the better the SNR and the more coils used the better the SNR. Several types of coil are currently used in MR imaging, including (but are not limited to):

- volume coils (generally used to accommodate a 'volume' of tissue)
  - body coil (saddle configuration)
  - birdcage coils (head coils)
  - solenoid coils (tube shaped for vertical field systems)

- surface (or local) coils (generally placed on or in the surface)
  - linear coils (simple surface coil or local coil configuration)
  - quadrature coils (with coils (or electronics) configured perpendicular)
  - Helmholtz pair (two coils combined with B_1 fields in the same direction)
  - Maxwell pair (two coils combined with B_1 fields in the opposite direction)
  - phased array (multiple coils elements and multiple receivers)
  - multi-coil elements (multiple elements, multiple receivers for parallel imaging).

Volume coils

Volume coils can be configured in a solenoidal, saddle and/or birdcage configuration. A volume coil can both transmit RF and receive the MR signal and is often called a transceiver. It encompasses the entire anatomy and can be used for head, extremity or total body imaging. Head and body coils of a type known as the birdcage configuration are used to image relatively large areas and yield uniform SNR over the entire imaging volume. However, even though volume coils are responsible for uniform excitation over a large area, because of their large size they generally produce images with lower SNR than other types of coils. This tends to be more noticeable when there is a mismatch between the size of the field of view and the size of the coil. As an example, if one were to image a knee using the integral body coil, the signal would originate from a thin slice having a small field of view, but the noise would originate from the entire volume of the coil.

SNR can be improved by the use of more than one element in a coil. Quadrature detection by a circularly polarized coil uses two elements offset by 90°. Each element acts as an individual coil detecting signal returning from the region of interest. The SNR is not doubled, however, as each element also receives noise. The improvement of SNR is due to the fact that noise is random – tending to average out of the picture – whereas signal is non-random and is reinforced in the final image.

Modern coils take this concept further by using multiple elements, each having its own channel.

Surface coils

Coils configured with a simple loop of wire and other components are known as **linear coils**. These coils typically offer a high SNR because they only detect noise from a small area, and they are positioned close to the area of interest. SNR can be further improved by the use of quadrature detection as described in the previous section.

Surface coils are used to improve the SNR when imaging structures near the surface of the patient (such as the temporo-mandibular joint). Generally, the nearer the coil is situated to the structure to be imaged, the greater the SNR. This is because the coil is closer to the signal-emitting anatomy, and only noise in the vicinity of the coil is received, rather than the entire body. Surface coils are usually small and specially shaped so that they can easily be placed near the anatomy to be imaged with little or no discomfort to the patient. However, signal (and noise) is received only from the sensitive volume of the coil that corresponds to the area located around the coil. The size of this area extends to the diameter of the coil and at a depth into the patient equal to the diameter of the coil ×0.75.

The sensitivity of the coil is related to its size. The volume of tissue that can be imaged by a particular coil is determined by a factor known as the sensitivity profile of the coil. For a circular surface coil, this can be imagined as a slightly elongated half-sphere extending from the diameter of the coil into the patient. Specifically, the signal that is detected by a particular RF coil is related to the diameter of the coil: the sensitivity profile provides signal from the anatomy located across the diameter of the coil and to a depth of 75% of the diameter. For this reason, coils need to be placed in close proximity to the anatomy of interest.

The limits in the area associated with the sensitivity profile create challenges when imaging anatomic structures that are located deep within the patient. For example, if a coil with a diameter of 10 cm is used, then the field of view that can be imaged is also 10 cm, to a depth of 7.5 cm. Therefore, there is a *fall-off* of signal as the distance from the coil is increased in any direction. Signal fall-off often occurs when imaging tissues deep within the patient (such as the prostate gland in the male patient). To obtain optimal signal quality in tissues and anatomic structures deep within the patient, intra-cavity coils can be used (such as endorectal, endovascular, endovaginal, urethral and esophageal coils). For example, since anatomically the rectum is located directly posterior to the prostate gland, MR imaging of the prostate gland can be improved by placing a coil within the rectum. RF coils formerly known as surface coils have come to be known as local coils.

Multiple coils

Generally, the range of the area that can be imaged is limited by the size of the coil. Manufacturers have addressed this issue with the introduction of phased array coils. Historically the use of multiple coils was limited to the application of a pair of coils, perhaps in wrist or shoulder imaging, where one coil was placed on each side of the anatomy. Known as a Helmholtz pair, this configuration is a primitive way of obtaining fairly uniform signal across a volume of tissue. Another less popular configuration involved the use of three coils combined into one spherical arrangement known as a Maxwell coil.

These coils have now evolved into phased array systems, having multiple receive coils each responsible for acquiring signal from a particular volume of tissue within the region of interest.

Phased array coils consist of multiple coils and multiple receivers whose individual signals are combined to create one image with improved SNR and increased coverage. The smaller the RF coil, the better the SNR, and the more coils used the higher the SNR. Unfortunately, the smaller the coil, the smaller the area of coverage. In an attempt to get both good SNR and large coverage, manufacturers have combined multiple small coils with multiple receivers. This is known as phased array coil technology. Phased array coils are now widely used. Phased array coils can be configured with a number of coils arranged in a line (for spine imaging). This configuration is known as a linear array. Coils can also be configured where coils are positioned on both the anterior and the posterior of the patient allowing for coverage within the patient. This configuration is known as a volume array. Coil arrays began with four to six coils arranged in a line (linear) or a volume for increased coverage and SNR. For example, in a four-coil array, four coils and receivers can be grouped together in a line to increase longitudinal coverage (for spine imaging). The same four-coil array can also be configured with two coils positioned anterior (on top of the patient) and two posterior (below the patient) for body imaging. During data acquisition, each individual coil receives signal from its own small, usable FOV. The signal output from each coil is separately received and processed, but then combined to form one single, larger FOV. As each coil has its own receiver, the amount of noise received is limited to its small FOV, and all the data can be acquired in a single sequence rather than four individual sequences. Phased array coils can be increased from four-coil arrays up to 128-coil elements.

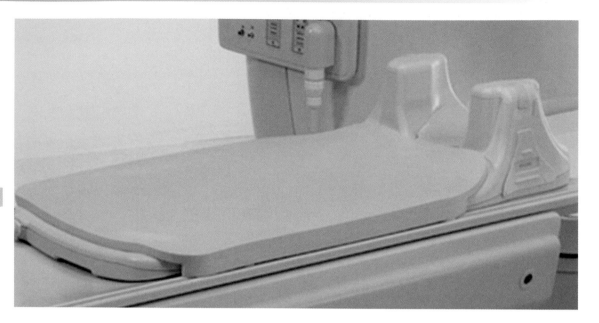

Figure 9.20 Spinal phased array coil.

Several types of phased array coils are now available. These include:

- spine phased array (linear array) (Figure 9.20)
- pelvic phased array (volume array)
- breast coil phased array (volume array)
- cardiac array (volume array)
- temporomandibular joint phased array (volume array)

At first, receiver coils were used to detect signal. Now coil elements called encoding coil elements can detect and, to a certain extent, also encode MR signal. These coil elements are required for parallel imaging techniques (*see* Chapter 5). These techniques use coils to detect a sensitivity map (related to the sensitivity profile previously mentioned) of the signal near the coil (Figures 9.21 and 9.22). Some manufacturers have coil systems with as many as 32 coil elements to produce images in much shorter scan times than conventional imaging.

SNR and resolution

As the SNR is enhanced when using local coils, greater spatial resolution of small structures can often be achieved. Remember though, coils do *not* provide high resolution, but rather high signal. This high signal, obtained by the use of local coils can be 'traded' for higher resolution (small FOV, thin slice thickness and/or large imaging matrix). When using local coils, a body coil is generally used to transmit RF and the local coil is used to receive the MR signal unless the local coil is also a transmitter.

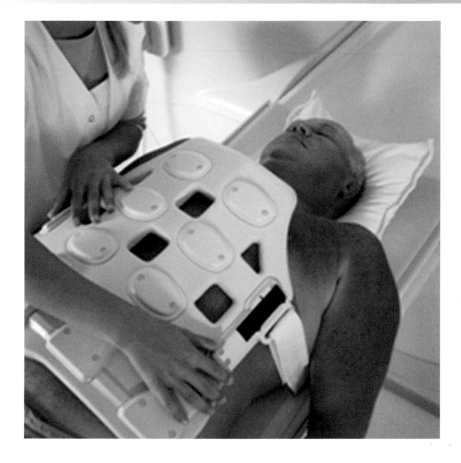

335

Figure 9.21   Parallel imaging coils.

Summary

Large coil

- large area of uniform signal reception
- increased likelihood of aliasing with small FOV
- positioning of patient not too critical
- lower SNR only allows for lower resolution
- used in examinations of torso where signal coverage is necessary (chest, abdomen)

Small coil

- small area of signal reception
- less likely to produce aliasing artefact
- positioning of coil and patient critical
- high SNR can be traded for higher resolution
- used in examinations of small body parts (wrist, spine, knee)

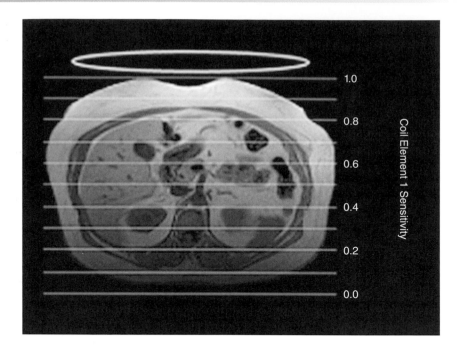

Figure 9.22 Sensitivity encoding in parallel imaging.

Coil safety

There are a few basic rules to ensure the safe operation of RF coils. Coil safety includes consideration of the hardware (cables and coils) and the RF absorption (heating and localized RF burns). RF safety will be discussed in Chapter 10.

Coils are connected to the system by cables, which must consist of a conductive material so that the RF power can be delivered to the coil and the signal can be sent to the image processor. They therefore have the capacity to transmit the heat that occurs during normal operation. However, under certain circumstances, this heat may burn the patient or the insulating material of the cable. To prevent such an occurrence, always make sure the cables are not looped and do not touch the patient or the bore of the magnet. Also cables should not be positioned near other wires or cables, such as ECG leads and the like.

Coil cables should be inspected regularly and should not under any circumstances be used if the insulation is damaged. To receive optimum signal from the patient, the coils must be correctly tuned. In the past, each RF coil had to be manually tuned for each scan. Today, RF coils are auto-tuned. Each manufacturer achieves this in a different way.

RF shielding

In MRI, shielding is important not only for the magnetic field but also for the RF field. RF shielding can be accomplished by the use of copper shielding, which is also known as a Faraday cage. The Faraday cage consists of copper shielding within the scan room walls, copper screening within scan room windows and copper 'teeth' (known as door seals) along the door frame of the room. If RF shielding is compromised, RF artefacts (zipper artefacts or buzz artefacts) can result. (For more information about artefacts, refer to Chapter 7.)

Patient transportation system

All systems use a hydraulically or mechanically driven couch (or patient table) to lift the patient up to the level of the bore and to slide them into the bore of the MR imaging system. This is usually achieved by pedals or buttons that move the couch up or down, and in or out of the bore. The table should be comfortable for the patient and allow for the attachment of coils and immobilization devices. There should also be a mechanism for evacuating the patient rapidly from the bore in an emergency. Some systems enable the couch to be undocked (removed) from the magnet so that patients can be transported out of the room in an emergency without moving them on to another trolley first. All couches must, of course, be magnetically safe and contain no metal parts. The patient transport system has become more sophisticated to allow automated rapid movement of the patient between scanning positions during contrast enhanced MRA.

New configurations of MR scan couch have included those where the RF coil is placed *within* the table (rather than on top of it). This configuration has become popular for breast imaging, where prone patient positioning in larger patients has limitations. When the patient is positioned prone (on top of the breast coil) even a 70 cm bore scanner can be limiting. Imagine a 70 cm bore scanner, where the patient table is located in the center of the bore, this leaves 35 cm of space for the patient (from table to the top of the bore) and approximately 35 cm of useless space below the table surface. For breast imaging, the coil is placed on top of the table and patient positioned on top of the coil. This results in limited space for the patient. In many cases, when the patient is positioned on top of the coil apparatus, with breasts positioned in the coils themselves, the patient's back can be very close to or even touching the top of the bore of the imager. If, however, the coil is positioned within the patient table, the patient is essentially lying at the 35 cm location (within the 70 cm bore), with their back above and their breasts below. This configuration is efficient for positioning patients for breast imaging in MR, particularly for larger patients and/or large-breasted patients.

MR computer systems and the user interface

Now that many of the individual components of the MR imaging system have been described, it is time to discuss the computer systems and user interface components. The magnet, RF system, gradient system and associated components do not function without 'direction'. To make MR images, all these components need to be directed or programmed to function properly. This direction is offered by a computer system and overseen by the programmer, and then implemented by the user. System functionality is initially set up or programmed by the computer programmer (or pulse programmer) and the systems are then operated on a day-to-day basis by the technologist, radiographer or the physician. MRI computer systems vary with manufacturer. Most consist of:

- the computer system (a minicomputer, with expansion capabilities)
- pulse control unit
- an array processor for Fourier transformation

- an image processor that takes data from the array processor to form an image
- hard disc drives for storage of raw data and pulse sequence parameters
- a power distribution mechanism to distribute and filter the alternating and direct current
- the operator console for user interface.

The computer system

When MR imaging systems were initially developed (in the 1970s), computer systems consisted of an entire room full of computer components. In addition to the computer itself, the computer room housed other system components such as gradient amplifiers, RF amplifiers, power distribution units and image storage capabilities. Today, as computer systems have become more efficient, most MR systems can be operated by a computer much like a desktop computer. For the most part, MR computers are programmed at the system manufacturer by pulse programmers, who pre-program pulse sequences, scan parameters and image processing functions. They are generally programmed such that the order and timing of RF and gradient pulses are 'set' based on the parameters and options 'set' by the 'system user' (technologist). For example, as the technologist selects the resolution parameters (FOV, thickness and matrix), the pulse programmer has selected the appropriate strength, duration and timing of gradient pulses to be applied. This occurs during image acquisition or scanning.

Image acquisition or scanning

During MR image acquisition, a sequence of RF and gradient pulses are applied to a patient within the MR scanner. This sequence of RF and gradient pulses is known as a pulse sequence. Current passed through the gradient coils and RF coils is switched on and off very rapidly at precise times during the pulse sequence. This allows for **gradient pulses** and **RF pulses**. The strength, order and timing of the gradient pulses determines MR image resolution (mainly related to FOV, thickness and matrix). The strength, order and timing of the RF pulses determines MR image contrast (T1 weighing, T2 weighting, PD weighting). The **pulse control unit** oversees or controls the order and timing of RF and/or gradient pulses, and the pulse programmer assigns or programs these pulses based on the technical factors selected by the user.

The pulse control unit

During image acquisition gradient coils are switched on and off rapidly (creating gradient pulses), while the pulse sequence occurs. These gradient pulses allow for MR signals to be spatially localized along the three axes of the magnet (X, Y and Z), and the strength, order and timing of the pulses determines MR image resolution (mainly related to FOV, thickness and matrix). For example, the amplitude (and duration) of the slice selection gradient is related to slice thickness. The strength and duration of the phase and frequency encoding gradients is related to the FOV and imaging matrix. Gradients are also used to rewind or spoil transverse magnetization and/or to rephase magnetization (to create gradient echoes). Since the same three gradients (X, Y and Z) perform all these tasks (spatial encoding, control resolution and refocus MR signals) accurate pulsing of the gradient coils is essential. Gradient amplifiers supply the power to the gradient coils. The pulse control unit co-ordinates the functions of the gradient amplifiers and the coils so that they can be switched on and off at the appropriate times and for the appropriate duration of time.

The pulse control unit is also responsible for co-ordinating the transmission and amplification of the RF. RF at the resonant frequency is transmitted by the RF transceiver to the RF amplifier and then through an RF monitor, which ensures that safe levels of RF are delivered to the patient. The strength, order and timing of the RF pulses determines image contrast RF amplifiers oversee the power to the RF transmitter coils. The pulse control unit co-ordinates the functions of the RF amplifiers and the coils so that they can be switched on and off at the appropriate times and for the appropriate duration of time.

Operator interface

The operator interface is located in a control room adjacent to the scan room. The flat-panel monitor displays a graphical user interface allowing the input of scan parameters and also allows for the graphical positioning of the slices.

In addition to data acquisition and viewing the recently acquired images, the operator console provides access to a whole host of image manipulation techniques. These include:

- scan functions – scan set-up, scanning
- image manipulation – viewing, post processing and reformatting images.

MR systems are operated on a day-to-day basis by the technologist, radiographer or physician. For scanning, the technologist selects a pre-prescribed protocol or manually selects a protocol for imaging. Each protocol consists of scan factors for optimal image acquisition to include: image contrast (TR, TE, TI, flip angle), resolution (FOV, thickness, matrix) and scan time (NSA, BW, matrix), and a number of other factors. These factors have been programmed by the pulse programmer and are stored in the system's host computer. Once images are acquired, the MR image data are stored on the hard drive, PACS, CD, DVD drive and/or by filming.

MR image storage

Today, filming of MR images is uncommon. Generally, if a permanent copy of images is required, they can be stored on a CD or DVD. If film storage of MR image data is required, the images can be permanently stored from the image console on to single emulsion film similar to that used in computed tomography. However, filming MR images can be somewhat tricky, because the bright-ness and contrast settings vary with each image. These brightness and contrast settings are referred to as window and level settings. Window is the number of shades of gray and the level is related to the brightness of the image. Unlike CT, in which window and level settings are 'fixed' and rely on Hounsfield units, MR images are viewed with window and level settings set by 'eye', based on the anatomy and pathology. Therefore, images with high intrinsic signal may require different window and level settings so that important anatomic and pathologic findings may be visualized adequately on the MR image.

For permanent storage, data may be archived either on to magnetic tape (rarely used), DAT tape, optical disk, CD or on PACS systems (generally the method of choice today). This archive function can also be accessed through the operator's console. Images are stored so that cases can be retrieved for further manipulation and imaging in the future. They may also be used for comparison when repeat examinations are performed on the same patient.

Now that each component of the equipment has been described, it is appropriate to discuss the safe operation of this equipment. This is the subject of the next chapter.

 For questions and answers on this topic please visit the supporting companion website for this book: www.wiley.com/go/ mriinpractice

10

MRI safety

Introduction

To date, there have been no known long-term adverse biological effects associated with extended exposure to the magnetic fields used in MR imaging. However, on review of the individual components of the magnetic resonance imaging process several reversible effects of magnetic field, gradient and radio frequency fields can be observed. Much of the research into MR safety has been carried out in the USA, where most of the literature on safety originates. In February 1982, the Food and Drug Administration (FDA) issued guidelines to hospitals' Investigational Review Boards (IRBs) in *Guidelines for evaluating electromagnetic exposure risks for trials of clinical NMR*. This was later followed up with an evaluation of potential risks and hazards. As in any medical procedure, risks are always a possibility. When considering safety for the patient in the MR environment, critical decisions must be made. As in any medical procedure, the decision to scan or

MRI in Practice, Fourth Edition. Catherine Westbrook, Carolyn Kaut Roth, John Talbot.
© 2011 Blackwell Publishing Ltd. Published 2011 by Blackwell Publishing Ltd.

not to scan is a medical one, and any medical decision is to be made on a case-by-case basis by the physician and determined on a risk versus benefit basis.

Even though there are no known biological effects associated with MRI, there have been a number of accidents that have occurred in the MR environment. MR imaging has been used clinically since the mid-1980s. Unfortunately, during the 30-plus years that MR has been performed, there have been a significant number of reported accidents and near misses, including burns, device failures, contrast reactions and even death during MR procedures, for healthcare employees, patients and patient families within the MR environment. Reported accidents (and adverse events) are not limited to ferromagnetic metal objects flying into the magnetic field. Many incidents associated with the radiofrequency fields, the gradient fields and contrast media have also been reported.

Government guidelines

In 2001, a tragedy occurred when a 6-year-old child was killed by a ferromagnetic oxygen tank while in the MRI scanner. At that time, no formal MRI safety standards had been published. This tragedy prompted the American College of Radiology (ACR) to develop a Blue Ribbon Panel of MR experts including radiologists, physicians, PhDs, technologists, and representatives from corporate, FDA and the law profession. The panel's mission was to produce guidelines for MRI safety entitled *ACR Guidance Document for Safe MR Practices*. This document is known as the *White Paper on MRI Safety* and was published for the first time in 2002. By definition, 'A white paper is an authoritative report or guide that often addresses issues and how to solve them. White papers are used to educate readers and help people make decisions. They are often used in politics, business, and technical fields.' The MRI Safety white paper is intended to provide guidelines for MR imaging facilities for the development and implementation of safety policies and procedures. It has been reviewed, rebutted and updated periodically since its first publication in 2002. This chapter discusses safety considerations for MRI and the ACR white paper recommendations for many of these considerations.

ACR White Paper on MRI Safety

Although there are no formal standards for MRI safety, the ACR white paper offers guidelines for safe and effective operation of the MR imaging facility. It is divided into several sections, each of which takes into account the different aspects of MR imaging, and hence various considerations for MR safety.

ACR Guidance Document for Safe MR Practices

A   Establish, implement, and maintain current MR safety policies and procedures
B   Static magnetic field issues: site access restriction
   1   Zoning
   2   MR personnel and non-MR personnel

343

Current and up-to-date safety information

Due to the time it takes for printed material to be produced, books may be somewhat dated with respect to safety information that changes on a day-to-day basis. For current and up-to-date resources for MRI safety visit the following websites:

* www.mrisafety.com, MRI Safety website by Dr Frank Shellock
* www.imerser.com, Institute for Magnetic Resonance, Safety, and Education and Research.

Safety terminology

Formerly, when devices and materials were deemed safe for MRI they were considered to be 'MR compatible', or if the device was not safe for exposure to MRI it was considered 'not MR compatible' or 'MR incompatible'. In 2005, the American Society for Testing and Materials

(ASTM) International published *New Terminology with Regard to Magnetic Resonance Imaging (MRI) and Implants and Devices*. This documentation modified terms to better define the devices and their safety within the MR environment. MR safe, MR unsafe and MR conditional are now the accepted terms for defining devices in MRI. Definitions for these terms, quoted from the article, include:

MR safe: *'An item that poses no known hazards in all MRI environments.'*
MR unsafe: *'An item that is known to pose hazards in all MRI environments.'*
MR conditional: *'An item that has been demonstrated to pose no known hazards in a specified MRI environment with specified conditions of use. Field conditions that define the specified MRI environment include static magnetic field strength (B_0), spatial gradient, dB/dt (time varying magnetic fields), radio frequency (RF) fields (B_1) [in units of W/kg (watts per kilogram)/specific absorption rate (SAR)].*

Additional conditions, including specific configurations of the item, may be required to deem a device safe, unsafe or conditional in MRI. According to the website www.mrisafety.com, the **MR conditional** information has been sub-categorized to indicate specific recommendations for the particular object, as follows.

Conditional 1 – *The object is acceptable for the patient or individual in the MR environment, despite the fact that it showed positive findings for magnetic field interactions during testing. Notably, the object is considered to be 'weakly' ferromagnetic, only.*
Conditional 2 – *These particular 'weakly' ferromagnetic coils, filters, stents, clips, cardiac occluders, or other implants typically become firmly incorporated into the tissue six weeks following placement.*
Conditional 3 – *Certain transdermal patches with metallic foil (e.g. Deponit, nitroglycerin transdermal delivery system) or other metallic components, although not attracted to an MR system, have been reported to heat excessively during MR procedures.*
Conditional 4 – *This halo vest or cervical fixation device may have ferromagnetic component parts; however, the magnetic field interactions have not been determined. Nevertheless, there has been no report of patient injury in association with the presence of this device in the MR environment at the static magnetic field strength used for MR safety testing.*
Conditional 5 – *This object is acceptable for a patient undergoing an MR procedure or an individual in the MR environment only if specific guidelines or recommendations are followed (see specific information for a given object on this website and contact the manufacturer for further information).*
Conditional 6 – *This implant/device was determined to be MR conditional according to the terminology specified in the American Society for Testing and Materials (ASTM) International, Designation: F2503.*
Conditional 7 – *Important note: this device is not intended for use during the operation of an MR system for an MR procedure.*
Conditional 8 – *Note: this information pertains to an implant/device that has MRI labeling at 1.5 Tesla and 3 Tesla. For example, a particular device may be safe at 1.0 T but unsafe at 3.0 T (or visa versa).*

MR operator caution: unfortunately there seems to be a misunderstanding among the MR community that if a device is tested and deemed safe at high field (3.0 T) it is automatically safe at lower field strengths (0.5 T). Just because a particular implant (or device) is safe at 3.0 T it does

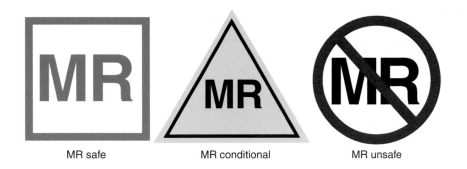

MR safe   MR conditional   MR unsafe

Figure 10.1   Standard labels associated with MR device testing.

not automatically make that device safe at high field (1.0 T), mid-field (0.5 T), low field (0.2 T) or even ultra-low field (0.01 T). Every implant or device *must* be tested under the exact conditions that it will experience during MR imaging, including *all* the components of MR imaging – static magnetic field strength (B_0), radio frequency (B_1), and gradient (strength and speed).

According to the website www.mrisafety.com, *'Terminology from the American Society for Testing and Materials (ASTM) International and utilized by the FDA (Food and Drug Administration) refers to **MR unsafe** as an item that is known to pose hazards in all MRI environments'*, as follows:

Unsafe 1 – *The object is considered to pose a potential or realistic risk or hazard to a patient or individual in the MR environment primarily as the result of movement or dislodgment of the object. Other hazards may also exist.*

Unsafe 2 – *This object displays only minor magnetic field interactions which, in consideration of the in vivo application of this object, is unlikely to pose a hazard or risk in association with movement or dislodgment.*

For a comprehensive explanation, see Shellock *et al.* (2009).

All devices used in MRI should be clearly marked for quick and easy identification. Labels have been developed such that devices can be easily identified, even at a considerable distance from the device (Figure 10.1).

Hardware and magnetic field considerations

To create MR images, a static magnetic field, a radio frequency field and a gradient field are required. The primary effect of the static field is associated with devices, implants and projectiles. Generally, the magnetic field associated with the magnetic field gradients is considered to be a TVMF, since it is switched on and off rapidly during image acquisition. The RF field is also considered to be a TVMF (according to the ACR guidelines for MR safety) since it is an oscillating (or alternating) magnetic field. Each of these types of magnetic field can pose very different safety considerations. This section discusses all the components of the imaging process to evaluate potential adverse affects and/or long-term biological effects relative to exposure to each different type of magnetic field.

Radio frequency fields

As discussed in Chapter 1, during the excitation phase of the sequence, a magnetic field oscillating at the Larmor frequency is applied by a transmit coil (see Chapter 9). In spin echo sequences at least one additional rephasing pulse is applied to rephase spins. This is another oscillating magnetic field and as the flip angle increases (from 90° to 180°) the energy of the RF pulse required increases four-fold. For this reason, fast spin echo sequences give the greatest concern for RF effects as they use a train of 180° RF pulses. This section describes the safety considerations for the RF fields.

The bioeffects of RF irradiation include:

- heating of tissues
- RF antennae effects
- thermal injuries.

These are measured as specific absorption rate (SAR) in units of watts per kilogram (W/kg) and temperature (core body temperature and peripheral body temperature).

Radio frequency irradiation

As the energy level of frequencies used in clinical MR imaging is relatively low and non-ionizing compared with X-rays, visible light and microwaves, the predominant biological effect of RF irradiation absorption is the potential heating of tissue. Although non-thermal effects have been reported, they have not yet been confirmed. As an excitation pulse is applied, some nuclei absorb the RF energy and enter the high-energy state. As they relax, nuclei give off this absorbed energy to the surrounding tissues, or lattice (*see* Chapter 2). RF heating is induced within the patient and is related to the frequency, the field strength and the patient size. In frequencies below 100 MHz, 90% of absorbed energy results from tissue currents (eddy currents in tissues) induced by the magnetic component of the RF field. As frequency is increased, absorbed energy is also increased, so heating of tissue is largely frequency dependent. For this reason, RF heating is less of a concern in MR systems operating below 1 T.

The majority of tissue heating is located at the periphery of the patient and can easily be dissipated. There are, however, areas of the body with considerable resistance. These areas can cause local (focal) heating and/or burns. According to IEC 60601-2-33 *Requirements for the Safety of MR Equipment for Medical Diagnosis* and the FDA *Guidelines for MR Diagnostic Devices*, limits for whole body heating include:

Normal mode limit (suitable for all patients) – 0.5°C or 2 W/kg
First level controlled mode (medical supervision) – 1.0°C or 4 W/kg
Second level controlled mode – greater than 1°C or 4 W/kg (requires IRB approval)

IEC/FDA limits for localized heating include:

Head normal mode limit – 38°C or 3.2 W/kg averaged over head mass
Torso normal mode limit – 39°C or 10 W/kg over any 10 g
Extremities normal mode limit – 40°C or 10 W/kg over any 10 g
No first level for head, torso or extremities

346

Specific absorption rate (SAR)

The biologic effect of RF absorption is tissue heating. It is therefore necessary to monitor RF absorption. The FDA limit for RF exposure is measured either as an increase in body temperature or the specific absorption rate (SAR). This is manifested as tissue heating and the patient's ability to dissipate excess heat. The FDA limit for temperature is an increase of 1.0°C in the core of the body. In the periphery, higher increases to 38°C in the head, 39°C in the trunk and 40°C in the extremities are permitted. Since the measurement of patient temperature, particularly core temperature, poses practical considerations (i.e. placing a temperature probe onto/or within the patient during imaging), there is a more efficient means for the measurement of RF absorption. It can be measured in units of watts per kilogram (W/kg) and expressed in terms of SAR. SAR, is a quantity that depends on the RF pulse characteristics (watts), including induced electric field and pulse duty cycle, and patient characteristics (kg), including tissue density, conductivity and the patient's size. Therefore, the patient's weight and the pulse sequence parameters selected are important factors when monitoring SAR.

Care must therefore be taken in recording the patient's correct weight to ensure the SAR does not exceed the permitted levels. SAR can be used to calculate an expected increase in body temperature during an average examination. Also, SAR limits are calculated over time. As of July 2004, limits have been increased. In the USA the recommended SAR level for imaging used to be 4.0 W/kg (whole body averaged over 15 min), 3.2 W/kg (head averaged over 10 min), 8 W/kg (head or torso, per gram of tissue over 5 min) and 12 W/kg (extremities, per gram of tissue over 5 min). Current SAR limits are shown in Table 10.1.

The FDA has reclassified MRI facilities. Sites that are studying the safety of scanning at SAR values above 4.0 W/kg whole body average are no longer required to limit their capabilities for proton imaging. Sites using research software may still require approval. The FDA also permits an attenuate criterion relying on temperature of the tissues. This is what most sites adhere to. For non-investigational MR sites, new modifications have been established to allow more slices per scan on body imaging. The FDA has acknowledged MR as an established diagnostic tool with recognized risks that are well controlled by the design and use of the equipment.

RF antennae effects

Radio frequency fields can be responsible for significant burn hazards because of the electrical currents that are produced in conductive loops. MRI equipment such as ECG leads and surface coils should therefore be used with extreme caution. When using a surface coil, the operator must

Table 10.1. SAR limits in the USA.

Area	Dose	Time (minutes)	SAR (W/kg)
Whole body	averaged over	15	4
Head	averaged over	10	3
Head or torso	per gram of tissue	5	8
Extremities	per gram of tissue	5	12

be careful to prevent any electrically conductive material (i.e. the cable of the surface coil) from forming a conductive loop with itself or with the patient. Tissue or clothing could potentially be ignited by uninsulated cables. Coupling of a transmitting coil to a receive coil may also cause severe thermal injury. The site's engineer should perform routine checks of surface coils to ensure proper function. At a conference in which they presented the biological effects and safety aspects of NMR, the New York Academy of Science recommended that wires used in MR imaging systems should be electrically and thermally insulated.

Thermal injuries

There have been a number of burns and even fires associated with exposure to the RF fields in MRI. Several types of tattoo have been reported to exhibit heating which has resulted in burns in patients who have undergone MRI. However, many of the second- and third-degree burns were reported to have been associated with the cables from the coils and contact with patient skin. In addition, some localized thermal injuries to patients have been noted after imaging where there was no wire in close proximity to the injury. Recently, the FDA released a public health advisory about the risk of burns associated with medication skin patches (metallic drug delivery patches). In the FDA report on MR-related injuries there was a report of a patient who was imaged with metallic foil on one leg, resulting in sparks and flames. For these reasons, the ACR white paper recommends:

> When electrically conductive materials (such as metals, wires, ferromagnetic inks from tattoos, etc.) are required to be within the bore of the MR scanner with the patient during imaging, care should be taken to place thermal insulation (including air, pads, etc.) between the patient and the electrically conductive material, while simultaneously attempting (as much as feasible) to keep the electrical conductor from directly contacting the patient during imaging.

Summary

There are some types of scans (FSE, TSE and some scan options (MTI – magnetization transfer imaging) that have higher concerns for RF effects. Remember, as the flip angle is doubled (for example from 90° to 180° flip angles), the power increases by a factor of four (or four times the power). When acquiring FSE (or TSE) scans where there is a train of 180° pulses there is considerably more power than with a spin echo acquisition with one single 90° pulse followed by one 180° pulse. The good news is that studies show that patient exposure up to 10 times the recommended levels produces no serious adverse effects, despite elevations in skin and body temperatures. As body temperature increases, blood pressure and heart rate also increase slightly. Even though these effects seem insignificant, patients with compromised thermoregulatory systems, hypertension or cardiovascular disease may not be candidates for MR. In addition, those areas of the body with an inability to handle or dissipate heat (the orbits and the testicles) have been evaluated independently, and in standard pulse sequences have shown no significant increase in temperature. Corneal temperatures were shown to increase from 0° to 1.0°C. However, as some faster imaging sequences are developed which increase RF deposition to the patient, these areas may need to be re-evaluated.

Gradient magnetic fields

As discussed in Chapter 3, gradients are used to spatially encode signal. In some sequences they are also used to generate echoes (*see* Chapters 2 and 5). Gradients create a time-varying magnetic field (TVMF) that result in unique safety considerations different from those associated with the RF and static field.

TVMF effects include:

- peripheral nerve stimulation
- magneto-phosphenes
- acoustic noise.

349

Time-varying magnetic fields

Biological effects associated with changing magnetic fields (TVMF) include induction of voltage within the conductor (or within the human body). These voltages result in several phenomena, including peripheral nerve stimulation and magneto-phosphenes. Many studies have looked at the biological effects of TVMF, because they exist around power transformers and high-voltage lines. The health consequences are not related to the strength of the gradient field, but rather to changes in the magnetic field that cause induced currents. In MR, there is concern about nerves, blood vessels and muscles, which act as conductors in the body. Faraday's law of induction states that changing magnetic fields (ΔB) induce an electrical voltage (ΔV) in any conducting medium. Induced currents are proportional to the material's conductivity and the rate of change (or change in time, Δt) of the magnetic field.

$$\Delta B / \Delta T = \Delta V$$

where

ΔB = change in magnetic field (caused by switching gradients)
Δt = change in time
Δv = change in voltage.

In MR, this effect is determined by factors such as pulse duration, wave shape, repetition pattern and the distribution of the current in the body. The induced current is greater in peripheral tissues because the amplitude of the gradient is higher away from the magnetic isocenter.

Peripheral nerve stimulation

TVMF effects vary with the strength, speed and duration of the gradient pulses. Biological effects that vary with current amplitude include reversible alterations in vision, irreversible effects of cardiac fibrillation, alterations in the biochemistry of cells and fracture union. As gradient amplitude and speed increase, TVMF effects increase. For this reason, there are particular pulse sequence types (EPI sequences such as perfusion, diffusion and **blood oxygen level dependent**, **BOLD**) that pose an increased risk of TVMF effects. Effects occasionally experienced during MRI examinations using echo planar techniques include mild cutaneous sensations and involuntary muscle contractions. This phenomenon is known as peripheral nerve stimulation.

The FDA limit for gradient fields used to be 6T/s for all gradients. In this case, therefore, ΔB is 6T and ΔT is 1s. In addition, the FDA used to limit axial gradient fields to 20 mT/m/s and gradient rise times to 120 (µs) microseconds. EPI sequences pose the greatest concern for TVMF effects as strong gradients are switched rapidly during EPI acquisition. As of July 2004, these limits have been increased so that gradient strengths are limited to those below that *'sufficient to produce severe discomfort or painful nerve stimulation'*.

Magneto-phosphenes

On occasion, patients will note unusual visual disturbances during MR scanning. Visual effects may occur when retinal phosphates are stimulated by induction from TVMF. This phenomenon is known as magneto-phosphenes and is described as 'stars in one's eyes' or presents as light flashes. It is thought to be due to stimulation of the retina by an external magnetic field.

Acoustic noise

As current is passed through the gradient coils during image acquisition, a significant amount of acoustic noise is created. Although noise levels on most commercial systems are considered to be within recommended safety guidelines, noise can cause some reversible and irreversible effects. These effects include communication interference, patient annoyance, transient hearing loss and – in patients who are susceptible to hearing impairment – permanent hearing loss.

The ACR recommends that:

> all patients, volunteers, family members, and healthcare workers (essentially anyone who intends to enter the scan room during image acquisition or during scanning) should be offered and encouraged to use hearing protection prior to undergoing any imaging in the MR scanners.

Hearing protection can be provided in the form of earplugs or headphones. Earplugs are an acceptable and inexpensive way of providing hearing protection and should be used regularly. Generally speaking, simple foam earplugs can attenuate the acoustic noise by 10 dB to 20 dB. Many imaging systems include headphones so that the patient can listen to music during the MRI scan. These headphones are generally anti-noise headphones, where the patient hears music rather than gradient noise. Unfortunately, some of these anti-noise headphones are large relative to the size of the head coil. The technologist should therefore pay particular attention to the fit of the headphone apparatus within the head coil to ensure that the headphones cover the ears properly.

Manufacturers are also improving quiet gradient systems where there is a significant reduction in gradient noise during image acquisition As this alternative is a hardware upgrade and is located within the scanner itself, it can be an expensive option. This anti-noise or destructive noise apparatus is also known as the quiet gradient system. These quiet gradient systems reduce noise and at the same time allow for better communication between the operator and the patient. These options describe the ACR recommendations for clinical imaging (FDA approved imaging sequences). However, according to the ACR guidelines:

MR scan sequences that have not yet been approved by the FDA are to have hearing protective devices in place prior to the initiation of any MR sequences. Without hearing protection in place, MRI sequences that are not FDA-approved should not be performed on patients or volunteers.

Summary

There are some types of hardware alternative (high speed gradients), scans (EPI, perfusion, diffusion, BOLD) and scan options (high resolution (small FOV, thin slice thickness and high matrix) combined with rapid imaging) that produce increased TVMF effects. In addition, since gradient strength increases as we move away from the isocenter, it is the periphery of the body that is most susceptible to TVMF effects associated with gradient magnetic fields. According to the ACR, there are types of patient who require additional caution with respect to gradient field (TVMF) effects associated with EPI sequences (perfusion, diffusion, functional MRI, MRA), including: *'Patients with implanted or retained wires in anatomically or functionally sensitive areas (e.g. myocardium or epicardium, implanted electrodes in the brain). Therefore, the decision to limit the dB/dt (rate of magnetic field change) and maximum strength of the magnetic field of the gradient subsystems during imaging of such patients should be reviewed by the level 2 MR personnel/designated attending radiologist supervising the case or patient.'*

The main magnetic field

The main magnetic field (static field known as B_0) is responsible for the alignment of nuclei. In solenoid electromagnets the field is usually horizontal, while in permanent magnets the field is generally vertical (Figure 10.2). Unlike the fields previously described (RF and gradient fields),

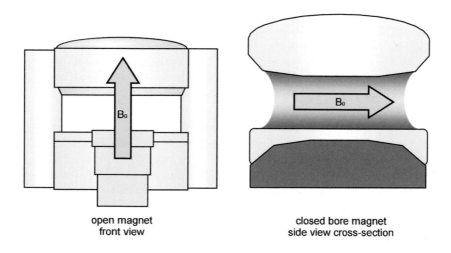

open magnet
front view

closed bore magnet
side view cross-section

Figure 10.2   Static field directions in a permanent and superconducting system.

the main magnetic field is a static or unchanging field. Although there are no known long-term biological effects associated with exposure to the static magnetic field, there are non-biological safety issues, primarily due to ferromagnetic projectile hazards and malfunction of implanted devices. The FDA limit for static magnetic field strength used to be 2.0 T for clinical imaging. As of July 2004, these limits have been increased to 4.0 T for babies and infants up to one month of age and 8.0 T for adults and children (over one month of age). Higher field strengths are permitted for research with informed consent. This section will describe safety considerations associated with the static magnetic field.

Biological effects of the static magnetic field

In the field of diagnostic imaging, a major concern is the possibility of potential biological effects. In nature, the magnetic field associated with the Earth has significant effect on lower life forms. The orientation of magnetotactic bacteria and the migratory patterns of birds (as well as migratory aquatic mammals and some fishes) are influenced by the 0.6 G magnetic field that surrounds the Earth. In MRI, small electrical potentials have been observed in large blood vessels that flow perpendicular to the static magnetic field. Most studies show no effects on cell growth and morphology at field strengths below 2 T. Data accumulated by the National Institute for Occupational Safety, the World Health Organization and the US State Department show no evidence of leukemia or other carcinogenesis. However, the *New England Journal of Medicine* reported an increase in leukemia in men exposed to electrical and magnetic fields in Washington State from 1950 to 1979. In these cases the electromagnetic fields were produced by alternating currents, which resulted in changing magnetic fields. Although similar effects were detected in New York in 1987, no evidence of adverse effects has been noted in people working with linear accelerators who are exposed to static magnetic fields. The few reports of potential carcinogenesis seem controversial, since many of the study methods have been criticized.

Static fields below 2.0 T

Although no biological effects have been observed in human subjects at field strengths below 2 T, reversible effects have been noted on ECGs at these field strengths. An increase in the amplitude of the T wave can be noted on an ECG due to the magneto-hydrodynamic effect. This is produced when conductive fluid such as blood moves across a magnetic field. This phenomenon is related to Faraday's law of induction (previously discussed). This phenomenon is proportional to the strength of the magnetic field. Despite this effect, no serious cardiovascular effects have been observed in patients undergoing MR.

This hemodynamic effect is considered reversible as the ECG tracing returns to normal when the patient is removed from the magnet. This is generally not a clinical issue (in which the patient is injured by the effect) but rather a practical nuisance (with cardiac gating altered). The magneto-hemodynamic effect can present problems when cardiac gating, particularly at higher field strengths. In cardiac gating, scans are timed to the patient's heartbeat and triggered by the R wave. When the amplitude or height of the T wave increases, the system can trigger from the elevated T wave rather than the R wave. The result of inappropriate triggering is degradation in image quality and/or an increase in overall scan time (*see* Chapter 8). As a remedy to this gating inaccuracy, many manufacturers have modified the ECG gating systems to reduce this elevated T wave effect. However, any modification to the ECG tracings can produce false readings if used to monitor the patient. Therefore, it is recommended that the ECG gating leads are not used for patient monitoring. For this reason, when patient monitoring is required, pulse oximetry should be used.

Static fields above 2.0 T

Some reversible biological effects have been observed on human subjects exposed to 2.0 T and above. These effects include fatigue, headaches, hypotension and irritability. Another potential problem at these higher field strengths is the effect of magnetic interaction energy and cell orientation. Certain molecules (such as DNA) and cellular sub-units (such as sickled red cells) have magnetic properties that vary with direction. This effect is biologically important at a field strength of 2.0 T because of the twisting force or torque that is exerted on these molecules. For this reason, many facilities are reluctant to image patients in sickle cell crisis.

Quench

In Chapter 9, superconducting magnets and cryogens were discussed. Superconducting magnets are generally solenoidal electromagnets that have been super-cooled with cryogens (in a cryogen bath). Liquid helium is generally used as the cryogen with very low temperatures of 4 K (Kelvin) where 4 K is approximately −269°C (−450°F) and close to absolute zero (0 K). Helium is stable as a gas, and is lighter than air. To create liquid helium, the gas must be compressed. As stated in Chapter 8, it requires 748 liters of helium gas to make just one liter of liquid. In a scanner with a cryostat volume of 1500 liters, a spontaneous helium boil-off would liberate over 1 000 000 liters of gas. This event is known as a quench (due to the fact that the magnetic field is rapidly stifled) and can cause serious safety issues.

Helium may escape from the cryogen bath accidentally or the process can be manually instigated (by pressing a button) in the case of an emergency. As the helium is vented from the cryostat, the windings of the main magnet cease to exhibit superconductivity, and resistance in the conductor causes the current to stop flowing. This in turn reduces the electromagnetic field to zero in the space of a few minutes. Quenching may cause severe and irreparable damage to the superconducting coils, so a manual quench should only be performed when there is a clear danger to life or limb.

In the event of a fire, it is important that firefighters are not permitted to enter a magnet room until it can be proven that the magnetic field has been fully quenched. Breathing tanks can be ferromagnetic and cause serious injury. All systems should have helium-venting equipment, which removes the helium to the outside environment in the event of a quench. If this fails, helium will vent into the room and replace the oxygen. For this reason, all scan rooms should contain an oxygen monitor that sounds an alarm if the oxygen falls below a certain level. Under these circumstances immediate evacuation of the patient and personnel is necessary.

If there is a quench pipe failure, an inwardly opening magnet room door may become sealed shut by the sudden pressure differential between the magnet room and the control room. This is the result of a high volume of helium gas being vented into the magnet room. The pressure difference may be equalized in an emergency situation by breaking the control room window. To expedite this process, many systems have been equipped with 'pop-out' windows that are designed to separate from their frame in the event of an increase in pressure in the MR scan room. The scan room door can then be opened as usual and the patient evacuated. In such a case

353

the patient should be immediately evacuated and evaluated for asphyxia, hypothermia and ruptured eardrums. These are all possible side effects from a sudden drop in oxygen level, reduced
room temperature and dramatic increase in air pressure.

Ultra-high field imaging

Approximately 85% of MR scanners used for clinical imaging worldwide are 1.5 T imaging systems,
however there has been an increase in the distribution of ultra-high field (3.0 T and above) imaging
systems. Many of these systems have been distributed for improved SNR. SNR is linearly proportional to the square of the field strength. Signal induced in the receive coil increases as the square
of B_0, so a 4T system would have double the signal of a 1T.

There are several safety considerations that are unique to field strengths higher than 1.5 T. They
include the following.

- An increase in the RF power (SAR) at higher field strengths.
- The lack of research and testing (of implants and devices) at higher field strengths.
- Limited clinical experience at these field strengths.
- Limited experience in protocol optimization on humans and/or animals.

It may be advisable to avoid imaging (in situations such as pregnancy and/or implants that may
be contraindicated) at these ultra-high field strengths until more research has been done or more
clinical experience has been gained. Remember, MR imaging in patients with MR conditional
implanted devices, should be scanned *only* if the device has been tested at the specific field
strength in which it will be scanned. For example, if the device has been tested and deemed MR
safe at 1.5 T, it should only be scanned at 1.5 T. This particular device may *not* be MR safe at higher
field strengths (3.0 T) or even at lower field strengths (e.g. 1.0 T). So, various implanted devices
should be scanned only at the field strength at which they were tested. *All* MR imaging is a medical
decision, to be made by the physician, case by case and on a risk versus benefit basis.

Fringe fields

The magnetic field outside the bore of the magnet is known as the stray field or **fringe field** (Figure
10.3). Under certain circumstances the fringe field can cause fatalities – in one documented case
by the torque on a ferromagnetic aneurysm clip. Hazards of fringe fields are associated with the
siting of MR systems. The static magnetic field has no respect for the confines of conventional
walls, floors or ceilings. For this reason, magnetic field shielding is required. Active shielding
ensures that the 5 gauss line is now usually contained within the magnet room.

Forces in the MR environment

Two forces cause ferromagnetic materials and devices to move when in the proximity of a static
magnetic field. These forces are known as the translational force and the rotational force.

The rotational force is responsible for the aneurysm clip moving or twisting when entering the
bore of the magnet. This torque on the clip can result in devastating consequences, such as an

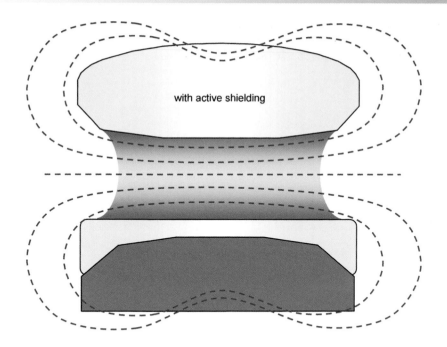

with active shielding

Figure 10.3   The fringe field.

intracranial hemorrhage and death. The rotational force on a particular device is greatest as the device approaches isocenter.

The translational force is responsible for ferromagnetic objects being violently attracted into the MRI scanner. The translational force increases as the object (such as a paperclip) approaches the magnetic isocentre.

Projectiles

Ferromagnetic metal objects can become airborne as projectiles in the presence of a strong static magnetic field. This is known as the **missile affect**, where an object (such as an oxygen tank) becomes a missile. Remember, small objects such as paper clips and hairpins, have a terminal velocity of 40 mph when pulled into a 1.5 T magnet, and pose a serious risk to the patient and anyone else present in the scan room. The force with which projectiles are pulled towards a magnetic field is proportional to the strength of the magnetic field, the distance from the magnet, the mass of the object and the material from which the device is made. There are many medical devices and instruments that can inadvertently enter the MR scan room. Even surgical tools such as hemostats, scissors and clamps, although made of a material known as surgical stainless steel, are strongly attracted to the main magnetic field (Figure 10.4).

Oxygen tanks are also highly magnetic and should *never* be brought into the scan room. However, there are non-ferrous oxygen tanks available, which are MR safe and/or MR conditional. Immobilization bags should be tested with a hand-held magnet, as some of these are filled with highly ferromagnetic steel shot rather than sand. To avoid tragedies in the MR scan room from projectiles, all devices should be tested and deemed safe prior to entering the MR scan room.

356

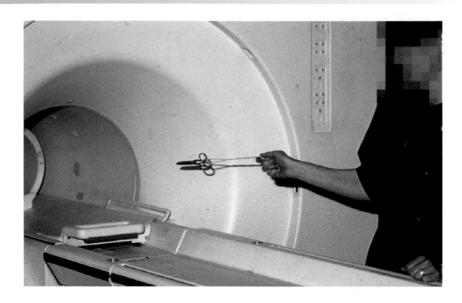

Figure 10.4   The translational force is responsible for attracting ferromagnetic items such as stainless steel scissors.

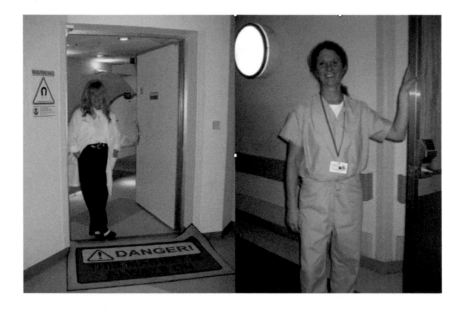

Figure 10.5   Zone III (known as the 'warm zone') and Zone IV (known as the 'hot zone') shown on the photograph of a 1.5T scanner.

Siting considerations

The decision to purchase and site a new MR system can be daunting. The architectural structure must be considered, as well as the dimensions, costs, materials, mechanical and electrical components, and all under the careful consideration of MRI safety. This section will describe siting and zoning considerations for MRI.

Site planning

There are many difficult decisions to be made when installing a magnet system. Safety considerations such as magnetic field location, system weight and power requirements will be discussed within this section. Additional architectural and planning considerations for system siting include:

- appropriate power source (and power restrictions for a particular area)
- air conditioning
- shielding for the RF and static field
- room venting
- surrounding structures in the vicinity of the imaging facility.

Certain sites may have noise and power restrictions. These locations would be sub-optimal for system siting. In addition, locations that have large metal components (or moving metal components) could also pose significant challenges for a safe and effective MR facility. For example, a location in which a subway train runs under the site could provide variations and inhomogeneities in the static magnetic field and hence poor image quality (depending on the train schedule). Although these notions seem nonsensical, careful consideration of these before a magnet is purchased prevents unnecessary expenditure and wastage. Architectural requirements include:

- structural reinforcement
- spatial dimensions
- mechanical and electrical components
- magnetic field considerations (static field strength and fringe field)
- zones.

The primary consideration associated with siting a new MR system is whether to house it in an existing building or to construct a new one. The cost implications for new construction are considerable. Very often the field strength of the magnet, along with the resulting fringe field, is a limiting factor. At present, there are no real guidelines for determining the 'perfect' field strength. In fact, the optimal field strength depends on the patient populous and clinical indications that an imaging center hopes to serve. Each facility has to evaluate the purpose of the system, along with the local site considerations, to decide on the optimal field strength. For example, in many cases a low field (0.3 T) system is adequate for imaging purposes. However, if high-speed imaging, high-resolution imaging and/or spectroscopy are required, a high field system of at least (1.5 T) is necessary. The field strength is important, because as field strength increases, the size of the fringe field generally increases (depending on the magnet configuration). Shielding can control this, but also adds significantly to the cost of the unit.

Safety for devices within and outside the scan room

In addition to structures *within* the scan room, the safety of personnel, equipment, structures and monitors *outside* the unit must be considered. The static field is three-dimensional and extends above and below the magnet and to the sides. The magnetic field strength decreases with the cube of the distance from the magnet, therefore any monitoring and computer devices should be located beyond the 5 G line. In addition, the entrance to the unit and the area surrounding the building must be free from magnetic field effects, to avoid people with pacemakers (or other MR unsafe implanted devices) inadvertently walking into the field. Walls built around the building usually suffice.

Mobile MR units located in trucks have additional safety considerations. They must comply with road traffic regulations (such as weight and wheel base area) and also consider the magnetic fringe field. In addition, the site where the truck is parked must have an appropriate power source, level ground, and a parking location that is structurally strong enough to take the standing weight of the truck and its contents.

At any site, cooling and air conditioning requirements for the computer and its components should be assessed. Helium venting in the event of a quench, power supply, and adequate door and room dimensions need to be taken into account. Adequate RF shielding should be installed and checks made to ensure that monitors and computers located in the vicinity do not interfere with the image. The floor plan of the scan room and the control room should be designed so that there can be rapid straight-line evacuation to an area where emergency equipment can function properly.

In short, the entire facility should be designed with the safety of the patients and personnel in mind. Magnetically controlled security doors located at all entrances to the magnetic field are often the best way of achieving this. Routine preventive maintenance checks by the service engineer and continuing education are also important. Education and safety training is important for MR healthcare employees, but also for ancillary personnel, including hospital workers, maintenance workers, housekeeping staff, fire fighters, police, medical emergency workers and/or anyone who might inadvertently enter the MR environment. Careful planning and diligent upkeep of an MR facility can provide a safe environment for patients and employees.

MRI facility zones

Since the inception of MR imaging, there have been a number of devastating and fatal accidents in the MR environment. For this reason, the International MR Safety Committee issued recommendations for areas near and within the MR scan room.

In an attempt to provide consistent safety from facility to facility, the ACR white paper recommends that each facility has clearly delineated 'zones' (Figure 10.6). The goal is to control access to the MRI system and the magnetic field, and to prevent devastating mishaps in this magnetic environment. The 'zones' are defined as follows.

- Zone I
  - includes all areas that are freely accessible to the general public
  - generally includes the parking lot, the general hallway, etc.
  - all personnel are permitted in Zone I.
- Zone II
  - is the interface between the publicly accessible uncontrolled Zone I and the strictly controlled Zone III

ZONE I: general public - negligible MRI Hazard

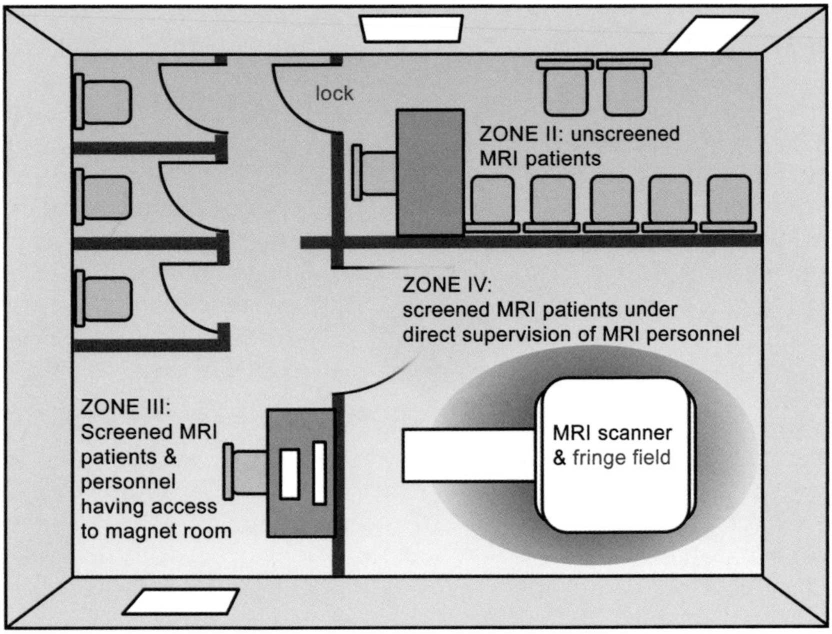

lock

ZONE II: unscreened
MRI patients

ZONE IV:
screened MRI patients under
direct supervision of MRI personnel

ZONE III:
Screened MRI
patients &
personnel
having access
to magnet room

MRI scanner
& fringe field

Figure 10.6   The 'zoning' recommended by the ACR *White Paper on MRI Safety*. Note that there should be locked access between Zone II and Zone III.

- there should be a lock and warning signs (even lighted signs and placards) between Zone II and Zone III
- generally pertains to the patient waiting room
- all personnel are permitted in Zone II; however, there should be a MR trained 'gate-keeper' to keep patients (non-MR personnel) from inadvertently wandering into Zone III and Zone IV.
- Zone III
  - all access to at least Zone III is to be strictly restricted, with limited access
  - is the region in which free access by unscreened non-MR personnel and/or ferromagnetic objects and equipment can result in serious injury or death
  - generally pertains to the dressing room and/or the console area; this area should be strictly monitored as it is the interface to Zone IV
  - only Level 2 personnel can escort Level 1 personnel into this zone. Level 2 personnel should also keep visual and/or verbal contact with Level 1 personnel at all times while in Zone III and IV.
- Zone IV
  - is only suitable for screened patients under direct constant supervision of MRI staff as there is a risk of patient heating, RF antenna effects, missile effects and anoxia due to quench pipe failure
  - only Level 2 personnel can escort Level 1 personnel into this zone. Level 2 personnel should also keep visual and/or verbal contact with all Level 1 personnel at all times while in Zone III and IV.

Safety education

Over the years it became clear that there was limited uniformity in the level of training among MR personnel. In an attempt to provide adequate safety training to appropriate MRI healthcare workers, the ACR has 'labeled' healthcare workers based on their level of safety training in MRI. Today, it has become the accepted standard to provide safety training and education for anyone who could access the MRI scan room, including all those persons directly involved in MR imaging such as technologists, radiographers, radiologists, radiology nurses and other healthcare workers in MRI. There are also a number of ancillary persons who work indirectly with MRI, including receptionists, patient transporters, maintenance workers, house-keeping staff, etc. Many hospital-based imaging sites provide safety training for the entire hospital system during employee orientation. In addition, it is advised that all patient nursing, housekeeping, fire department, emergency, police and anyone who may be exposed to the magnetic environment are educated about the potential risks and hazards of the static magnetic field (at the very least to Level I).

Levels of personnel

The level of training denotes the access the person gains in the MR environment. To identify those persons who have had more extensive training to the broader aspects of MRI safety, the ACR white paper recommends 'levels' of personnel with respect to MRI safety. It is these 'levels' of training that will define the tasks that are acceptable within the MR environment.

- *Non-MR personnel* – essentially no MRI training (includes patients, visitors or facility staff who do not meet the criteria of Level 1 or Level 2 MR personnel).
- *Level 1* – individuals who have passed minimal safety educational efforts to ensure their own safety as they work within Zone III regions (e.g. MRI department office staff, patient aides).
- *Level 2* – individuals who have been more extensively trained and educated in the broader aspects of MR safety issues, including issues related to the potential for thermal loading/burns, direct neuromuscular excitation from rapidly changing gradients, etc. (e.g. MRI technologists, radiologists, radiology department nursing staff).

Protecting the general public from the fringe field

It is recommended that the general public (those persons who have not been properly educated and screened for the effects of magnetic fields) are not exposed to magnetic field strengths in excess 5 G. For this reason, many imaging facilities are situated so that public areas (Zone I) are below this strength, and areas above are either inaccessible (locked) or clearly marked (with signs). This section will discuss safety considerations for the patient, patient screening and screening devices.

Patient and personnel screening

Patient and personnel screening is the most effective way to avoid potential safety hazards to patients. For this reason, *all* patients and personnel must be screened, as if they were having the procedure themselves, before entering the scan room (Zone IV). Patients and MR employees with questionable ferromagnetic foreign objects either in or on their bodies should be rigorously examined to avoid any serious health risks and accidents. This controlled environment can be maintained by carefully questioning and educating all patients and personnel. This screening is usually achieved via a questionnaire (or screening form) completed and documented by all persons entering the magnetic field. The International Society for Magnetic Resonance in Medicine (ISMRM; www.ismrm.org), the ACR (www.acr.org), the safety website mrisafety.com and the Institute for Magnetic Resonance Safety, Education, and Research (IMRSER) have all published questionnaires (and screening forms) that can be downloaded and should be used as a guideline for facility screening forms. In fact, it is recommended that the form be downloaded and used without any modification so as not to omit important information.

Screening must include anyone who enters the scan room (Zone IV), including patients, those accompanying patients for their examinations, staff and visitors. The international MR safety committee IMRSER also recommends that this screening is performed by 'trained professionals' (Level 2 personnel) and that each individual should be screened more than once (once by completing a screening form and at least once by a verbal and one visual interview). Also, *everyone* should be screened *every* time they enter the scan room and this screening should be documented.

According to the ACR white paper warning signs should be attached at all entrances to the magnetic field (including the fringe field) to deter entry into the scan room with ferromagnetic objects. Signs should include those at the entrance of Zone II and also between Zone II and Zone III. It is also recommended that a lighted sign be posted at the entrance to Zone III stating 'the magnetic field is on', in red light.

Screening devices (hand-held magnets and metal detectors)

Metal detectors and hand-held magnets are used as an adjunct to verbal screening. It should be noted that the sensitivity of such devices may not guarantee that there is no metal present, or that a device having negligible attraction to a hand-held magnet will not have considerable attraction to a 3T magnet.

These devices should therefore be used with caution.

Implants and prostheses

Metallic implants pose serious damaging effects, which include torque, heating and artefacts on MR images. Before imaging patients with MR, any surgical procedure that the patient has undergone before the MR examination must be identified. This section provides a brief overview of a few types of implant and prosthesis, and is intended as an introduction to a few common implants and their effects in the magnetic field. Furthermore, as implant and device information changes on a daily basis, it is recommended that prior to MR imaging every technologist refers to an up-to-date list of MR implants. For a complete, and up-to-date list of MR compatible implants and prostheses, visit the MRI safety web page at www.mrisafety.com.

It is also important to understand that if an implanted device has been tested and deemed safe for a given field strength, it may be imaged at that field strength only – not lower and not higher. Each device must only be scanned using the specific conditions under which it was tested. For example, if a device has been tested at 1.5 T then it can be scanned at 1.5 T, not at 1.0 T and not at 3.0 T. Testing includes, but is not limited to the following characteristics:

- torque and heating
- functionality of the device
- device interference with image quality
- artefacts
- safety associated with particular devices.

Torque and heating

Some metallic implants have shown considerable torque when placed in the presence of a magnetic field. The force or torque exerted on small and large metallic implants can cause serious effects, as unanchored implants can potentially move unpredictably within the body. The type of metal used in such implants is one factor that determines the force exerted on them in magnetic fields. While non-ferrous metallic implants may show little or no deflection to the field, they could cause significant heating, due to their inability to dissipate the heat caused by radio frequency absorption. However, heating experiments have not shown excessive temperature increases in implants. However, that if a particular implanted device (such as the MR conditional deep brain stimulator) has specific criteria by which it should be scanned (specific field strength, specific RF coil configuration, specific SAR limit, specific gradient limitation and specific static field strength) these criteria *must* be adhered to. Cases of deep brain burns have been reported in cases where criteria were ignored.

Artefacts from metallic implants

Although artefacts cannot be considered as a biological effect of the MR process, misinterpretation of MR images can yield devastating consequences. The size of the metallic implant, the type of metal (more or less ferromagnetic), the pulse sequence and some of the imaging parameters used determine the size of the artefact shown on the MR image. Note that the artefact on the right-hand image (Figure 10.7) is markedly larger than the artefact on the left-hand image, even though the aneurysm clip is the same size in both patients. In this case the artefact is more marked on the right-hand image as the GE sequence used is more sensitive to magnetic susceptibility than spin echo. This type of clip is contraindicated and the patient should not have been referred for an MRI examination.

Intracranial vascular clips

Some intracranial aneurysm clips are absolute contraindications to MR imaging. Clip motion may damage the vessel, resulting in hemorrhage, ischemia and/or death. Intracranial clips made of titanium have been used, and have proved safe for MR. Today many intracranial vascular clips are considered to be MR conditional. IMRSER recommend that MR imaging in patients with intracranial clips is unsafe unless the clip is *'known to be safe'*. For these reasons, all implanted devices, particularly intracranial vascular clips should be properly identified before they enter the MRI scan room.

Intravascular coils, filters and stents

A number of intravascular devices have been tested and have proved to be MR conditional. Although they have shown deflection in the magnetic field, these devices usually become imbed-

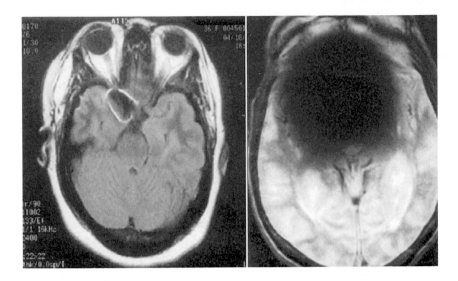

Figure 10.7   Axial images of the brain in a patient with intracranial vascular clips acquired with spin echo (left) and gradient echo (right) sequences. Susceptibility artefact is much greater in the gradient echo image.

ded in the vessel wall after several weeks and are unlikely to become dislodged. Therefore it is considered safe to perform MR imaging on most patients with intravascular devices, provided a reasonable period of time has elapsed after implantation. Like any other device they must be reviewed on a case-by-case basis, prior to MRI.

Extra-cranial vascular clips

Several carotid artery vascular clamps have been tested, and each showed deflection in the magnetic field. However, the deflection was mild when compared with the pulsatile vascular motion within the carotids. Extra-cranial clips tend to be surrounded by fibrous tissue or scar after surgery. Many facilities recommend that MR is delayed until 4–6 weeks after surgery, but in an emergency situation imaging can probably be performed sooner and all studies should be evaluated on a case-by-case basis.

Vascular access ports

Only a few of the many implanted vascular access ports tested showed measurable deflection in the magnetic field. These deflections are thought to be insignificant to the applications of such ports. Therefore, it is probably safe to image patients with implanted vascular access ports.

Heart valves

A number of heart valve prostheses have been evaluated for magnetic susceptibility and have shown negligible deflection to the magnetic field. The deflection is minimal compared with normal pulsatile cardiac motion. Therefore, although patients with most valvular implants are considered MR conditional, careful screening for valve type is advised because there are valves whose integrity could be compromised.

Dental devices and materials

Many dental implants have been tested and 12 of these have shown measurable deflection to the magnetic field. However, most are thought to be safe for MR imaging. Although most devices are not significantly affected by the magnetic field, susceptibility artefacts can adversely affect image quality in MR, especially in gradient echo imaging. Some dental devices are magnetically activated and therefore can pose potential risks for MR imaging, and for the device itself.

Penile implants

Only one of nine penile implants tested showed measurable deflection to the magnetic field. This, the Dacomed Omniphase, is unlikely to cause severe damage to the patient but may become uncomfortable, so an alternative imaging procedure may be considered. Most of today's penile implants are made of plastic.

Otologic implants

Three cochlear implants tested were attracted to the magnetic field and were magnetically or electronically activated. They are therefore definitely contraindicated for MRI. Some patients with otologic implants have been issued a card warning them to avoid MR imaging.

Ocular implants

Several implants were tested and two were deflected by a 1.5 T static magnetic field. The Fatio eyelid spring could cause discomfort and the retinal tack could injure the eye because it is made from a ferromagnetic form of stainless steel.

Intra-ocular ferrous foreign bodies

Intra-ocular ferrous foreign bodies are a cause of major concern in MR safety. It is not uncommon for patients who have worked with sheet metal to have metal fragments or slivers located in and around the eye. Since the magnetic field exerts a force on ferromagnetic objects, a metal fragment in the eye could move or be displaced and cause injury to the eye or surrounding tissue. Small intra-ocular fragments could be missed on a standard radiograph. However, a study demonstrated that metal fragments as small as $0.1 \times 0.1 \times 0.1$ mm can be detected on standard radiographs. In addition, metal fragments from $0.1 \times 0.1 \times 0.1$ mm to $0.3 \times 0.1 \times 0.1$ mm were examined in the eyes of laboratory animals in a 2.0 T magnet. Only the $0.3 \times 0.1 \times 0.1$ mm fragments moved, but they did not cause any discernible clinical damage. Therefore, although computed tomography

(CT) is more accurate in detecting the presence of small foreign bodies, plain film radiography should be adequate in screening for intra-ocular ferrous foreign bodies that have sufficient size to cause ocular damage.

The ISMRM screening form asks the patient: 'Have you ever been hit in the eye by metal?' This is worded to imply that even if they once had metal in their eye and thought it had been removed they should still be screened with plain X-rays. It is also recommended that two views are obtained for evaluation of the orbits. Such views include a 20° posterior–anterior (Water's view) and a lateral or two Water's views with the eyes looking up and down. The ACR white paper still recommends plain film radiography (two views).

Bullets, pellets and shrapnel

When considering imaging patients who could potentially have some type of ammunition (bullets, pellets, shrapnel) within their body, there are two main considerations: what and where? For obvious reasons, it is imperative to know what material the bullet is made of. According to the ACR *White Paper on MRI Safety*:

> *Many types of bullets (pellets and shrapnel) were tested and few demonstrated ferromagnetic properties. Of the 21 that were tested, only four demonstrated significant deflection in the magnetic field. Of these, three were made outside the USA, and two were reported to contain copper or copper-nickel-jacketed lead. Although these bullets did possess ferromagnetic properties, and clearly moved within the magnetic field, they did not cause further injury to the patient as they were located in regions of the body that were not vital organs or structures.*

Regardless of the material, it is almost more important to know where the bullet is located. In some cases where the patient has been shot in the gluteal muscle, and the bullet is lodged well within the muscle itself, deflection of the bullet is unlikely to cause further damage to the patient. If, however, the bullet is lodged near the spinal cord, even slight deflection could result in serious complications. *'It is advisable to take extreme caution in imaging patient with bullets or shrapnel, and to be aware of the location of such metal within the body.'*

Another consideration for any metallic implanted device includes the possibility of susceptibility (or metal) artefacts on MR images. Artefact size varies with type of metal, size of metal, type of scan and scan parameters. In ammunition that has a ferromagnetic alloy, artefacts can compromise image quality. As we might suspect, non-ferromagnetic bullets demonstrate mild to moderate artefacts whereas ferromagnetic bullets demonstrate more severe artefacts on MR images. In an attempt to avoid further injury to the patient, or suboptimal image quality, each patient should be considered on a case-by case basis.

Orthopedic implants, materials and devices

Each of 15 orthopedic implants tested showed no deflection within the main magnetic field. However, a large metallic implant such as a hip prosthesis can become heated by currents induced in the metal by the magnetic and radio frequency fields. It appears that such heating is relatively low. Most orthopedic implants have been imaged with MR without incident.

Surgical clips and pins

Abdominal surgical clips are generally safe for MR because they become anchored by fibrous tissue, but they produce artefacts in proportion to their size and can distort the image. It is recommended that, if possible, the MR procedure is delayed until 4–6 weeks post-operative, although this may not be necessary. As always, patients should be evaluated on a case-by-case basis. According to the ACR white paper:

> Skin staples and superficial metallic sutures: patients requested to undergo MR studies in whom there are skin staples or superficial metallic sutures (SMS) may be permitted to undergo the MR examination if the skin staples or SMS are not ferromagnetic and are not in the anatomic volume of RF power deposition for the study to be performed. If the nonferromagnetic skin staples or SMS are within the volume to be RF-irradiated for the requested MR study, several precautions are recommended including warning the patient, and cold compresses placed on the skin staples.

Halo vests and other similar externally applied devices

Halo vests pose several risk factors, which include deflection and subsequent dislodging of the halo, heating due to RF absorption, electrical current induction within the halo rings, electrical arcing and severe artefactual consequences that could render the imaging acquisition useless. Non-ferrous and non-conductive halo vests that are MR conditional are commercially available. Therefore, in the light of the potential risks and hazards associated with halo vests, it is advisable to identify the halo vest before proceeding with MR imaging.

Electrically, magnetically or mechanically activated or electrically conductive implanted devices

Certain implanted devices are contraindicated or precautions for MR imaging because they are magnetically, electrically or mechanically activated. Each device should be evaluated on a case-by-case basis. These implants include:

- cardiac pacemakers
- cochlear implants
- tissue expanders
- ocular prostheses
- dental implants
- neurostimulators
- bone growth stimulators
- implantable cardiac defibrillators
- implantable drug infusion pumps.

The function of such implants is impaired by the magnetic field, so patients with such devices should not be examined using MR. Also, devices that depend on magnetization to affix themselves to the patient (such as magnetic sphincters, magnetic stoma plugs, magnetic dentures and magnetic prosthetic device), could be demagnetized and may be contraindicated for MR.

Devices and monitors in MRI

There are specific criteria by which ancillary devices are deemed MR safe or MR conditional. Such criteria recommended by the ISMRM include:

- FDA approval
- manufacturer declaration
- prior testing.

It is probably prudent to trust no one and test each device yourself before risking patient safety.

Pacemakers

Until recently *all* cardiac pacemakers were considered to be an absolute contraindication for MRI. Even field strengths as low as 5 G may be sufficient to cause deflection, programming changes and closure of the reed switch that converts a pacemaker to an asynchronous mode. In addition, patients who have had their pacemaker removed may have pacer wires left within the body. These could act as an antenna and (by induced currents) cause cardiac fibrillation. For this reason, there used to be limits for scanning such patients with implanted pacer wires.

Today, it *may* be acceptable to scan some patients with implanted pacer wires (patients whose pacemaker has been removed) as long as the wires are cut close to the skin and not looped outside the chest. As with any implanted device this should be evaluated on a case-by-case basis. If the benefit outweighs the risk, MR imaging may be acceptable. For specific questions about imaging of such patients, post questions on www.mrisafety.com. Warning signs should be posted at the 5 G line to prevent the exposure of anyone with a pacemaker or other electronic implants.

Scanning patients with contraindicated cardiac pacemakers

Some facilities have imaged non-dependent pacemaker patients without incident. If a given site is intending to scan a patient who has a cardiac pacemaker, there are specific criteria that they should observe, including:

- the patient is a non-dependent pacer patient
- the patient is clinically fit to undergo the exam
- there is a radiologist, cardiologist and representative from the pacer company available before, during and after the MR examination.

To err on the side of caution, however, most imaging facilities still do not image pacemaker patients.

Scanning patients with MR conditional cardiac pacemakers

Recently, new MR conditional cardiac pacemakers have been approved by the FDA. However, this particular implanted device has specific criteria under which it should be scanned (specific SAR limit, specific gradient limitation and specific static field strength). These criteria *must* be adhered to. In addition, there are pacemaker settings and imaging criteria that *must* be observed during the scan.

For a complete and up-to-date report on cardiac pacemakers and scanning, visit the MRI safety web page at www.mrisafety.com.

Patient conditions

Pregnant patients

As yet, there are no known biological effects of MRI on the fetus. However, a number of mechanisms could potentially cause adverse effects as a result of the interaction of electromagnetic fields with developing fetuses. Cells undergoing division, which occurs during the first trimester of pregnancy, are more susceptible to these effects.

The FDA requires labeling of MR systems to indicate the safety of MR when used to image the fetus and infant. The current recommendation by the FDA states: 'If non-ionizing imaging (like sonography) is suboptimal, or if the information to be gained by MR would have required more invasive testing (like radiography, CT, angiography to name a few), MRI is acceptable.' In the light of the high-risk potential for pregnant patients in general, many facilities prefer to delay any examination of pregnant patients until after the first trimester and then have a written consent form signed by the patient before the examination. In addition, the American College of Obstetricians and Gynecologists recommends that pregnant patients should be reviewed on a case-by-case basis. The Society of Magnetic Resonance Imaging Safety committee suggests that: 'Pregnant patients or those who suspect they are pregnant should be identified before undergoing MRI to assess the relative risks vs the benefits of the examination.'

Due to the exquisite intrinsic soft tissue contrast and high resolution of MR images and the low safety considerations, MR has become more common for the evaluation of the fetus and/or for the pregnant patient. MR can be used in cases where there is suspicion of abnormality of the fetus or the mother and other non-ionizing forms of diagnostic testing (such as ultrasound) are inadequate. Single shot FSE sequences can be acquired for the evaluation of the fetus, the placenta, uterus, fallopian tubes (for torsion), the uterus, cervix and other female pelvic structures. In some cases, fetal MRI has diagnosed lesions within the fetus, which has allowed for surgery to be performed *in utero* (before the baby was born) and the delivery of a healthy baby.

In the United Kingdom, the National Radiological Protection Board (NRPB) guidelines specify that: 'It might be prudent to exclude pregnant women during the first three months of pregnancy.' However, many fetuses have undergone MRI since 1983 without any abnormalities at birth or after four years of age.

Most imaging uses field strengths up to and including 1.5 T. There has been an increase in the distribution of ultra-high field imaging systems (3 T and above). However, for many safety reasons – including pregnancy – there has been little or no research on humans or animals at these field strengths. Therefore, it may be advisable to avoid imaging at ultra-high field until more research has been done or more clinical experience gained.

Gadolinium enhancement is at present best avoided when examining a pregnant patient. Studies performed in pregnant baboons have shown that gadolinium does cross the placenta and enter the amniotic fluid. In this case, the gadolinium within the fluid is ingested by the fetus, passed via the urinary tract and ingested again. Since there are no research data about the safety of gadolinium chelates and their ability to stay intact (gadolinium molecules with chelates) it is prudent to avoid the administration of gadolinium chelates during pregnancy. Although fetal imaging has become more commonplace, it is still recommended to avoid gadolinium in pregnant patients. Pregnant patients, like all patients are screened for the possibility of renal disease prior to the administration of gadolinium. For more information on gadolinium safety, nephrogenic systemic fibrosis and acceptable glomerular filtration rates refer to Chapter 11.

Pregnant employees

MR facilities have established individual guidelines for pregnant employees in the MR environment. The safety committee of the ISMRM determined that pregnant employees can safely enter the scan room, but should leave while the RF and gradient fields are employed (during the time the scanner is running). Some facilities, however, recommend that the employee stays out of the magnetic field entirely during the first trimester of pregnancy.

A survey showed no increased incidence of spontaneous abortions among MR radiographers and nurses (the natural incidence of spontaneous abortions is about 30%). Following this survey, the unit that carried out the study changed its in-house policy from one in which radiographers were kept out of the magnetic field during pregnancy to a policy that allows pregnant radiographers and technologists to set up the patient, but not to remain during image acquisition.

It has been suggested that informed workers make their own decision. In the US, this recommendation was influenced by a legal decision on the rights of pregnant workers in hazardous environments. Each person must make their own decision to either stay in the unit or, if possible, rotate back into a nearby radiology department. However, to leave an environment that is probably safe and move into one that is known to be hazardous may be inadvisable. These suggestions may change as the use of ultra-high field systems increases.

Medical emergencies

As in any medical facility, the MR suite should be equipped with emergency medical supplies on a crash cart. However, caution is required as many of these supplies can be incredibly dangerous in an MR environment. For this reason, in any critical situation, it is recommended that the patient is rapidly removed from the magnetic field before resuscitation begins and/or while resuscitation is being administered.

Patient monitoring

The ISMRM Safety Committee recommends that all patients are monitored 'verbally and visually'. Patients who cannot be contacted verbally and visually require more rigorous monitoring by pulse oximetry. These patients include those who are not responsive, those who are comatose, unconscious, sedated or hearing impaired, those who have weak voices or speak another language, and pediatric patients. The ECG used for cardiac gating is not acceptable for monitoring the patient as it has been modified to compensate for the magneto-hemodynamic effect.

Safety policy

The ACR white paper on MRI safety makes the following recommendations for every MRI facility.

Establish, implement, and maintain current MR safety policies and procedures

1 All clinical and research MR sites, irrespective of magnet format or field strength, including installations for diagnostic, research, interventional, and/or surgical applications, should maintain MR safety policies.

2 These policies and procedures should also be reviewed concurrently with the introduction of any significant changes in safety parameters of the MR environment of the site (e.g. adding faster or stronger gradient capabilities or higher RF duty cycle studies) and updated as needed. In this review process, national and international standards and recommendations should be taken into consideration prior to establishing local guidelines, policies, and procedures.

3 Each site will name an MR medical director whose responsibilities will include ensuring that MR safe practice guidelines are established and maintained as current and appropriate for the site. It is the responsibility of the site's administration to ensure that the policies and procedures that result from these MR safe practice guidelines are implemented and adhered to at all times by all of the site's personnel.

4 Procedures should be in place to ensure that any and all adverse events, MR safety incidents, or 'near incidents' that occur in the MR site are reported to the medical director in a timely fashion (e.g. within 24 hours or 1 business day of their occurrence) and used in continuous quality improvement efforts. It should be stressed that the Food and Drug Administration states that it is incumbent upon the sites to also report adverse events and incidents to them via their MedWatch program. The ACR supports this requirement and feels that it is in the ultimate best interest of all MR practitioners to create and maintain this consolidated database of such events to help us all learn about them and how to better avoid them in the future.

Safety tips

Here are some tips for maintaining a safe environment for patients and their relatives.

- Before sending the patient an appointment, check with them – or the referring clinician – that they do not have a pacemaker or other contraindicated implants; or if all else fails, a skull and chest radiograph will show an intracranial aneurysm clip and cardiac pacemaker.
- When sending out the appointment include any relevant safety information and details of the examination – this will allay the patient's fear of the unknown.
- Try to ensure that the waiting area is calming and pleasant.
- Carefully screen the patient and anyone else accompanying the patient into the scan room. This should include questions about surgical procedures, metal injury to the eye and pacemakers.
- Ensure that the patient and relatives/friends remove all credit cards, loose metal items, keys, jewelry, etc.
- Check for body piercing (any body part can be pierced).
- Tattoos can heat up during image acquisition. A cool wet cloth placed over the tattoo acts as a good heat dissipater. Tattooed eyeliner may be contraindicated as heat can cause ocular damage.
- Bras and belts should also be removed even if they are non-ferrous and are not in the imaging field. They may still heat up and reduce image quality by locally altering the magnetic field.

- Ask the patient to change into a gown for all examinations, as this is really the only way of ensuring that the patient has removed all dangerous objects.
- Always re-check the patient before they are taken into the magnetic field, regardless of how many times they have been checked before. It is the radiographer's responsibility to keep the MR environment safe.
- Remember that patients are likely to know nothing about magnetism and the potential hazards.
- Anxious and sick patients especially cannot be trusted to give you correct information. Be extra vigilant with these types of patient. If you are in any doubt about their safety, *do not take them into the magnetic field*.

As in any medical procedure, the decision to scan or not to scan is a medical decision. Any medical decision is to be made on a case-by-case basis by the physician and should be based on a risk versus benefit basis.

371

 For questions and answers on this topic please visit the supporting companion website for this book: www.wiley.com/go/ mriinpractice

Reference

Shellock FG, Woods TO, Crues JV (2009) MRI labeling information for implants and devices: explanation of terminology. *Radiology* **253**: 26–30 (available as a pdf file on www.IMRSER.org).

11

Contrast agents in MRI

Introduction

Image contrast and the parameters that control this in MRI have been discussed in detail in Chapter 2. Since water has a high signal intensity in T2 weighted images, pathology is commonly evaluated using this type of weighting. Pathological tissue often has a large number of free water spins and therefore T2 weighted images display a good intrinsic contrast between pathology and normal tissue. However there are some pathologies in which the high intrinsic contrast provided by T2 weighted images may be insufficient to detect lesions accurately. To increase contrast, enhancement agents may be introduced that selectively change T1 and T2 relaxation times of certain tissues.

Parameters

Several parameters influence inherent image contrast in MRI. These parameters include: **intrinsic contrast parameters** (those over which there is no control, such as T1, T2 relaxation times and the relative proton density of the tissue) and **extrinsic contrast parameters** (those that can be controlled, such as TR, TE, TI and flip angle) (*see* Chapter 2).

MRI in Practice, Fourth Edition. Catherine Westbrook, Carolyn Kaut Roth, John Talbot.
© 2011 Blackwell Publishing Ltd. Published 2011 by Blackwell Publishing Ltd.

Mechanism of action of contrast agents

In MR images, it is the relaxation mechanisms that determine image contrast. Tissues with long relaxation times appear differently to those with short relaxation times. In MRI, contrast media are based on the ability of the agent to affect the local magnetic field and hence the T1 and T2 relaxation times of tissues. For this reason contrast media in MRI consist of agents with varying magnetic susceptibilities. The most commonly used contrast agents are gadolinium based. As an element, gadolinium (Gd) is ferromagnetic; however, when used as a contrast agent, gadolinium is *bound* or chelated to other chemicals. As a ferromagnetic element, gadolinium is highly toxic; however, gadolinium can be made safe for use by binding or chelating the gadolinium to other molecules (to be discussed later in this chapter). At body temperature, gadolinium chelates are paramagnetic and have a low, positive effect on the local magnetic field. As a result, gadolinium agents shorten T1 relaxation and create bright lesions on T1 weighted images (Figure 11.1). These are known as T1 agents. However, gadolinium agents also shorten T2 relaxation times and can produce dark areas on T2 weighted images. Historically superparamagnetic iron oxide agents were used for liver imaging but they are now not commonly used. Therefore this chapter focuses on the use of gadolinium-based contrast agents only.

Although intrinsic parameters cannot be changed, they can be influenced. Influences to intrinsic parameters can be made by alterations in static field strength and temperature. As the patient temperature changes, T1 relaxation and T2 decay change. In addition, as B_0 is increased T1 increases and T2 decreases. Also, modifications in local magnetic fields (within tissues) alter the T1 and T2 relaxation times, and hence image contrast in MRI. Both T1 recovery and T2 decay are influenced by the magnetic field experienced within the nucleus. The local magnetic field responsible for these processes is caused by:

- the main magnetic field
- the fluctuations caused by the magnetic moments of nuclear spins in neighboring molecules.

These molecules rotate or tumble, and the rate of rotation of the molecules is a characteristic property of the solution, and depends on:

- the viscosity of the solution
- the temperature of the solution.

Gadolinium contrast agents can affect both T1 and T2 relaxation times. Therefore, if T1 is shortened then T2 is also shortened, and visa versa. Therefore, gadolinium can be administered to shorten both T1 and T2 relaxation times. A 50% reduction in the T1 relaxation time (originally 2000 ms in water) for example results in a 1000 ms reduction in the T1 time. When an agent appears to have greater affect on T1 weighted images, we know this agent as a T1 agent. Gadolinium is an example of such an agent. However, gadolinium also causes a shortening of T2*. This is, however, much smaller than its T1 shortening effects and, as T2* occurs so rapidly, these effects can only be seen transiently when the contrast agent first passes through the capillary bed (see Perfusion imaging, Chapter 12).

Molecular tumbling

During any discussion of the principles of MRI, the spinning (precession and/or wobbling) of the nucleus is described (*see* Chapter 1). In fact, the entire molecule tumbles in the presence of a

374

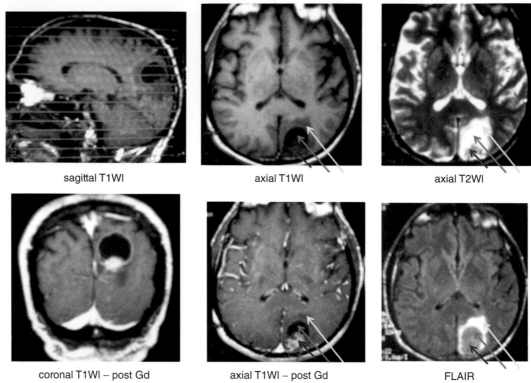

sagittal T1WI   axial T1WI   axial T2WI

coronal T1WI – post Gd   axial T1WI – post Gd   FLAIR

Figure 11.1   Various types of MR image contrast. Top left (Sagittal T1), top middle (Axial T1), Top right (Axial T2) Bottom left (Coronal T1 – post Gd), Bottom middle (Axial T1-post Gd), Bottom right (FLAIR). Note the lesion on the posterior portion of the brain has several components (tumor, cyst and edema). On the T1 weighted image the entire lesion appears dark, whereas on the T2 weighted image the entire lesion appears bright. The three arrows demonstrate the three components of this particular lesion. The red arrow indicates the tumor (enhanced with gadolinium, Gd), the blue arrow (indicates the cystic component of the lesion) and the yellow arrow (indicates the edema surrounding the cystic component). Note that the acquisition of various image contrast, combined with contrast enhancement, provides different information for this complex lesion. Note also the contrast enhancement of the lesion on the axial T1 weighted image post Gd is different from the enhancement on the coronal T1 weighted image post Gd. The axial image was acquired first after injection and then the coronal was acquired. The increased enhancement on the coronal imaging is likely due to the relative delay after injection. For this reason, it is recommended to acquire two acquisitions (in different planes) post Gd administration, particularly for CNS lesions. Two views are acquired for the evaluation of the architecture of the lesion and for the hemodynamics of the lesion. Architecture of the lesion (viewed by orthogonal planes) provides information about the shape of the lesion and hemodynamics provides information about enhancement characteristics (blood flow to the lesion).

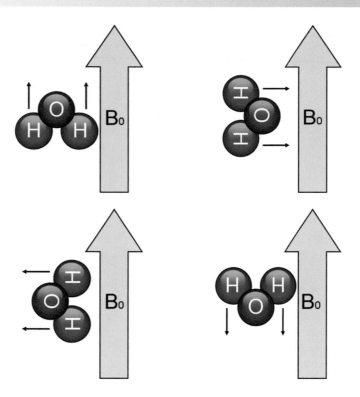

375

Figure 11.2   Tumbling of water molecules. Top left (time 1), top right (time 2), bottom left (time 3), bottom right (time 4).

magnetic field (not *just* the nucleus). When a particular molecule (such as CH_3, fat, or H_2O, water) tumbles at a rate precisely at or near the Larmor frequency, T1 relaxation is efficient, or short. For example, the fat molecule tumbles very close to the Larmor frequency and therefore has a short T1 relaxation time.

Tumbling molecules create fluctuations in the local magnetic field. Figure 11.2 illustrates the tumbling of water molecules. In the illustration on the left, where the water molecule is in the magnetic field, during 'time #1', the magnetic moments (μ) of the hydrogen nuclei add to B_0, during 'time # 2' there is no net effect as the magnetic moments lie perpendicular to B_0, and at 'time #3' they impose B_0 and therefore subtract from (or yield a negative effect on) the applied field B_0, During 'time # 4' there is no net effect as the magnetic moments lie perpendicular to B_0. This tumbling therefore results in local fluctuations in the magnetic field (higher field at 'time #1', no change at 'time #2', lower field at 'time #3' and no change at 'time #4'. . . and so on). To slow down the tumbling rate, and hence reduce the relaxation times, gadolinium can be introduced.

Dipole–dipole interactions

Water tumbles much faster than the Larmor frequency, resulting in inefficient relaxation and a long T1 relaxation time (dark on T1 weighted images). If a tumbling molecule with a large magnetic moment is placed in the presence of water spins, local magnetic field fluctuations occur.

In the case of a gadolinium chelate molecule, these fluctuations are near the Larmor frequency, and so T1 relaxation times of nearby spins can be reduced (bright on T1 weighted images). This is the effect that occurs when enhancement agents with large magnetic moments come into contact with spins in water. The T1 relaxation time of the water is reduced so enhancing lesions (such as tumors associated with free water) appear bright on a T1 weighted image.

Magnetic susceptibility

When evaluating suitable enhancement agents, their magnetic susceptibility must be considered. Magnetic susceptibility is a fundamental property of matter and is defined as the ability of the external magnetic field to affect the nucleus of an atom and/or magnetize it. Magnetic susceptibility effects include diamagnetism, paramagnetism, superparamagnetism and ferromagnetism. As discussed in Chapter 9:

- diamagnetic substances such as gold and silver show mild negative effects on the local magnetic field within the nucleus
- paramagnetic substances such as gadolinium chelates have a positive effect on the local magnetic field
- superparamagnetic substances such as iron oxides have large magnetic moments, have a positive susceptibility (greater than paramagnetic substances) and create large disruptive changes in local magnetic fields
- ferromagnetic substances such as iron have high positive susceptibilities, acquire large magnetic moments when placed in a magnetic field and retain this magnetization even when the external field is removed.

T1 agents

As paramagnetic substances have positive magnetic susceptibilities, they provide a suitable choice for an enhancement agent in MRI. Gadolinium (Gd), a trivalent lanthanide element (a rare earth metal ion), is ideal because it has seven unpaired electrons and the ability to allow rapid exchange of bulk water. Unpaired electrons have a magnetic moment (μ) that is 500 000 times that of a hydrogen proton. It is this large magnetic moment that creates fluctuations in the local magnetic fields.

Water within the body (such as free water associated with tumors) tumbles much faster than the Larmor frequency resulting in inefficient relaxation (long T1 and T2 relaxation times).

When molecular tumbling creates fluctuations in a magnetic field near the Larmor frequency, the T1 relaxation time of nearby water spins is reduced. This results in an increased signal intensity of water in T1 weighted images. For this reason, gadolinium is known as a **T1 enhancement agent**. Other T1 enhancement agents include manganese – an intravenous agent used in liver imaging, and hyperpolarized helium – a T1 ventilation agent used for the evaluation of the lungs (*see* Figure 11.7).

Although some lesions can be visualized without contrast agents, it is difficult to visualize all lesions without contrast enhancement. In Figure 11.3, the image in the top row is unenhanced and the image on the bottom left is enhanced with gadolinium (single dose). The larger metastatic lesion (identified with the red arrow – located on the patient's left posterior region of the brain) is relatively conspicuous even without contrast. However, the conspicuity of the smaller metastatic

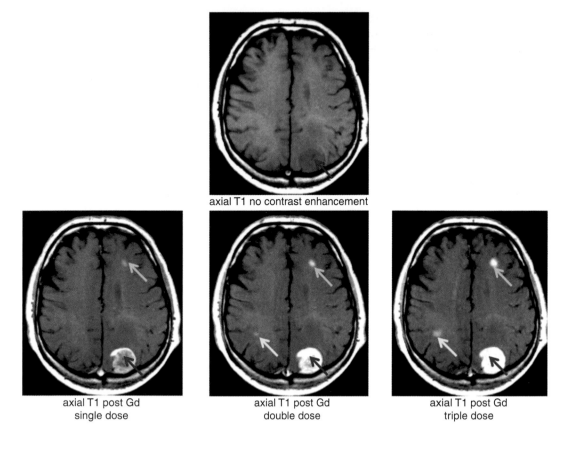

axial T1 no contrast enhancement

axial T1 post Gd
single dose

axial T1 post Gd
double dose

axial T1 post Gd
triple dose

Figure 11.3   This image demonstrates axial T1 weighted images of the brain in a patient with metastatic disease.

lesions (identified with the blue arrow – located in the patient's left frontal lobe, and yellow arrow – in the patient's right parietal lobe) are virtually invisible on the unenhanced image. To enable the visualization of the smaller metastatic lesions required double dose (bottom middle image). For better visualization, triple dose (bottom right image) might be required. Contrast dosage will be discussed later in this chapter.

T2 agents

Although we consider gadolinium to be a T1 agent, it can also be used to shorten T2, and particularly T2*. For this reason gadolinium can also be used as a **T2 enhancement agent**. When paramagnetic gadolinium is administered during dynamic brain imaging (acquired as a T2* image), perfusion information can be gleaned from the images. Perfusion, by definition, is blood supply into a volume of tissue. The degree of perfusion can be assessed by tracking the uptake of contrast media in the tissue under investigation (*see* Chapter 12).

Relaxivity

When contrast agents are used in MRI, it is not the agent itself but the effects of the agent that are measured. In MRI, it is the function of the agent on the related tissues that determines image enhancement.

The effect of a substance on relaxation rate is known as its **relaxivity**. As previously discussed, water tumbles much faster than the Larmor frequency resulting in inefficient relaxation and persistence of phase coherence. T1 and T2 times are directly affected by local magnetic fields and any substance that affects T1 also affects T2. Since *short T1* and *long T2* relaxation times both increase signal intensity, and since these are *opposing* effects, it would seem difficult to find a substance that both shortens the T1 time and, at the same time, lengthens the T2 time.

Relaxivity is expressed in the following equations:

$$\text{(1/T1)observed} = \text{(P) (1/T1)enhanced} + \text{(1} - \text{P) (1/T1)bulk water}$$

and

$$\text{(1/T2)observed} = \text{(P) (1/T2)enhanced} + \text{(1} - \text{P) (1/T2)bulk water.}$$

The relaxivity equations show that the inverse of T1 in bulk water combined with an enhancement agent results in a new relaxivity, (1/T) enhanced. P is the fraction or concentration of the substance, and therefore as the concentration is increased the effect of the agent is also increased. The equation also demonstrates that T1 and T2 are equally affected by enhancement agents. However, since the T2 relaxation time of biological fluids (approximately 100 ms) is much shorter than the T1 relaxation time (approximately 2000 ms), a higher effective concentration of the enhancement agent (or a high susceptibility imaging sequence) is needed to produce significant shortening of T2. Although it seems impossible for a tissue to possess both short T1 and long T2 (as these are opposing affects), it may be possible for a given tissue to have various substances within that do possess these characteristics. For example, methemaglobin (a component of hemorrhage) has such short T1 and long T2 relaxation times. For this reason, methemaglobin appears bright on T1 weighted image and also bright on T2 weighted image.

High relaxivity agents

Historically, most of the gadolinium agents introduced to the market have exhibited similar relaxivity properties, determined by the amount of gadolinium present. Recently, there have been new gadolinium agents introduced to the market having a higher relaxivity for the same dose. These high relaxivity agents have been developed to allow for better visualization of pathology and/or the ability to use lower doses. One such agent, Gd-BOPTA (brand name of MultiHance) has been used for a number of years and was approved by the FDA for use in the United States. When using high relaxivity agents, such as Gd-BOPTA, the relaxivity is essentially twice that of the standard relaxivity agents. This has the benefit of providing greater lesion conspicuity at a given dose, or in MRA a higher signal from small vessels (Figure 11.4).

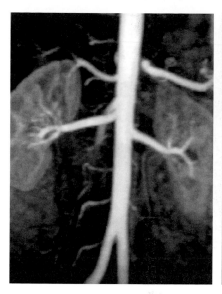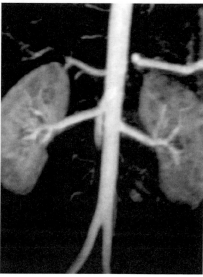

Figure 11.4 Images were acquired for the renal arteries. The image on the left was acquired with the new (higher relaxivity) agent with 20 ml. The image on the right with standard gadolinium with a standard MRA (40 ml) dose.

Gadolinium administration/dose

The recommended dosage of gadolinium is 0.1 millimoles per kilogram (mmol/kg) of body weight, (0.2 ml/kg). Several specific agents have been approved for up to 0.3 mmol/kg or three times the dose as compared with the majority of gadolinium agents. The lethal dose, (LD_{50} – the dose required to kill half of the study population) determined in rat studies is between 6 and 20 mmol/kg. This is never approached in the clinical situation.

In addition to safety, dose should be considered for clinical evaluation as well. As dose increases (to a point), the ability to visualize structures and lesions also increases. With standard gadolinium the optimal dose is weight-based. Higher relaxivity agents can, in some cases, create an increase in signal intensity that would otherwise require a double dose of standard agent (Figure 11.4). Care should be taken to calculate dose, the type of contrast used and to document dose and agent for the clinician to provide optimal diagnostic value for the patient.

Some facilities opt to inject every patient with a standard dose of, for example, 10 ml. This is an *unacceptable* method of contrast enhancement. When considering the affect of dose on enhanced MR images, review the images illustrated in Figure 11.3. The image on the top is unenhanced, and the image on the bottom left is enhanced with gadolinium (single dose), bottom middle (double dose) and bottom right (triple dose). Imagine a patient with a weight of 90 kg. If this patient is injected with 10 ml, the effective dose is essentially one half the recommended dose. In this case, several lesions could be missed on enhanced imaging. Note the difference in visualization of lesions for single, double dose and triple dose of standard gadolinium. For these reasons, it is essential to calculate dose (by weight) and document the dose (and type) of the contrast that has been administered.

It is acceptable for the technologist/radiographer to inject contrast agents in radiology (X-ray, CT, MRI). However, according to the ACR White Paper on MRI Safety:

> The ACR approves of the injection of contrast material and diagnostic levels of radiopharmaceuticals by certified and/or licensed radiologic technologists and radiologic nurses under the direction of a radiologist or his or her physician designee who is personally and immediately available, if the practice is in compliance with institutional and state regulations

To comply with these ACR recommendations, a facility must have a doctor present during an injection of any contrast agent.

Gadolinium safety

Gadolinium is a rare earth metal (lanthanide) more commonly known as a heavy metal. Heavy metals in nature include lead and mercury and can be lethal to humans. Metal ions with free electrons tend to accumulate in tissues with a natural affinity for metals (binding sites). Sites within the body that bind $Gd+3$ include membranes, transport proteins, enzymes and the osseous matrix (and/or the reticuloendothelial system: lungs, liver, spleen and bone). As the body is unable to excrete these metals, they can remain in the tissues for a long period of time. Gadolinium in its native state is highly toxic and a cumulative poison.

Fortunately there are substances with a high affinity for metal ions. These substances are known as chelates. The chelate (from the Greek word *khele*, meaning 'claw') binds some of the available sites of the metal ion. The first chelate that proved effective for MR contrast media was diethylene triaminepentaacetic acid (DTPA). DTPA binds eight of the nine binding sites of the gadolinium ion leaving the ninth free for close approach of water molecules to the paramagnetic material. In binding the gadolinium ion to a chelate such as this the toxicity is greatly reduced and the product can be readily excreted by the body. In a patient with normal renal function, the biological half-life of gadolinium is less than 2 hours. This time is extended, however, in patients with impaired renal function. As each type of gadolinium agent is different, anyone administering contrast agents must read the manufacturer's literature for information on possible side effects, reactions and contraindications.

There are a number of paramagnetic gadolinium agents that are approved for use within the US and worldwide (Figure 11.5 and Table 11.1). The difference between the agents varies with the chelate. Some agents are linear molecules and others are macrocyclic molecules, some agents are ionic others non-ionic. The majority of these agents are excreted by the kidneys. There is yet another gadolinium chelate, gadobenate dimeglumine, known as Gd-BOPTA, that has been in use in Europe for several years and has recently become available in the US. It has shown promise for use in the liver as it is excreted by the renal and also (to a small extent) by the hepatobiliary system. This agent has a higher relaxivity than the standard gadolinium agents. Due to this higher relaxivity, Gd-BOPTA administered at standard dose (0.1 mmol/kg), provides the enhancement of double dose (0.2 mmol/kg) of standard gadolinium agents. If, however, Gd-BOPTA is administered at half dose (0.05 mmol/kg), enhancement will be similar to standard dose (0.1 mmol/kg) of standard gadolinium (Figure 11.4). The brand name for this agent is MultiHance. There are three ionic linear agents (Gd-BOPTA, Gd-EOB-DTPA and Gadofosveset) that are cleared by both renal and hepatobiliary mechanisms to varying degrees.

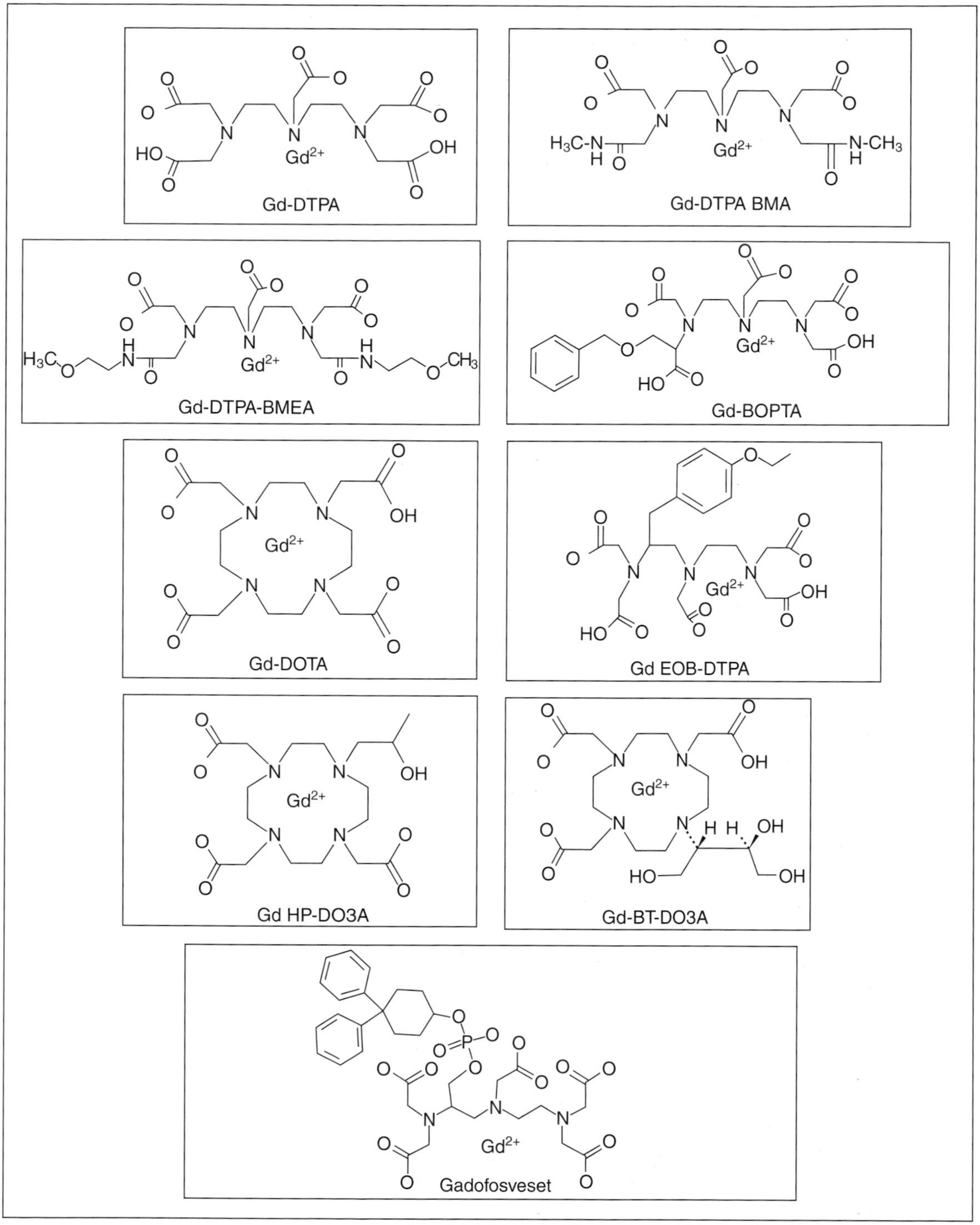

Figure 11.5 Paramagnetic gadolinium agents. The 'circular molecules' such as Gd-DOTA, Gd HP-DO3A and Gd-BT-DO3A are known as 'macrocyclic' molecules. The others are known as 'linear' molecules.

Table 11.1   Comparison of the types of gadolinium chelate that are used in the US and worldwide, with generic name, brand name, molecular structure and charge.

Within the US				
Chemical	**Generic name**	**Brand name**	**Molecular structure**	**Charge**
Gd-DTPA	gadodentetic acid	Magnevist	linear molecule	ionic
Gd-HP-DO3A	gadoteridol	Prohance	macrocyclic molecule	non-ionic
Gd-DTPA	gadodiamide	Omniscan	linear molecule	non-ionic
Gd-DTPA-BMEA	gadoversetamide	Optimark	linear molecule	non-ionic
GD-BOPTA	gadobentetic acid	MultiHance	linear molecule	ionic
Gd-EOB-DTPA	gadoxetic acid	Eovist (known as Primovist outside the US)	linear molecule	ionic
Gd-DTPA	gadofosveset trisodium	Vasovist	linear molecule	ionic
Outside the US				
Gd-BT-DO3A	Gadobutrol	Gadovist (approved in Canada)	macrocyclic molecule	ionic
Gd-DOTA	gadoteric acid	Dotarem	macrocyclic molecule	ionic

Unlike iodinated agents there are few safety considerations associated with gadolinium contrast agents. One such consideration is the stability of the gadolinium chelate. As discussed, gadolinium element is a heavy metal and therefore toxic. To make gadolinium safe for use as a contrast agent, it is bound or chelated to a molecule that binds with the gadolinium. The stability of the bind is an important safety consideration. It stands to reason that if the molecule is not stable (i.e. the gadolinium easily comes apart from the chelate), this leaves only gadolinium element within the body. Additional safety considerations will be discussed in the next section.

Whenever contrast agents are administered during imaging (X-ray, CT or MRI), there is a risk of an adverse event. Adverse events can be considered as a side effect or a reaction and can be classified as mild, moderate or severe.

Nephrogenic systemic fibrosis

Prior to the FDA approval for gadolinium contrast agents, studies have shown that approximately 80% of gadolinium is excreted by the kidneys in 3 h and 98% is recovered by feces and urine in one week. As the result of these studies, it became clear that gadolinium contrast is excreted from the body through the urine. Until recently, it was thought that the use of gadolinium was indicated and deemed safe for all patients, including patients with poor renal function. In 2006, a Danish study prompted serious concern about the use of gadolinium contrast agents for MRI and MRA procedures in patients who suffered from renal insufficiency. These patients contracted a condition known as nephrogenic systemic fibrosis (NSF).

Patients who were in renal failure and received gadolinium developed a 'bark-like' skin condition, which was misdiagnosed as scleroderma. On additional review, the condition became known as nephrogenic fibrosing dermopathy (NFD). Further investigation revealed that this condition not only affected the skin, but the organ system as well. At this point the condition became known as nephrogenic systemic fibrosis (NSF). NSF is a fatal condition with virtually no cure. Although treatment does help, it must be administered immediately. Unfortunately, many NSF symptoms do not reveal themselves for several days to several weeks after contrast administration. To date, no cases of NSF have been reported in patients with normal renal function. For these reasons, gadolinium is a contraindication and a relative precaution for patients in renal failure.

Other contrast agents

Gadolinium is not the only element that could be considered as a contrast agent in MRI. Other elements such as manganese and iron oxide have been shown to produce alterations in T1 and T2 relaxation times. For this reason, they can be used as contrast agents in MRI. This section provides a brief overview of other agents currently used as contrast media in MRI.

Other T1 agents

Although they are not commonly used, there are a few other agents that are used as T1 contrast agents in MRI. These additional agents include manganese, used for liver imaging, and hyperpolarized helium gas for inhalation imaging for the lungs. Such agents shorten T1 and therefore appear bright on T1 weighted images. Manganese is taken up by the Kupffer cells in the liver. In this case the normal liver will enhance and lesions remain darker (Figure 11.6). Enhanced lung images are shown in Figure 11.7, and demonstrate 'ventilation' information.

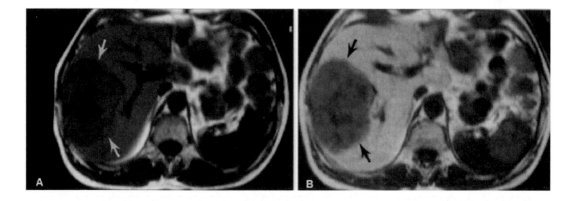

Figure 11.6   Axial T1 weighted image of the liver without (left) and with (right) manganese contrast (Teslascan) agent administration. Note that the enhanced image (right) demonstrates enhancement of the normal portions of the liver, rendering the liver lesion dark relative to the normal liver parenchyma.

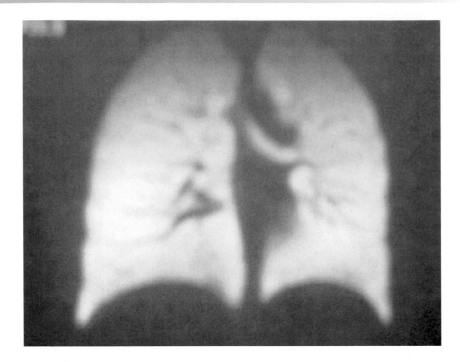

Figure 11.7   T1 weighted gradient echo image of the lungs after inhalation of hyper-polarized helium gas. Th helium gas provides increased signal enhancement on T1 gradient echo images and therefore provides ventilation information.

Oral and rectal enhancement agents

Gastrointestinal contrast agents are not as widely used as intravascular agents at present but may increase in use in the future. Oral contrast agents have been researched for bowel enhancement. Iron oxides (dark on T2 weighted images) and fatty substances (bright on T1 weighted images) have been used orally to try to enhance the gastrointestinal tract effectively (Figure 11.8). However, due to constant peristalsis, positive agents (those agents that make bowel bright) enhance bowel motion artefacts. The use of antispasmodic agents helps to retard peristalsis and/or ultra-fast imaging techniques to reduce these artefacts.

Formerly, there was an agent called Perflubron (perfluorocarbon) that rendered bowel black in T2 weighted images. Perfluorocarbon is a substance that holds oxygen, and therefore it is used as a blood replacement agent during transplantation. For a period of time this agent was approved as a contrast agent for MRI. However, since the agent was rarely utilized, it is no longer available for use as a contrast agent. Today, there are facilities that use juices such as blueberry and mango juice (to make bowel dark on T2 weighted images) as enhancement agents. Also, agents such as dilute gadolinium are used (to make bowel bright on T1 weighted images) to enhance bowel. In addition, agents such as dilute barium solutions can be used to make bowel contents appear dark. Air has also been used as an effective negative contrast agent in the rectum. By showing a signal intensity void in the distended rectum, the prostate in males and the uterus in females can be more clearly demonstrated when imaging the pelvis.

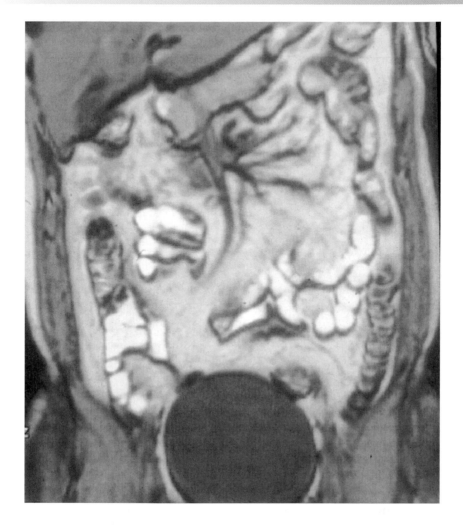

Figure 11.8   Coronal image of the abdomen with bowel contrast enhancement.

Current applications of gadolinium contrast agents

When gadolinium contrast agents became available in the early 1990s, many people were of the impression that contrast media was not necessary for MRI because of the high soft tissue contrast provided by MR images. In reality, contrast media has found its way into day-to-day clinical usage. Today, clinical indications for the brain, spine and body for gadolinium include (but are not limited to):

- tumors pre- and post-operation
- pre- and post-radiotherapy

- infection
- infarction
- inflammation
- post-traumatic lesions
- post-operation lumbar disc.
- contrast-enhanced MRA.

Head and spine

Like other contrast agents, gadolinium cannot cross the *intact* blood–brain barrier (BBB). However, gadolinium has proven invaluable in imaging the central nervous system (brain and spinal cord) because of its ability to pass through *breakdowns* in the BBB. Since lesions are associated with breakdowns in the BBB, these lesions will enhance with gadolinium. For this reason, gadolinium is commonly used to evaluate lesions of the CNS both within and outside the BBB.

The brain

Lesions outside the BBB are known as extra-axial lesions, and as they are outside the BBB, they demonstrate normal enhancement. These areas include the falx cerebri, choroid plexus, pineal gland, pituitary gland (hypophysis) and the pituitary stalk (infundibulum). Other normal enhancing structures include slow-flowing vessels, sinus mucosa and muscular structures. Areas with slow-flowing blood, such as the cavernous sinus and the venous drainage system, may also demonstrate enhancement. Therefore, fat and slow-flowing blood can often be mistaken for blood products. These normal enhancing structures should be recognized by the technologist so as not to misinterpret them as abnormalities. The diagnosis of other extra-axial lesions such as acoustic neuromas and meningiomas has been facilitated by the use of gadolinium (Figures 11.9 and 11.10). In the pituitary gland a macro-adenoma enhances rapidly. Conversely, due to the densely packed cells associated with a pituitary micro-adenoma, the micro-adenoma appears dense compared with the normal enhancement of the normal pituitary gland (a vascular organ). In addition since the pituitary gland rapidly enhances, images should be acquired rapidly after contrast enhancement.

Intra-axial lesions such as infarcts and tumors of the brain enhance due to the breakdown in their BBB (Figure 11.12). Generally, peri-infarctal edema does not enhance. Although recent infarctions do not enhance until the BBB has been disrupted, some evidence suggests that arterial vessels in the brain enhance and therefore any occlusion or slow flow in these vessels can be demonstrated. Since some lesions of the brain enhance more slowly than others it is recommended to acquire at least two acquisitions (often in orthogonal imaging planes) after the administration of gadolinium contrast.

Metastatic disease can be demonstrated with the use of gadolinium. Studies have shown that at higher doses, gadolinium can make metastatic lesions appear more conspicuous. As patient management (and treatment) changes according to the number of intracranial metastatic lesions, the ability to demonstrate these lesions is essential.

In Figure 11.3, the image in the top row is unenhanced and the image on the bottom left is enhanced with gadolinium (single dose). The larger metastatic lesion (identified with the red arrow – located on the patient's left posterior region of the brain) is relatively conspicuous even without

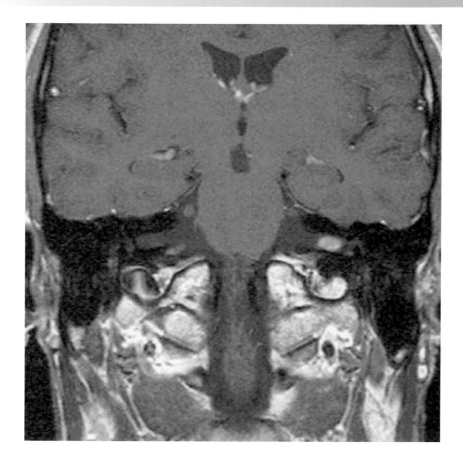

Figure 11.9   Coronal T1 weighted image of a small acoustic neuroma after administration of gadolinium.

contrast. However, the conspicuity of the smaller metastatic lesions (identified with the blue arrow – located in the patient's left frontal lobe, and yellow arrow – the patient's right parietal lobe) are virtually invisible on the unenhanced image. To enable the visualization of the smaller metastatic lesions required double dose (bottom middle image). For better visualization, triple dose (bottom right image) might be required.

Perfusion is microcirculation or the delivery of blood to tissues. Perfusion imaging is the measurement of blood volume in these areas. This measurement, however, is complicated because fewer than 5% of tissue protons are intravascular. To measure perfusion the signal intensity in perfusing spins may be suppressed or increased. This can be achieved either by the introduction of additional pulses (known as spin tagged perfusion) or by introducing enhancement agents (*see* Chapter 12). Agents such as gadolinium may be localized in the capillary bed and produce large magnetic moments in the capillary network, creating magnetic fields that extend into the adjacent tissues. This results in perfusion information in patients with ischemia in brain parenchyma, liver parenchyma and in myocardial infarction.

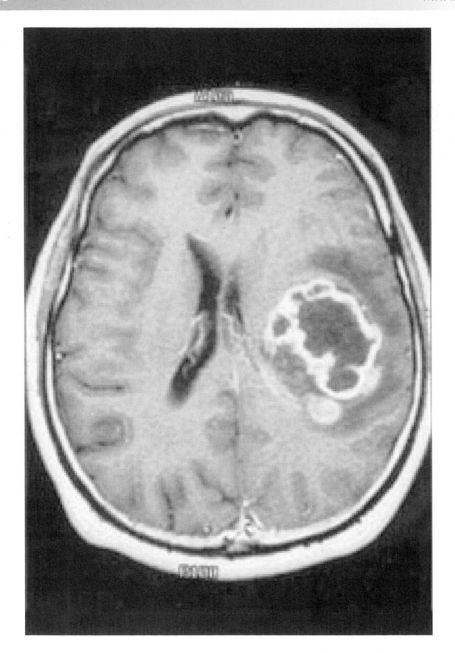

Figure 11.10   Axial I1 weighted image of a cerebral tumor after administration of gadolinium.

The spine

Lesions within the spinal cord lesions can be visualized with the use of gadolinium (Figure 11.11). Although lesions can sometimes be detected without the use of gadolinium, they are better delineated with gadolinium enhancement agents. In addition, gadolinium can demonstrate the

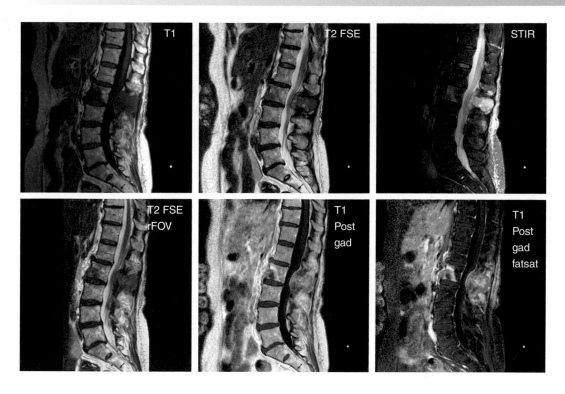

Figure 11.11   Sagittal images of the lumbar spine with bone metastases, showing T1 weighted image (upper left), T2 weighted image (upper middle), STIR (upper right), T2 weighted image with rectangular FOV (lower left), T1 weighted image post Gd (lower middle) and T1 weighted image post Gd with fat saturation (lower right).

presence of other anomalies such as a syrinx. Lesions such as multiple sclerosis (MS) and other inflammatory disorders including AIDS and/or abcesses enhance with the use of gadolinium. Enhancing MS plaques may indicate activity within the plaque.

When symptoms recur in patients who have had discectomy surgery, it is recommended that patients receive contrast-enhanced MRI of the lumbar spine, which can differentiate between scar tissue and recurrent herniated disc. Subtle enhancement can be shown in the scar in post-operative discectomy patients. In post-operative patients, initially scar enhances and disc does not. However, after approximately 30 min, disc matter shows signs of enhancement. For this reason, it is advisable to scan immediately after injection in cases where scar is suspected.

Metastatic lesions of the bone have been more clearly delineated by the use of gadolinium, and bone lesions of the spine can be well visualized with the use of gadolinium (Figures 11.12 and 11.13). Enhancement can raise the signal intensity of the bone lesion to that of normal marrow making the lesion isointense with normal bone. If bony lesions are to be evaluated with gadolinium on T1 weighted images, fat suppression techniques should be used. Since the gadolinium makes the signal from the lesion bright and the fat in the marrow is also bright, the lesion is difficult to visualize. Therefore the use of fat suppression suppresses the signal from fat in the marrow allowing for the visualization within the bone.

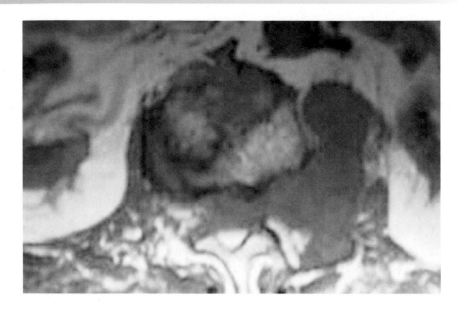

Figure 11.12   Axial T1 weighted image of a lumbar vertebra without gadolinium. Bony metastases are seen.

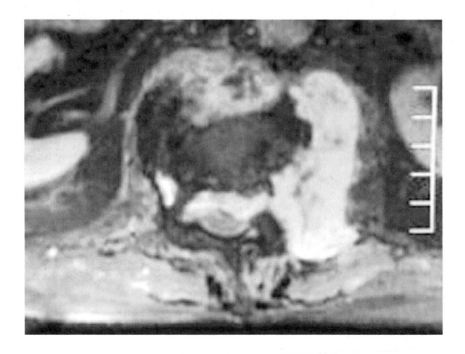

Figure 11.13   The same patient as in Figure 11.12 after gadolinium. Enhancement is clearly seen.

The body

Many lesions in the body can be demonstrated on T1 and also on T2 weighted sequences without the use of relaxation enhancing agents. However, it is the enhanced images of the visceral structures of the abdomen, acquired dynamically, that typically help to finalize the diagnosis. The use of gadolinium in body imaging is increasing. Even though contrast does not enhance all lesions within the body, gadolinium has shown some promising effects.

MRI of the abdomen

In MR imaging of the abdomen, gadolinium has been used for perfusion studies of the kidneys, liver, spleen, pancreas, adrenals, vascular structures and pelvic structures. Since the liver, spleen and kidneys are vascular organs, contrast enhances these structures almost immediately after injection (Figure 11.14). For this reason, rapid imaging is recommended. Dynamic enhancement and rapid imaging can be used to evaluate visceral and vascular structures in the abdomen.

When MR imaging is acquired for the evaluation of liver lesions, timing is essential (Figure 11.15). The majority of liver lesions are arterially fed. In this case, the first pass will demonstrate enhanced liver lesions. For this reason, malignant lesions will be demonstrated on the first pass after injection. As 85% of the liver's blood supply comes from the portal vein, the second pass will wash in the liver paryenchyma and therefore hide the appearance of liver lesions. By the

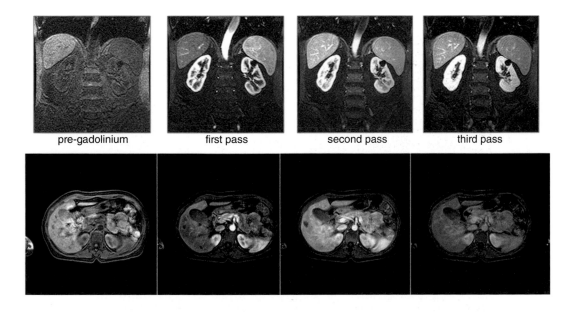

| pre-gadolinium | first pass | second pass | third pass |

Figure 11.14 Timing is essential for optimal abdominal imaging. Optimal enhancement characteristics can be visualized on the first-pass imaging sequence when spleen is brighter than liver; spleen appears mottled in enhancement and only the cortex of the kidneys is enhanced. By the second pass, liver and spleen are isointense (the same color gray) and the kidneys are perfused. By the third pass the visceral structures are beginning to 'wash out'.

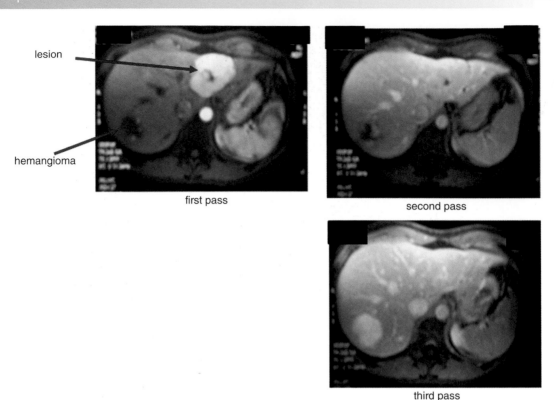

first pass

second pass

third pass

Figure 11.15   MR images of the abdomen (liver) during three phases after injection. Note that in the first phase (first pass) the liver lesion is enhanced. This represents a rapidly enhancing liver cancer. During the second phase (second pass) the liver and the lesion are isointense. By the third phase (third pass) another lesion enhances. This lesion represents a late enhancing, benign hemangioma.

second pass, both the normal liver and pathology will be enhanced, and therefore will appear isointense on MR images.

MRA of the body

Arterial flow in abdominal vessels can be visualized by acquiring MR images with contrast enhanced MRA (CE-MRA) 3D T1 gradient echo breath-hold acquisitions after gadolinium (Figures 11.16, 11.17 and 11.18). Peak enhancement differences occur shortly after injection, and by two minutes after injection lesions begin to enhance so that they are isointense with normal organ paren-chyma. For this reason, rapid imaging acquisitions should be used when imaging the abdomen to maximize the enhancement effect. For vascular lesions, 3D rapid imaging is essential.

In cardiac imaging, myocardial infarctions (MI) have been shown to enhance. This can be best visualized by cardiac perfusion sequences. These sequences are acquired dynamically with gado-linium enhancement for the evaluation of MIs during rest and during physical or pharmacologic induced stress (see Chapter 8).

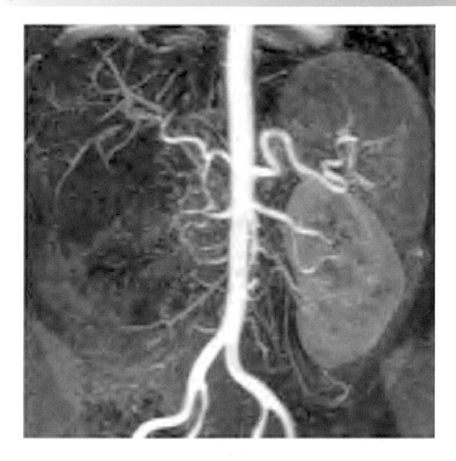

Figure 11.16   Abdominal vessels after gadolinium administration – arterial phase.

In breast imaging, the use of gadolinium followed by repeated rapid acquisitions (acquired with fat saturation and/or followed by subtraction techniques) is proving to help determine the nature of suspicious lesions within the breast tissue (Figure 11.19). Breast imaging requires high-resolution imaging (to evaluate architecture) of the lesion and rapid imaging (to evaluate hemodynamics). Lesions that have a spiculated architecture are likely to be malignant. Lesions that 'wash-in' (enhance) rapidly and 'wash-out' rapidly are thought to be malignant. Therefore, many rapidly enhancing and/or spiculated enhanced lesions are thought to be malignant. In addition, this technique seems to demonstrate multi-focal lesions that are not always apparent on plain mammography.

Conclusion

Overall examination time may lengthen with the use of intravenous contrast in MRI because additional sequences are performed (post contrast). In most cases T1 and T2 weighted sequences should be performed before the use of gadolinium, followed by contrast administration and one or more T1 weighted series. Multiple T1, post contrast sequences can be used in dynamic imaging of the breast, abdomen and chest, and multiple sequences are also useful for the evaluation of

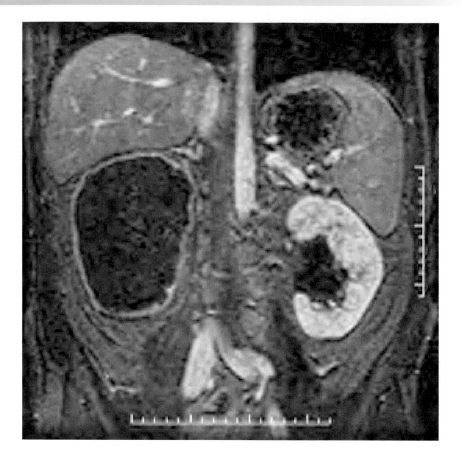

Figure 11.17   Abdominal vessels after gadolinium administration – intermediate phase.

brain lesions in different imaging planes. Gadolinium has improved the visualization of lesions in many cases and it has enabled a more precise delineation of lesions in T1 weighted images.

The increased use of enhancement agents has placed a large responsibility on the system operator. The operator should be aware of dosage, timing and potential imaging artefacts associated with enhancement agents. The technologist or radiographer should understand that lesions (as well as normal structures such as slow-flowing vessels and other structures) can be enhanced by contrast agents. Flow motion artefacts increase with the use of gadolinium and should therefore be anticipated and compensated for by the operator, especially when imaging vascular areas of the body. In addition, gadolinium should be used in conjunction with fat-suppression techniques in areas where it is suspected that the increased signal from enhancement will become isointense with fatty tissues. Finally, different concentrations of gadolinium will affect image contrast and produce a layering effect in the bladder.

 For questions and answers on this topic please visit the supporting companion website for this book: www.wiley.com/go/ mriinpractice

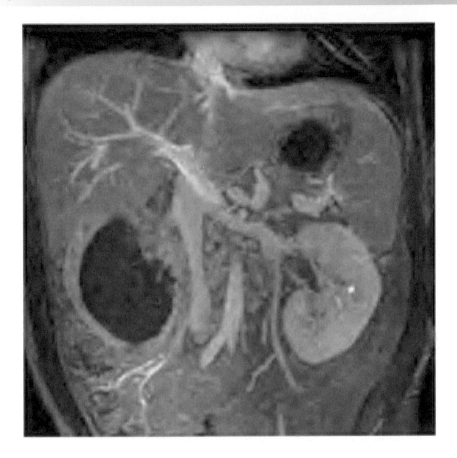

Figure 11.18   Abdominal vessels after gadolinium administration – venous phase.

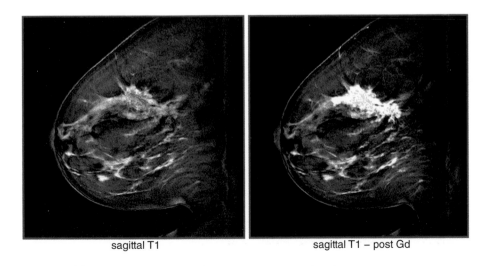

sagittal T1   sagittal T1 – post Gd

Figure 11.19   Sagittal T1 weighted images of the breast were acquired (without, left) and (with, right) gadolinium enhancement. Note that the lesion is enhanced on the post Gd image (right).

12

Functional imaging techniques

Introduction

The previous chapters introduce the basis for MRI by describing fundamental pulse sequences and image formation. Technical developments in system hardware and software have allowed for ultra-fast imaging sequences in the order of milliseconds. Ultra-fast imaging sequences permit an almost unlimited range of applications that were never possible with conventional MR imaging sequences. Most of these are now collectively called **functional imaging techniques** because they allow MRI to be used to assess function and physiology as opposed to merely conventional structural imaging.

Such applications include:

- diffusion weighted imaging (DWI)
- perfusion imaging
- functional brain imaging (fMRI)
- real-time imaging of cardiac motion and perfusion (described in Chapter 8)
- spectroscopy (MRS)
- whole body imaging
- MR microscopy (MRM).

This chapter describes these functional imaging techniques and their applications.

MRI in Practice, Fourth Edition. Catherine Westbrook, Carolyn Kaut Roth, John Talbot.
© 2011 Blackwell Publishing Ltd. Published 2011 by Blackwell Publishing Ltd.

Diffusion weighted imaging (DWI)

Diffusion is a term used to describe the movement of molecules in the extra-cellular space due to random thermal motion. This motion is restricted by boundaries such as ligaments, membranes and macromolecules (Figure 12.1). Sometimes restrictions in diffusion are directional, depending on the structure of the tissues, and diffusion is also restricted in pathology. The net displacement of molecules diffusing across an area of tissue per second is called the **apparent diffusion coefficient (ADC).** In areas of restricted diffusion the ADC is low, whereas in areas of free diffusion it is high. A sequence can be sensitized to this motion by applying two gradients on either side of

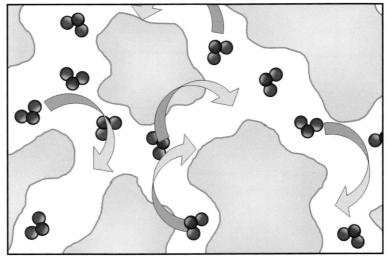

freely diffusing water

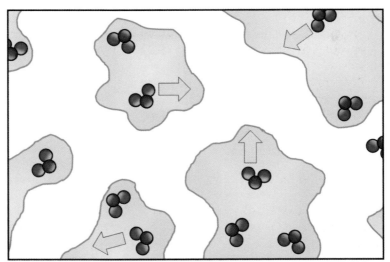

restricted water

Figure 12.1   Free and restricted diffusion in water.

180° RF pulse. This works in a similar way to phase contrast MRA (*see* Chapter 8) in that stationary spins will acquire no net phase change after the gradients have been applied. Moving spins, however, will acquire this phase change and result in a signal loss. In diffusion imaging, normal tissue that exhibits a high ADC has lower signal intensity than abnormal tissue that has a low ADC as the molecules within it are free to move, while diffusion becomes restricted when pathology is present.

Refer to animation 12.1 on the supporting companion website for this book: www.wiley.com/go/mriinpractice

Learning point: diffusion is another type of weighting

The signal change depends on the ADC of the tissue and the strength, duration and interval of the gradients (collectively known as the **b factor/value**, which is similar to the VENC in phase contrast MRA, *see* Chapter 8). In Chapter 2 we discussed how extrinsic contrast parameters such as the TR and TE control how much an intrinsic contrast parameter such as T1, T2 and PD contribute to the overall image contrast. For example, TE controls how much T2 contrast is displayed in the image. In diffusion imaging an extrinsic contrast parameter (b factor) controls how much a tissue's ADC contributes towards image weighting. If the TE and TR are long and b = 0 then the image is T2 weighted.

If we then increase the b factor the image weighting changes from T2 to diffusion weighting. By this we mean that areas will have a high signal not because they have a long T2 time, but because they have a low ADC. This is why this technique is called **diffusion weighted imaging (DWI)**. It is, in fact, another type of weighting. 'b' is expressed in units of s/mm^2. Typical 'b' values range from $500\,s/mm^2$ to $1500\,s/mm^2$.

DWI and directional effects

The diffusion gradient discussed above can be applied along all three axes, either individually or together. Individual acquisitions with different gradients sensitize the sequence to restricted diffusion along a particular axis. This is useful when imaging areas that have a directional difference in diffusion. The best example of this is in white matter, where white matter tracts take specific courses through the brain and spinal cord. Using DWI with a particular gradient applied allows us to see these white matter tracts in separate images. Tissues that display this characteristic are called **anisotropic**; tissues where this does not occur (such as gray matter) are called **isotropic**.

DWI and sequences

In DWI, spin echo sequences are commonly used where gradients are applied on either side of a 180° RF to sensitize the sequence to changes in diffusion. Usually very fast types of spin are used, such as SS-SE-EPI (*see* Chapter 5). This is not because diffusion happens particularly quickly, but because we need to reduce other types of motion such as flow, so that only motion from diffusion is measured. Typically single or multi-shot SE-EPI is used to acquire images in a few seconds. However, conventional spin echo can be used in areas with few motion artefacts.

There are two types of DW images.

- *Diffusion or trace* images are those where damaged tissue that has restricted diffusion (low ADC) is brighter than normal tissues where diffusion is free (high ADC). This is because spins in restricted tissue are refocused as they stay in the same place during the application of both gradients. However, in normal tissue where diffusion is random, refocusing is not complete and signals cancel. If motion varies rapidly, diffusion attenuation occurs and signal is lost in that area. Hence abnormal tissue is brighter than normal tissue.
- *ADC maps* are acquired via post-processing by calculating the ADC for each voxel of tissue and allocating a signal intensity according to its value. Therefore restricted tissue, which has a low ADC, is darker than free diffusing areas that have a high ADC. The contrast is therefore the mirror of the trace images. This is useful when **T2 shine through** is a problem.

T2 shine through occurs when lesions or areas with a very long T2 decay time remain bright on the DW or trace image. It is therefore difficult to know whether they represent an area of restricted diffusion or not. By producing ADC maps it is possible to differentiate between areas with a low ADC and those with a long T2 decay time. Look at Figures 12.2 and 12.3. On the trace image the infarcted tissue is bright, while on the ADC map it is dark. The ADC map enables differentiation of this area from the other high signal intensities seen on the ADC map. These areas represent tissues with a long T2 decay time, not those with a low ADC.

DWI uses

The most common use of DWI is in the brain after infarction. In early stroke, soon after the onset of ischemia but before infarct or permanent tissue damage, cells swell and absorb water from the extra-cellular space. Since cells are full of large molecules and membranes, diffusion is restricted and the ADC of the tissue is reduced. These areas appear bright on trace images and these changes can be seen within minutes of infarction as opposed to hours or days using conventional MRI techniques. Diffusion MRI can show irreversible and reversible ischemia lesions, so has a potential to discriminate salvageable tissues from irreversibly damaged tissues before a therapeutic intervention. However, timing of diffusion MRI is important – it can only visualize fresh lesions as water diffusion is decreased several days after stroke onset.

DWI can also be used to differentiate malignant from benign lesions, and tumor from edema and infarction. This is because these disease processes have different ADC values. In addition, DWI is proving a useful tool to image neonatal brains where it is sometimes difficult to discriminate between infarction and myelinating brain. DWI has also been used to map out myelination patterns in pre-term infants to assist in our understanding of this process and how hypoxic events cause certain types of brain damage. The anatomy of white matter tracts can be mapped using strong multidirectional gradients in **diffusion tensor imaging (DTI)** (Figure 12.4). This has enabled very detailed imaging of white matter in vivo and may enable the use of DWI to image certain white matter diseases.

Several studies are exploring the use of DWI in other areas and pathologies. So far these include:

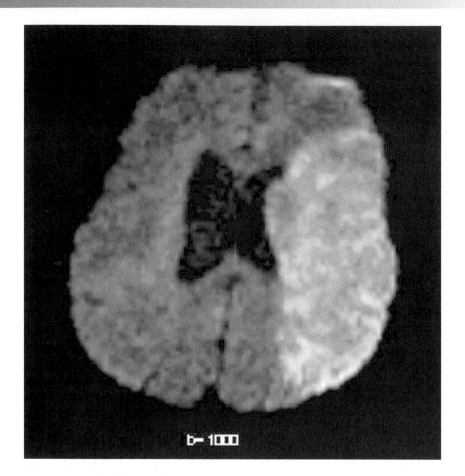

Figure 12.2   Axial trace image. Abnormality returns a higher signal than normal brain.

- characterizing liver lesions such as hepatocellular carcinoma, metastases and hemangiomas
- differentiating between mucin-producing pancreatic tumors and other tumors
- characterizing breast and prostate tumors
- imaging skeletal muscle injury
- imaging left ventricular damage after myocardial infarction
- discriminating between pathological and traumatic fractures
- overlaying DWI onto T1 weighted images to combine structural with functional data
- assessing bone bruising.

It is clear that DWI has applications in many areas of the body and that its use will increase in the future.

Perfusion imaging

Clinical perfusion measurements can be made with radio tracers, but as MRI is a non-ionizing technique with high spatial and temporal resolution that can be co-registered with anatomic

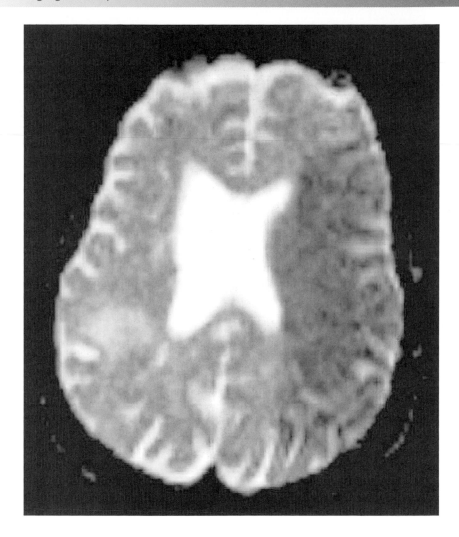

Figure 12.3   ADC map. Area of abnormality now has a low signal as it has a low ADC.

information, there is much interest in perfusion MRI studies. Perfusion is the regional blood flow in tissues and is defined as the volume of blood that flows into one gram of tissue. Perfusion is a measure of the quality of vascular supply to a tissue, and since vascular supply and metabolism are usually related, perfusion can also be used to measure tissue activity.

Perfusion is measured using MRI by tagging the water in arterial blood during image acquisition. Tagging can be achieved by either a bolus injection of exogenous contrast agent such as gadolinium, or by saturating the protons in arterial blood with RF inversion or saturation pulses. As the difference between tagged and untagged images is so small, ultra-fast imaging methods are desirable for reducing artefact. In their simplest form, perfusion images can be acquired with fast scanning acquisitions before, during and after a bolus injection of intravenous contrast. In this case several ultra-fast incoherent gradient echoes are acquired during breath hold at the same slice location. Since gadolinium shortens T1 recovery, visceral structures with high perfusion

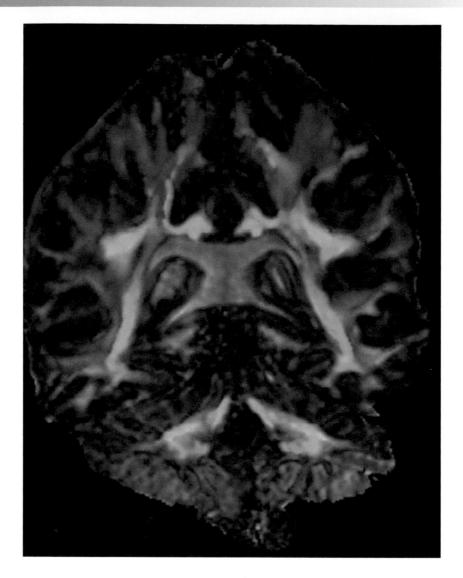

Figure 12.4 Diffusion tensor image showing white matter tracts.

appear bright on T1 weighted fast gradient echoes. This technique is useful for the evaluation of visceral structures such as the kidneys, liver and spleen.

Another technique to evaluate perfusion uses a bolus injection of gadolinium administered intravenously during ultra-fast T2 or T2* acquisitions. In this case, the contrast agent causes transient decreases in T2 and T2* decay in and around the microvasculature perfused with contrast. SS-GE-EPI sequences are usually used as they produce the required temporal resolution to measure such transient changes (Figure 12.5). Gradient echo EPI, especially when used with echo shifting (where the TE is longer than the TR), maximizes the susceptibility effects. After data acquisition, a signal decay curve is used to ascertain blood volume, transient time and measurement of

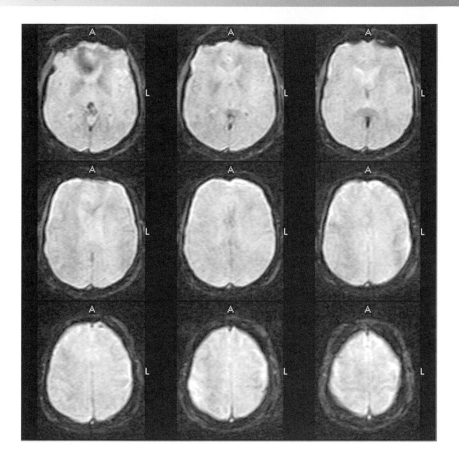

Figure 12.5 Perfusion imaging.

perfusion. This curve is known as a **time intensity curve**. Time intensity curves for multiple images acquired during and after injection are combined to generate a cerebral blood volume (CBV) map.

Perfusion imaging with arterial spin tagging is another perfusion technique. With continuous arterial spin labeling (CASL), arterial spins are attenuated by inversion or saturation pulses outside the FOV. An untagged image is also acquired as a reference image. In this technique the reference image is subtracted from the tagged image. Spin tagging is a non-invasive alternative to the introduction of exogenous contrast agents that is potentially quantitative.

Perfusion imaging uses

These techniques can be used to evaluate ischemia disease or metabolism at rest or during exercise. In addition, the malignancy of neoplasms can be reflected in increased tissue metabolism or perfusion. On the CBV map, areas of low perfusion appear dark (stroke) while areas of higher perfusion appear bright (malignancies). Such techniques show great potential in the evaluation of tissue viability and metabolism of vascular organs such as the heart, visceral structures and the brain. In particular, characteristic perfusion patterns are seen in hepatocellular carcinoma, metastases and hemangiomas. In renal imaging, acute focal changes can be seen in renal artery stenosis using perfusion techniques.

Susceptibility weighting (SWI)

Susceptibility weighting uses the susceptibility differences between tissues to generate contrast. Gradient echo sequences with a long TE are used and the signal from tissues with a different magnetic susceptibility become out of phase. This phase effect is used to generate image contrast.

SWI uses

SWI allows for small voxel imaging of blood vessels and iron-laden tissues and clinically is currently most useful in stroke and trauma.

Functional imaging (fMRI)

Functional MR imaging (fMRI) is a rapid MR imaging technique that acquires images of the brain during activity or stimulus and at rest. The two sets of images are then subtracted, demonstrating functional brain activity as the result of increased blood flow to the activated cortex. In the early days of this technique visualization of blood flow was achieved using contrast agents. More recently, blood has been used as an internal contrast.

The magnetic properties of blood are important in the understanding of this technique. Hemoglobin is a molecule that contains iron and transports oxygen in the vascular system as oxygen binds directly to iron. When oxygen is bound (oxyhemoglobin), the magnetic properties of iron are largely suppressed, but when oxygen is not bound (deoxyhemoglobin) the molecule becomes more magnetic. Therefore oxyhemoglobin is diamagnetic and deoxyhemoglobin is paramagnetic. Paramagnetic deoxyhemoglobin creates an inhomogeneous magnetic field in its immediate vicinity. This inhomogeneous magnetic field increases T2* decay and attenuates signal from regions containing deoxyhemoglobin.

At rest, tissue uses a substantial fraction of the blood flowing through the capillaries, so venous blood contains an almost equal mix of oxyhemoglobin and deoxyhemoglobin. During exercise, however, when metabolism is increased, more oxygen is needed and hence more is extracted from the capillaries. In muscle tissue the concentration of oxyhemoglobin in the venous system can become very low. The brain, however, is very sensitive to low concentrations of oxyhemoglobin and therefore the cerebral vascular system increases blood flow to the activated area. Blood oxygenation increases during brain activity and specific locations of the cerebral cortex are activated during specific tasks. For example, seeing activates the visual cortex, hearing the auditory cortex, finger tapping the motor cortex, etc. More sophisticated tasks, including maze paradigms and other thought-provoking tasks, stimulate other brain cortices.

The most important physiological effect that produces MR signal intensity changes between stimulus and rest is called **blood oxygenation level dependent (BOLD)**. BOLD exploits differences in the magnetic susceptibility of oxyhemoglobin and deoxyhemoglobin as a result of increased cerebral blood flow and little or no increase in local oxygen consumption that occurs during stimulation. Because deoxyhemoglobin is paramagnetic, vessels containing a significant amount

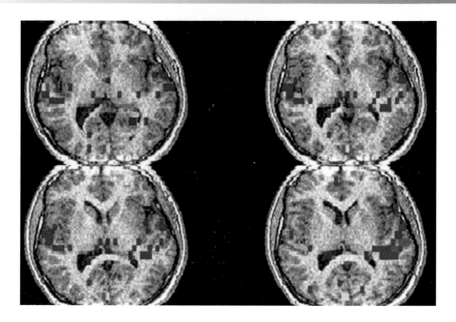

Figure 12.6   BOLD images of the brain. Functional areas shown in red.

of this molecule create local field inhomogeneities causing dephasing and therefore signal loss. During activity, blood flow to the cortex increases, causing a drop in deoxyhemoglobin, which results in a decrease in dephasing and a corresponding increase in signal intensity. These effects are very short lived and therefore require extremely rapid sequences such as EPI or fast gradient echo. To exploit T2* effects, BOLD images are usually acquired with long TEs (40–70 ms) while the task is modulated on and off. The 'off' images are then subtracted from the 'on' images and a more sophisticated statistical analysis is performed. Regions that were activated above some threshold level are overlaid on anatomical images (Figure 12.6). It is these regions that reflect brain activity. With EPI, images can be collected in a very short time and therefore, in principle, high temporal resolution is possible. However, the temporal resolution is limited by a blurred intrinsic hemodynamic response and a finite SNR.

Despite these limitations there is no doubt that this sophisticated technique develops our understanding of brain function and has several clinical applications, including the evaluation of stroke, epilepsy, pain and behavioral problems. There is also some potential in abdominal imaging. In particular, BOLD imaging has been used to predict tubular necrosis in the kidneys, and mesenteric ischemia.

Interventional MRI

MRI is now used for operative interventional procedures in some centers. The inherent safety and multi-planar facility of MRI makes it an ideal modality for some operative procedures. However, the development of this technique has required several modifications to existing hardware and software options.

Due to the restricted nature of conventional semi-conducting systems, a more open magnet design is required to permit easy access to the patient during the procedure. Low field permanent

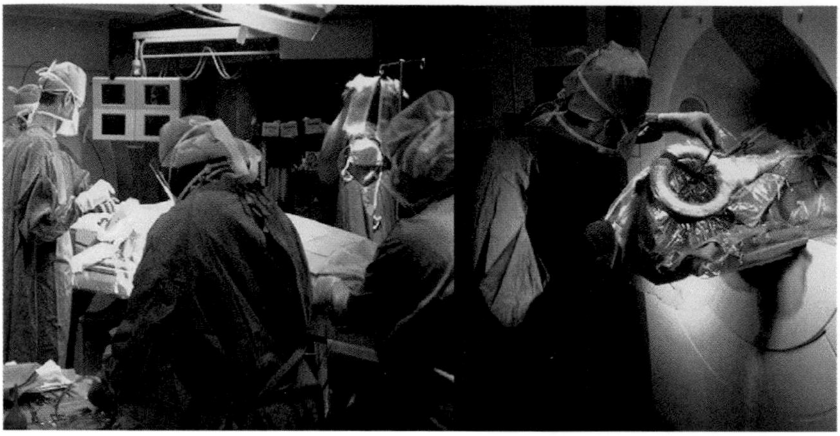

Figure 12.7   Interventional magnet system.

magnets are well suited from an access point of view, but image quality and acquisition times restrict their use to simple interventions. An interventional system uses a semi-conducting 0.5 T system shaped liked two doughnuts, which readily permits access to the patient and allows real-time image acquisition (Figure 12.7). This system permits:

- intra-operative acquisition of MR images without moving the patient
- online image-guided stereotaxy without pre-operative imaging
- 'real-time' tracking of instruments in the operative field registered to the MR images
- precise location of the area under examination (achieved via triangulation)
- continual monitoring of the procedure in three dimensions (using in-bore monitors).

This is an expensive technique, however. Flexible transmit and receive coils have been especially designed to fit around the operative area while allowing access for intervention. Endovascular coils have been developed to allow real-time tracking within vessels. In addition, all surgical instruments must be non-ferromagnetic and produce minimum susceptibility artefact so that they do not obscure the operating field. Anesthetic and monitoring equipment must also be MR safe.

Interventional MRI uses

Despite these design and safety implications, interventional MR has been used in many operative techniques including:

- liver imaging and tumor ablation
- breast imaging and benign lump excision
- orthopedic and kinematic studies
- congenital hip dislocation manipulation and correction
- biopsies
- functional endoscopic sinus surgery.

One important application is tumor ablation using either laser therapy (in which heat is used to ablate the tumor) or cryotherapy (when extreme cold is used for ablation). MRI is the only imaging technique that can discriminate tissue of different temperatures. Since T1 recovery and T2 decay are temperature dependent, temperature changes alter image contrast. For this reason, techniques such as laser and cryotherapy can be monitored using MRI.

Interstitial laser therapy (ILT) is a promising therapeutic technique in which laser energy is delivered percutaneously to various depths in tissue. Previously the extent of heat distribution from the laser was difficult to assess. The use of EPI sequences has enabled real-time monitoring of laser-induced therapy providing a non-invasive method for intra-operative assessment of heat distribution during ILT. Similarly, interventional MR has enormous potential in the evaluation of cryotherapy. This exciting technique may have profound influences on interventional radiology. It is likely that in the future, interventional vascular suites will be replaced by interventional MR systems and many surgical and interventional procedures will be carried out using MR technology.

MR spectroscopy (MRS)

MR spectroscopy produces a spectrum as opposed to an MR image. A spectrum is a plot of signal intensity vs frequency that shows the chemical shift or frequency difference between different elements. This chemical shift is caused by the electron shielding of a specific atom to create a difference in field strength and therefore frequency. Chemical shift is measured in parts per million in frequency (ppm). Chemical dispersion increases with field strength. Fluorine, carbon and sodium can be measured using MR spectroscopy, but hydrogen is the most widely used in clinical imaging. Table 12.1 shows the typical hydrogen or proton spectra available in human tissue.

A spectrum is located is located one of two ways. Both use an image for guidance.

- **Single voxel** techniques use three intersecting slices to locate a single voxel from which to measure the spectrum. Currently there are two types of single voxel technique:
  - stimulated echo acquisition mode (STEAM)
  - point resolved spectroscopy spin echo (PRESS).

Table 12.1   Typical hydrogen or proton spectra available in human tissue.

Spectrum	Abbreviation	Effect	Resonance
NAA-N-acetyl aspartate	NAA	neuronal marker	2.0 ppm
Lactate	Lac	product of anaerobic glycosis	1.3 ppm
Choline	Cho	present in cell membrane	3.2 ppm
Creatine	Cr-PCr		3.0 ppm
Lipids	Lip	result of cellular decay	0.9, 1.3 ppm
Myo-inositol	Ins	glial cell marker	3.5, 3.6 ppm
Glutamine/Glutamate	Glx	neurotransmitter	2.1, 3.8 ppm

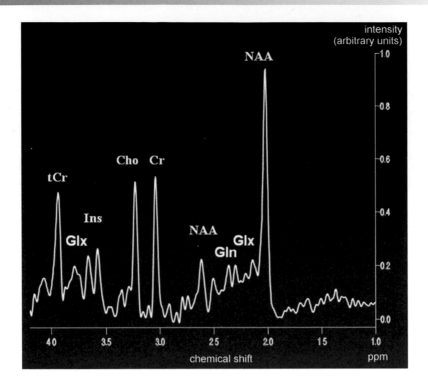

Figure 12.8   MR spectra of the brain.

- Both localize in a single acquisition but suffer from SNR and chemical shift artefacts. Motion is sometimes a problem if multiple TR periods are used.
- **Multi-voxel** techniques are more time efficient as they acquire multiple voxels by encoding in K space as in conventional imaging.

By viewing spectra from either single or multi voxels it is possible to compare the relative amounts of each to determine a disease process (Figures 12.8 and Figure 12.9). For example, elevations in the following are indicators for tumors:

- NAA drop indicates tumor cell invasion
- choline elevation indicates tumor growth
- lactate changes indicate anaerobic status
- lipid elevation indicates tumor necrosis.

MR spectroscopy uses

MRS is used in the following ways:

- to diagnose in conjunction with MRI
- to plan therapy (Figure 12.10)

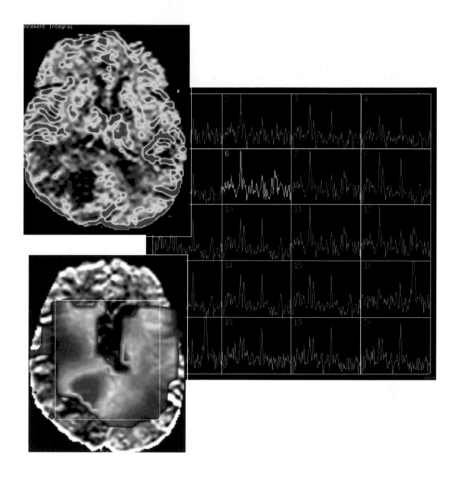

Figure 12.9   Multi-voxel MRS technique.

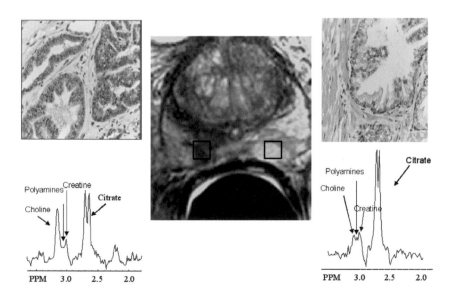

Figure 12.10   MRS for prostate imaging.

- biopsy guidance
- to aid in prognosis
- therapy monitoring.

In particular, MRS is useful in stroke and tumor staging, especially in the brain, breast and prostate. It may also have some use in the diagnosis and understanding of depression, epilepsy and schizophrenia.

Whole body imaging

This uses MRI to image the whole body in a single examination. This may be appropriate for screening patients for common diseases such as cancer and cardiovascular disease, and for skeletal surveys in patients with widespread bone disease. Most centers have devised protocols that image areas independently using fast imaging sequences such as EPI and turbo gradient echo.

Extra studies are performed in patients with a particular risk of disease. For example, breast imaging is added onto the standard protocol in patients with specific concerns over breast pathology. Manufacturers are developing hardware and software tools to enable fast imaging of the whole body in a single examination (not unlike CT scanning). This includes having multiple coil elements and independent receiver channels enabling a FOV of more than 200 cm.

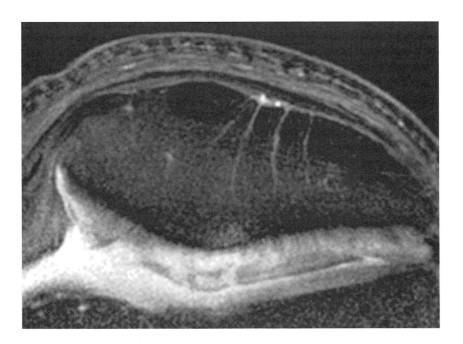

Figure 12.11 MR microscopy of the patellar cartilage. Voxels many, many times smaller than in conventional imaging are used.

MR microscopy (MRM)

Magnetic resonance microscopy (MRM) uses extremely fine resolution data to image structures with the same resolution as pathology sections. It is therefore an ideal research tool as it allows study in detail of very small areas of tissue. Pathologists can use MRM to examine tissue samples without conventional sectioning. With MRM, investigators can study models of disease, toxicology and the effects of drug therapies. Because of the SNR problems associated with very small voxels (*see* Chapter 4), very high fields and dedicated ultra-small coils are necessary to image in this manner. MRM is being used in many areas, but in clinical use the main application appears to be in bone and joint imaging, especially of hyaline cartilage (Figure 12.11).

For questions and answers on this topic please visit the supporting companion website for this book: www.wiley.com/go/ mriinpractice

Glossary

A

Acceleration factor	a term used in parallel imaging techniques to indicate the factor by which the scan time is reduced.
Acquisition window	*see* **sampling time**.
Active shielding	uses additional superconducting coils located at each end of the main magnet inside the cryostat to shield the system.
Active shimming	additional solenoid magnets to adjust field homogeneity.
Actual TE	the time between the echo and the next RF pulse in SSFP.
ADC map	post-processing in DWI that produces images where abnormal tissue is darker than normal tissue.
Aliasing	artefact produced when anatomy outside the FOV is mismapped inside the FOV.
Alnico	alloy used in making permanent magnets.
Angular momentum	the spin of MR active nuclei, which depends on the balance between the number of protons and neutrons in the nucleus.
Anisotropic	voxels that are not the same dimension in all three planes.
Anti-foldover	also called **no phase wrap**. Over-samples along the phase encoding axis by increasing the number of phase encodings performed.
Apparent diffusion coefficient (ADC)	the net displacement of molecules in the extracellular space due to diffusion.
Atom	a tiny element that is the basis for all things.
Atomic number	sum of protons in the nucleus – this number gives an atom its chemical identity.

B

B_0	the main magnetic field measured in tesla.
b factor	strength, interval and duration of the gradients in DWI and DTI.

MRI in Practice, Fourth Edition. Catherine Westbrook, Carolyn Kaut Roth, John Talbot.
© 2011 Blackwell Publishing Ltd. Published 2011 by Blackwell Publishing Ltd.

Bandwidth	a range of frequencies.
Black blood imaging	acquisitions in which blood vessels are black.
Blipping	used in EPI to step up or down through phase encoding steps.
Blood oxygen level dependent (BOLD)	a functional MRI technique that uses the differences in magnetic susceptibility between oxyhemoglobin and deoxyhemoglobin to image areas of activated cerebral cortex.
Blurring	the result of T2* decay during the course of a long echo train.
Bright blood imaging	acquisitions in which blood vessels are bright.

C

CASL	continuous arterial spin labelling – attenuates arterial spins by inversion or saturation pulses outside the FOV.
CBV	cerebral blood volume.
Central lines	area of K space filled with the shallowest phase encoding slopes.
Chemical misregistration artefact	(also known as out of phase artefact) artefact caused by the phase difference between fat and water.
Chemical shift	artefact caused by the frequency difference between fat and water.
Coarse matrix	a matrix with a low number of frequency encodings and/or phase encodings, and results in a low number of pixels in the FOV.
Co-current flow	flow in the same direction as slice excitation.
Coherent	see **in phase**.
Concatenation	see **interleaving**.
Conjugate symmetry	the symmetry of data in K space.
Contrast to noise ratio (CNR)	difference in SNR between two points.
Counter-current flow	flow in the opposite direction to slice excitation.
Cross-excitation	energy given to nuclei in adjacent slices by the RF pulse.
Cross-talk	energy given to nuclei in adjacent slices due to spin lattice relaxation.
Cryogen bath	area around the coils of wire in which cryogens are placed.
Cryogens	substances used to supercool the coils of wire in a superconducting magnet.

D

Data point	point in K space that contains digitized information from encoding.
Decay	loss of transverse magnetization.
Diffusion	the movement of molecules due to random thermal motion.
Diffusion tensor imaging (DTI)	uses strong multi-directional gradients to currently image white matter tracts and muscle.
Diffusion weighted imaging (DWI)	technique that produces images whose contrast is due to the differences in ADC between tissues.
Double IR prep	sequence in which two 180° pulses are used to saturate blood in black blood imaging.
DRIVE	driven equilibrium – a pulse sequence that achieves a very high signal intensity from water even when using short TRs.
Driven equilibrium Fourier transform	the generic term for **DRIVE**.
DS-MRA	digital subtraction MR angiography – contrast is selectively produced for moving spins during two acquisitions. These are then subtracted to remove the signal from the stationary spins, leaving behind an image of only the moving spins.
DTPA	diethylene triaminepentaacetic acid, a gadolinium chelate.

E

Echo planar imaging (EPI)	single or multi-shot acquisition that fills K space with data from gradient echoes.
Echo time (TE)	time in milliseconds from the application of the RF pulse to the peak of the signal induced in the coil – TE determines how much decay of transverse magnetization is allowed to occur.
Echo train	series of 180° rephasing pulse and echoes in a fast spin echo pulse sequence.
Echo train length	the number of 180° rephasing pulse/echoes/phase encodings per TR in fast spin echo.
Effective TE	the time between the echo and the RF pulse that initiated it in SSFP – also the TE used in FSE.
Electrons	particles that spin around the nucleus.
Encoding	once a slice is selected, the signal is located or encoded along both axes of the image.
Entry slice phenomenon	contrast difference of flowing nuclei relative to the stationary nuclei because they are fresh.

Even echo rephasing	technique that uses two echoes to reduce flow artefact.
Excitation	application of an RF pulse that causes resonance to occur.
Extremity coils	saddle configured coils used to image upper and lower extremities.
Extrinsic contrast parameters	those parameters that can be changed at the operator console.

F

Fast Fourier transform (FFT)	mathematical conversion of frequency/time domain to frequency/amplitude.
Fat saturation	technique that nulls signal from fat by applying an RF pulse at the frequency of fat to the imaging volume before slice excitation.
Field of view (FOV)	area of anatomy covered in an image.
Fine matrix	matrix where there are a high number of frequency encodings and/or phase encodings, and results in a large number of pixels in the FOV.
First order motion compensation	gradient moment nulling.
Flip angle	the angle of the NMV to B_0.
Flow encoding axes	axes along which bipolar gradients act in order to sensitize flow along the axis of the gradient used in phase contrast MRA.
Flow phenomena	artefacts produced by flowing nuclei.
Flow-related enhancement	decrease in time of flight due to a decrease in velocity of flow.
Foldover suppression	anti-phase aliasing software.
Fractional averaging	see **partial averaging**.
Fractional echo	see **partial echo**.
Free induction decay (FID)	loss of signal due to relaxation.
Frequency	the speed of a rotating object or the rate of change of phase per second.
Frequency encoding	locating a signal according to its frequency.
Frequency wrap	aliasing along the frequency encoding axis.
Fresh spins	nuclei that have not been beaten down by repeated RF pulses.
Fringe field	stray magnetic field outside the bore of the magnet.

Fully saturated	when the NMV is pushed to a full 180°.
Functional imaging techniques	techniques that allow MRI to be used to assess function and physiology.

G

Gd-BOPTA	gadobenate dimeglumine.
Gd-DOTA	gadoterate meglumine.
Gd-DTPA	gadopentetate.
Gd-DTPA-BMA	gadodiamide.
Gd-HP-DO3A	gadoteridol.
Ghosting	motion artefact in the phase axis.
Gibbs artefact	line of low signal in the cervical cord due to truncation.
Gradient amplifier	supplies power to the gradient coils.
Gradient echo	echo produced as a result of gradient rephasing.
Gradient echo-EPI (GE-EPI)	gradient echo sequence with EPI readout.
Gradient echo pulse sequence	one that uses a gradient to regenerate an echo.
Gradient moment nulling (rephasing)	a system of gradients that compensates for intra-voxel dephasing.
Gradient spoiling	the use of gradients to dephase magnetic moments – the opposite of rewinding.
Gradients	coils of wire that alter the magnetic field strength in a linear fashion when a current is passed through them.
GRASE	gradient echo and spin echo.
Gyromagnetic ratio	the precessional frequency of an element at 1.0 T.

H

Hahn echoes	echoes formed when any two 90° RF pulses are used in steady state sequences.
Half Fourier	*see* **partial averaging**.
High velocity signal loss	increase in time of flight due to an increase in the velocity of flow.
Homogeneity	evenness of the magnetic field.

417

Hybrid sequences	gradient echo and spin echo: 180° RF pulses are periodically applied to an EPI sequence to reduce susceptibility artefacts.
Hydrogen	the most abundant atom in the body.

I

ISMRM	International Society for Magnetic Resonance in Medicine.
IMRSER	Institute for Magnetic Resonance Safety, Education, and Research.
In phase	magnetic moments that are in the same place on the precessional path around B_0 at any given time.
Incoherent	*see* **out of phase**.
Inflow effect	another term for **entry slice phenomenon**.
Inhomogeneities	areas where the magnetic field strength is not exactly the same as the main field strength – magnetic field unevenness.
Interleaving	a method of acquiring data from alternate slices and dividing the sequence into two acquisitions – no slice gap is required.
Intra-voxel dephasing	phase difference between flow and stationary nuclei in a voxel.
Intrinsic contrast parameters	those parameters that cannot be changed because they are inherent to the body's tissues.
Ions	atoms with an excess or deficit of electrons.
Isotopes	atoms of elements that contain the same number of protons but a different number of neutrons.
Isotropic	voxels that are the same dimension in all three planes.

J

J coupling	causes an increase in the T2 decay time of fat when multiple RF pulses are applied as in fast spin echo.

K

K space	an area in the array processor where data about spatial frequencies are stored.

L

Larmor frequency	*see* **precessional frequency**.
Longitudinal plane	the axis parallel to B_0.

M

Magnetic field gradient	field created by passing current through a gradient coil.
Magnetic isocentre	the centre of the bore of the magnet in all planes.
Magnetic moment	denotes the direction of the north/south axis of a magnet and the amplitude of the magnetic field.
Magnetic resonance angiography (MRA)	method of visualizing vessels that contain flowing nuclei by producing a contrast between them and the stationary nuclei.
Magnetic susceptibility	ability of a substance to become magnetized.
Magnetism	a property of all matter that depends on the magnetic susceptibility of the atom.
Magnetization transfer contrast/ coherence (MTC)	technique used to suppress background tissue and increase CNR.
Magneto- hemodynamic effect	effect that causes elevation of the T wave of the ECG of the patient when placed in a magnetic field – this is due to the conductivity of blood.
Magnitude image	unsubtracted image combination of flow sensitized data.
Mass number	sum of neutrons and protons in the nucleus.
Maximum intensity projection (MIP)	technique that uses a ray passed through an imaging volume to assign signal intensity according to their proximity to the observer.
Molecules	where two or more atoms are arranged together.
MR active nuclei	nuclei that possess an odd mass number.
MR signal	the voltage induced in the receiver coil.
Multiple overlapping thin section angiography (MOTSA)	method combining a number of high resolution 3D acquisitions to produce an image that has good resolution and a large area of coverage.
Multi-shot	where K space is divided into segments and one segment is acquired per TR.
Multi-voxel	technique that acquires multiple voxels by encoding in K space in MR signal.

N

Net magnetization vector (NMV)	the magnetic vector produced as a result of the alignment of excess hydrogen nuclei with B_0.

Neutron	neutrally charged element in an atomic nucleus.
NEX (also known as number of signal averages or acquisitions depending on manufacturer)	number of excitations, the number of times an echo is encoded with the same slope of phase encoding gradient.
No phase wrap	anti-phase aliasing software.
Noise	frequencies that exist randomly in time and space.
Nucleons	particles in the nucleus.
Null point	the point at which there is no longitudinal magnetization in a tissue in an inversion recovery sequence.
Nyquist frequency	the highest frequency that can be sampled.
Nyquist theorem	states that a frequency must be sampled at least twice in order to reproduce it reliably.

O

Ohm's law	basic law of electricity – voltage (V) = current (I) x resistance (R).
Out of phase	when magnetic moments are not in the same place on the precessional path.
Out of phase artefact	see **chemical misregistration artefact**.
Outer lines	area of K space filled with the steepest phase encoding gradient slopes.

P

Parallel imaging	a technique that uses multiple coils to fill segments of K space.
Partial averaging	filling only a proportion of K space with data and putting zeros in the remainder.
Partial echo imaging	sampling only part of the echo and extrapolating the remainder in K space.
Partial voluming	loss of spatial resolution when large voxels are used.
Partially saturated	occurs when the NMV is flipped beyond 90° (91° to 179°).
Passive shielding	shielding accomplished by surrounding the magnet with steel plates.
Passive shimming	uses metal discs/plates at installation to adjust for large changes in field homogeneity.

Pathology weighting	achieved in IR pulse sequence with a long TE pathology appears bright even though the image is T1 weighted.
Permanent magnets	magnets that retain their magnetism.
Phase	the position of a magnetic moment on its precessional path at any given time.
Phase contrast angiography (PC-MRA)	technique that generates vascular contrast using the phase difference between stationary and flowing spins.
Phase encoding	locating a signal according to its phase.
Phase image	subtracted image combination of flow sensitized data.
Phase over-sampling	anti-phase aliasing software.
Phase wrap	aliasing along the phase encoding axis.
Point resolved spectroscopy spin echo (PRESS)	single voxel technique in MRS.
Polarity	the direction of a gradient, i.e. which end is greater than B_0 and which is lower than B_0. Depends on the direction of the current through the gradient coil.
Precession	the secondary spin of magnetic moments around B_0.
Precessional (Larmor) frequency	the speed of precession.
Precessional path	the circular pathway of magnetic moments as they precess around B_0.
Protium	the isotope of hydrogen used in MRI. Nucleus contains a single proton.
Proton	positively charged element of an atomic nucleus.
Proton density	number of mobile hydrogen protons per unit volume of that tissue.
Proton density weighted image	image that demonstrates the differences in the proton densities of the tissues.
Pseudo-frequency	frequency that is indirectly derived from a change of phase.
Pulse control unit	co-ordinates switching on and off the gradient and RF transmitter coils at appropriate times during the pulse sequence.
Pulse sequence	a series of RF pulses, gradient applications and intervening time periods.

Q

Quenching	sudden loss of the superconductivity of the magnet coils so that the magnet becomes resistive.

R

Radio frequency (RF)	low energy, low frequency electromagnetic radiation. Used to excite hydrogen nuclei in MRI.
Ramp sampling	where sampling data points are collected when the gradient rise time is almost complete – sampling occurs while the gradient is still reaching maximum amplitude, while the gradient is at maximum amplitude and as it begins to decline.
Readout gradient	the frequency encoding gradient.
Receive bandwidth	range of frequencies that are sampled during readout.
Recovery	growth of longitudinal magnetization.
Rectangular FOV	also known as asymmetric FOV – uses a FOV in the phase direction that is different to that in the frequency direction of the image.
Reduction factor	the factor by which the scan time is reduced using parallel imaging. Equals the number of coils used.
Relaxation	process by which the NMV loses energy.
Relaxivity	the effect of a substance on relaxation rate.
Repetition time, TR	time between each excitation pulse.
Residual transverse magnetization	transverse magnetixation left over from previous RF pulses in steady state conditions.
Resistive magnet	another term for solenoid magnet.
Resonance	a phenomenon that occurs when an oscillating object is exposed to a frequency having the same or similar oscillating frequency to the object.
Respiratory compensation	uses mechanical motion of air in bellows to order K space filling and reduce respiratory motion artefact.
Respiratory gating/ triggering	gates the sequences to chest wall movements to reduce respiratory motion artefacts.
Respiratory navigator echoes	monitors the signal intensity in a region of interest and acquires data only between prescribed boundaries.
Rewinders	gradients that rephase.
RF amplifier	supplies power to the RF transmitter coils.
RF pulse	short burst of RF energy that excites nuclei into a high-energy stage.
RF spoiling	the use of digitized RF to transmit and receive at a certain phase.

RF transmitter coil	coil that transmits RF at the resonant frequency of hydrogen to excite nuclei and move them into a high-energy state.
Rise time	the time it takes a gradient to switch on, achieve the required gradient slope and switch off again.
R to R interval	time between each R wave in gated studies.

S

Sampling interval	the time between samples taken during readout.
Sampling rate or frequency	rate at which samples are taken during readout.
Sampling time	the time that the readout gradient is switched on for.
SAR	specific absorption rate – a way of measuring the USA Food and Drug Administration limit for RF exposure.
SAT TR	time between each pre-saturation pulse.
Saturation	occurs when the NMV is flipped to a full 180°.
Sensitivity encoding	*see* **parallel imaging**.
Sequential acquisition	acquisition where all the data from each slice is acquired before going on to the next.
Shim coil	extra coils used to make the magnetic field as homogeneous as possible.
Shimming	process whereby the evenness of the magnetic field is optimized.
Signal to noise ratio (SNR)	ratio of signal relative to noise.
Signal voltage	induced in the receiver coil.
Single shot fast spin echo (SS-FSE)	a fast spin echo sequence where all the lines of K space are acquired during a single TR period.
Single voxel	techniques that use three intersecting slices to locate a single voxel in MRS.
Slew rate	the strength of the gradient over distance.
Slice encoding	the separation of individual slice locations by phase in volume acquisitions.
Slice selection	selecting a slice using a gradient.
Solenoid electromagnet	magnet that uses current passed through coils of wire to generate a magnetic field.
Spatial encoding	encoding or locating signal in spatial three dimensions of the imaging volume.

423

Spatial modulation of magnetization (SPAMM)	creates a saturation effect which produces a cross-hatching of stripes on the image; these can be compared with moving anatomy to determine its function.
Spatial resolution	the ability to distinguish two points as separate.
Spin-down	the population of high-energy hydrogen nuclei that align their magnetic moments anti-parallel to B_0.
Spin echo	echo produced as a result of a 180° rephasing pulse.
Spin echo-EPI (SE-EPI)	spin echo sequence with EPI readout.
Spin echo pulse sequence	one that uses a 180° rephasing pulse to generate an echo.
Spin lattice relaxation	process by which energy is given up to the surrounding lattice.
Spin–spin relaxation	process by which interactions between the magnetic fields of adjacent nuclei causes dephasing.
Spin-up	the population of low energy hydrogen nuclei that align their magnetic moments parallel to B_0.
Spoilers	gradients that dephase.
Steady state	condition where the TR is less than T1 and T2 relaxation times of the tissues.
Stimulated echo acquisition mode (STEAM)	single voxel technique in MRS.
Stimulated echoes	echoes formed when any two RF pulses are used in steady state sequences.
Superconducting magnet	solenoid electromagnet that uses super-cooled coils of wire so that there is no inherent resistance in the system the current flows, and therefore the magnetism is generated without a driving voltage.

T

T1 enhancement agent	a contrast agent that shortens T1 relaxation in tissues that take up the agent.
T1 recovery	growth of longitudinal magnetization as a result of spin lattice relaxation.
T1 relaxation time	time taken for 63% of the longitudinal magnetization to recover.
T1 weighted image	image that demonstrates the differences in the T1 times of the tissues.

T2*	dephasing due to magnetic field inhomogeneities.
T2 enhancement agents	agents that shorten T2 relaxation times in tissues that take up the agent.
T2 decay	loss of transverse magnetization as a result of spin–spin relaxation.
T2 relaxation time	time taken for 63% of the transverse magnetization to decay.
T2 shine through	when lesions remain bright on a trace image in DWI.
T2 weighted image	image that demonstrates the differences in the T2 times of the tissues.
tau	the time between the excitation pulse and the 180° rephasing pulse and the time between this and the echo. Sometimes used in STIR sequences as an alternative to the TI.
Thermal equilibrium	assumes patient's temperature is constant and therefore does not influence the thermal energy of hydrogen during the MR experiment.
3D volumetric acquisition	acquisition where the whole imaging volume is excited so that the images can be viewed in any plane.
Time from inversion (TI)	time from 180° inverting pulse to 90° excitation pulse in inversion recovery pulse sequences.
Time intensity curve	curve produced in perfusion imaging to show perfusion kinetics of a tissue.
Time of flight	rate of flow in a given time – causes some flowing nuclei to receive one RF pulse only and therefore produce a signal void.
Time of flight MR angiography (TOF-MRA)	technique that generates vascular contrast by using the inflow effect.
Time to echo (TE)	*see* **echo time**.
TR	*see* **repetition time**.
Trace image	image in DWI where abnormal tissue is brighter than normal tissue.
Transceiver	coil that both transmits RF and receives the MR signal.
Transmit bandwidth	range of frequencies transmitted in an RF pulse.
Transverse plane	the axis perpendicular to B_0.
Trigger delay	waiting period after each R wave – the time between the R wave and the beginning of data acquisition.
Trigger window	waiting period before each R wave in gated studies.
Truncation artefact	artefact caused by under-sampling so that edges of high and low signal are not properly mapped into the image.

425

Turbo factor   *see* **echo train length**.

2D volumetric   acquisition where a small amount of data is acquired from each slice
acquisition   before repeating the TR.

V

Volume coil   coil that transmits and receives signal over a large volume of the patient.

Voxel volume   volume of tissue in the patient.

W

Water saturation   technique that nulls signal from water by applying an RF pulse at the
                            frequency of water to the imaging volume before slice excitation.

Window levels and   settings that control brightness and contrast in MR images.
settings

Index

Numbers in **bold** type refer to tables. Numbers in *italic* type refer to figures.

MRI in Practice, Fourth Edition. Catherine Westbrook, Carolyn Kaut Roth, John Talbot.
© 2011 Blackwell Publishing Ltd. Published 2011 by Blackwell Publishing Ltd.

440